Diabetes and Endocrinology
Clinical Practice

CLINICAL PRACTICE SERIES

Series Editor: Professor A.C. Kennedy, MD, FRCP (Lond, Edin, Glas, Ire), FRSE, FACP (Hon), FRACP (Hon)

Formerly Muirhead Professor of Medicine, University Department of Medicine, Royal Infirmary, Glasgow

Diabetes and Endocrinology in Clinical Practice

W. Michael G. Tunbridge MA, MD, FRCP

and

Philip D. Home MA, DPhil, FRCP

Edward Arnold
A division of Hodder & Stoughton
LONDON   MELBOURNE   AUCKLAND

© 1991 W. Michael G. Tunbridge and Philip D. Home
First published in Great Britain 1991

British Library Cataloguing in Publication Data
Tunbridge, W. M. G.
  Diabetes and endocrinology in clinical practice.
  1. Medicine. Endocrinology
  I. Title II. Home, P. D.
  616.4

  ISBN 0-340-54561-5

All rights reserved. No part of this publication may be reproduced or transmitted in any form or by any means, electronically or mechanically, including photocopying, recording or any information storage or retrieval system, without either prior permission in writing from the publisher or a licence permitting restricted copying. In the United Kingdom such licences are issued by the Copyright Licensing Agency: 90 Tottenham Court Road, London W1P 9HE.

Typeset in Linotron Times
by Rowland Phototypesetting Limited, Bury St Edmunds, Suffolk
Printed and bound in Great Britain for Edward Arnold,
a division of Hodder and Stoughton Limited,
Mill Road, Dunton Green, Sevenoaks, Kent TN13 2YA
by St Edmundsbury Press Limited, Bury St Edmunds, Suffolk
and bound by Hartnolls Limited, Bodmin, Cornwall

SERIES EDITOR'S PREFACE

This new series is planned to give an account of current clinical practice with authoritative guidance on investigation, diagnosis and management. The series is aimed principally at candidates preparing for the MRCP(UK) or those who are gaining further experience in the speciality of their choice after acquisition of the MRCP(UK) diploma. I would hope that the texts would be useful to senior registrars and consultants who were seeking to keep themselves up to date across the various subspecialties in medicine and who prepare lectures and seminars for younger postgraduates. Some of the more precocious senior undergraduates may also be interested in consulting the books. These comments also apply to overseas postgraduates both while working in this country and after their return home. Most of the countries in the Middle East, Africa, India, Pakistan and the Far East are still very much in tune with the British practical clinical approach to patient management, finding highly technological approaches less appropriate to their local needs. The books are not extensively referenced since an important objective was to keep them to a size that is easily handled but lists of key references for further reading are provided.

Dr Tunbridge and Dr Home were invited to produce the third title in the series on Diabetes and Endocrinology in Clinical Practice. They are both active clinicians and teachers with well established reputations. They were encouraged to pursue a practical clinical approach based on a sound but not overelaborate base of relevant physiology and biochemistry and they have produced a text which should prove immensely useful in practice, providing authoritative guidance in diabetes and endocrinology. At the end of the book there is a selection of multiple choice questions which the reader should find helpful for self-assessment.

Glasgow, 1990   A.C. Kennedy

AUTHORS' PREFACE

The aim of this book is to provide practical guidelines for the investigation and management of patients with diabetes mellitus and endocrine disorders based on sound underlying physiological principles. It is intended for medical practitioners preparing for postgraduate qualifications but we hope that it will also be of interest to general physicians and to senior students who wish to keep abreast of the field. Suggestions for further reading on selected topics are included at the end of each chapter.

We make no apology for devoting half the book to diabetes mellitus which is an ageless, sexless and classless disease with high morbidity and increasing prevalence. Thyroid diseases are the commonest endocrine disorders but other rarer endocrine diseases are of importance because they may be life-threatening yet most are treatable and they present sporadically in various guises to all physicians.

We are pleased to express our gratitude to Dr Bill Simpson, Consultant Radiologist, Newcastle General Hospital, for the radiographs reproduced in Chapter 11; to Dr Keith Hall, Consultant Neuroradiologist for the radiographs and CT Scans used in Chapters 7 and 8, and to Mr Gordon Aylward of Novo-Nordisk (UK) for sponsoring the colour plates.

Newcastle upon Tyne, 1991
W.M.G. Tunbridge
P.D. Home

The illustration on the cover is of a pancreatic islet of Langerhans stained by immunohistochemistry for glucagon. The glucagon containing A-cells are visible around the periphery of the islet.

CONTENTS

Series Editor's Preface   v

Authors' Preface   vi

1 **What is Diabetes Mellitus?**   1
History   Classification of diabetes   Aetiology of diabetes
Pathogenesis and biochemistry of diabetes   Definition
of diabetes   Presentation of diabetes   Diagnosis and
differential diagnosis of diabetes   Assessment of the newly
presenting diabetic patient

2 **Late Tissue Damage in Diabetes Mellitus**   24
Prevalence and clinical significance of diabetic tissue
damage   Classification of late tissue damage of diabetes   Cause
of late tissue damage of diabetes   Is late tissue damage caused
by metabolic disturbance?   Pathological mechanisms of
microangiopathy   Diabetic eye disease   Diabetic renal
damage   Diabetic neuropathy   Musculo–skeletal problems in
diabetes   Diabetic dermopathy   Diabetic specific heart
disease   Cardiac and major vessel disease in diabetes   The
diabetic foot

3 **Delivering Optimal Care to the Patient with Diabetes**   61
Concepts underlying the organization of care   Targets for
therapy   Self-care, education and monitoring   The diabetes
service   The diabetes consultation   Audit of diabetes
care   Clinic monitoring of diabetic control

4 Treatment of Diabetes Mellitus 92
Introduction   Dietary management   Oral hypoglycaemic agents   Insulin therapy

5 Special Situations in Diabetes Management 134
Pregnancy in the diabetic woman   Diabetes in childhood   Diabetes in the elderly   Acute hyperglycaemic emergencies   Diabetes in patients undergoing surgery and other procedures   Dyslipidaemia in people with diabetes   Skin conditions in diabetes   Infections and diabetes

6 Gut Associated Peptide Hormones 159
The APUD system and multiple endocrine neoplasia   Insulin hypersecretion   Abnormalities of glucagon secretion   Abnormalities of somatostatin secretion   The Vipoma syndrome   Gastrinoma (Zollinger–Ellison) syndrome   Carcinoid syndrome

7 The Hypothalamus and Pituitary 175
Development and Anatomy   Physiology of hypothalamic–pituitary–target organ relationships   Anterior pituitary disorders   Acromegaly   Hyperprolactinaemia   Anterior pituitary failure   The neurohypophysis (posterior pituitary)   Diabetes insipidus   Inappropriate ADH section

8 The Thyroid 210
Development and anatomy   Physiology   Effects of iodine   Thyroid disease   Hyperthyroidism   Ophthalmopathy   Hypothyroidism   Thyroiditis   Goitre   Thyroid malignancy

9 The Adrenal Glands 244
Development and anatomy   Physiology of the adrenal cortex   Diseases of the adrenal cortex   Addison's disease   Secondary hypoadrenalism   Congenital adrenal hyperplasia   Cushing's syndrome   Conn's syndrome   Physiology of the adrenal medulla   Phaeochromocytoma

10 The Gonads 267
Development   The testis   The ovary   Pathological sexual disorders   Chromosomal abnormalities   Abnormal genitalia   Pubertal abnormalities   Hypogonadism in females   Virilization   Hypogonadism in males

11	**Calcium Metabolism, Parathyroid Hormone and Vitamin D**	**288**

Parathyroid hormone   Vitamin D   Calcium balance
Hypercalcaemia   Hypocalcaemia   Vitamin D
deficiency   Endocrine aspects of other bone disorders

12	**Multiple Choice Questions**	**308**
Index		**319**

1

WHAT IS DIABETES MELLITUS?

History

The first historical reference to what might be a description of the condition we know today as Diabetes Mellitus occurs in the *Ebers Papyrus*, a document from the 18th Egyptian Dynasty of about 1500 BC. Sweetness of urine was known in India some 1100 years later, and the term 'diabetes' is believed to have been used by the Greeks in the 3rd century BC. Aretaeus of Cappadocia, writing in the 1st century AD, was the first physician to describe the condition formally. He still largely defined the condition as the passing of copious amounts of urine and the loss of body flesh.

Although diabetes was recognized in various writings in the intervening centuries (including texts from China), it was Willis in 1674 who redescribed sweetness of the urine and made the deduction that this must be secondary to sweetness of the blood. Nevertheless, it was another 100 years before it was demonstrated that this sweetness was due to excess sugar, and a further 50 years before this was recognized as glucose.

It was the 19th century which saw the major advances in the description of diabetes, its dietary management, its biochemistry and the role of pancreatic pathology. Indeed a link between chronic pancreatitis and diabetes had already been noted at the end of the 18th century, but it was not until after the descriptions of glycosuria following pancreatectomy in dogs by von Mering and Minkowski (1890) that the suggestion of a missing pancreatic factor was made. The 19th century also saw the recognition that diabetes might not be a single disease, with a different natural history when presenting in childhood compared to late adulthood. The first clinical descriptions of coma in association with acidosis were also made at this time, and Bernard set the biochemical basis of the condition on its long road of discovery with his observations on the production of glucose by the liver.

Although descriptions of the treatment of diabetes appear in some of the very early documents, it is often difficult to appreciate whether the diets and herbal remedies offered represent specific therapies or whether they were merely parts of the regular therapeutic armoury available for serious disease at that time. Again it was nearly the 19th century before dietary management was formally introduced by Rollo, and throughout that

What is Diabetes Mellitus?

century a host of rather disparate dietary measures were suggested for the condition.

Towards the end of the 19th century the history of diabetes is dominated by the observations leading to the isolation of insulin, following the discoveries of Minkowski, and the demonstration by Opie of degeneration of the islets of Langerhans. Numerous attempts at insulin extraction were recorded after 1890, and some of the preparations (for example by De Witt, Zuelzer, Paulesco) appear to have had glucose lowering activity. While it seems likely that a therapeutic preparation would have been made in any case within a couple of years, it fell to the drive and ideas of Banting, the technical support of Best, the facilities and guidance of MacLeod and the biochemical expertise of Collip to produce an adequately pure and potent preparation of bovine insulin in 1922.

The following decades (Table 1.1) were most clearly marked by the development of the extended acting insulin preparations by Hagedorn and Hallas-Møller, and the accidental discoveries of the hypoglycaemic effects of the biguanide and sulphonylurea groups of drugs. It is as yet unclear whether the introduction of highly purified insulin preparations, glycosylated haemoglobin estimation, self-blood glucose monitoring, islet and pancreas transplantation, insulin infusion pumps and genetically engineered insulin will lead to history judging the period between 1973 and 1983 as the most significant yet in the understanding and management of diabetes.

Classification of Diabetes Mellitus

The clinical syndromes which together are termed diabetes are linked by some common features of their biochemical disturbance, resulting in common clinical manifestations. As discussed above diabetes was progressively recognized as polyuria, then glycosuria, then hyperglycaemia and more lately as

Table 1.1 Technical milestones in the management of diabetes

Year	Worker(s)	Milestone
1797	Rollo	Dietary management
1913	Allen	Severe calorie restriction
1921	Banting, Best, Collip MacLeod	Isolation and use of insulin
1936	Hagedorn and colleagues	Protamine–insulin complexes used
1939	Loubatières	Discovery of sulphonylureas
1970	Jørgensen and colleagues	Highly purified insulin available
1976	Sonksen and colleagues, Walford and colleagues	Self-blood glucose monitoring
1976	Koenig and colleagues	Glycosylated haemoglobin to monitor control
1979	Goeddel and colleagues	Genetically engineered insulin
1980	Many researchers	Microcomputers in diabetes management

relative or absolute hypoinsulinaemia with or without insulin insensitivity. The common defining characteristic of the disease has therefore always been, and remains, its metabolic disturbance. Indeed, diabetes is still officially defined by hyperglycaemia as if it was a single condition. This union is justified by the observations that not only are the symptomatic manifestations common to the different forms of diabetes (for example, polyuria, polydipsia, disposition to certain infections) as a result of their common metabolic cause, but also by the recognition that the long-term spectrum of tissue damage that occurs in people with diabetes (microangiopathy) is also common to all aetiological forms of the disease.

Terminology of Diabetes Classification

Type 1 ('insulin-dependent') and Type 2 ('non-insulin-dependent') diabetes

The best terminology for the classification of diabetes is currently a subject of dispute. As detailed below the majority of people with diabetes fall either into a group characterized by onset in childhood or early adulthood and who, within a few years, require insulin to avoid ketoacidosis even when well, or into a group with onset in the later years of life, often overweight, and with no requirement for insulin when well. These groups were known as 'juvenile onset' and 'maturity onset' diabetics (*sic*), respectively. It will be noted that both groups exclude diabetes due to pancreatic disease (or pancreatectomy), diabetes appearing during pregnancy or drug therapy and subsequently remitting, and some endocrine and tropical syndromes (Table 1.2).

These older terms fell into disuse with the observation of non-insulin-requiring diabetes presenting in childhood, and of insulin-requiring diabetes presenting throughout life. They were replaced by the terms insulin-dependent diabetes and non-insulin-dependent diabetes, but a consensus has never been reached on the exact meanings of these words. The greatest difficulties occur with the tendancy of many physicians to confuse insulin-treated diabetes with insulin-dependent diabetes, the latter strictly only being applicable to patients who develop ketoacidosis on insulin withdrawal when not under stress. Many patients with non-insulin-dependent diabetes are however improved with insulin therapy, and some will develop ketosis if not treated with insulin during acute illness. Furthermore, some patients who are dependent on insulin clearly have diabetes secondary to pancreatic disease, and many patients whose diabetes eventually evolves to complete insulin deficiency go through a period when insulin therapy can be withdrawn. The resulting confusion has caused widespread misuse of these terms in the literature on diabetes, where their appearance demands interpretation with care. For these reasons many authorities have now adopted an aetiological classification.

To avoid the nomenclature problems of the earlier terms the classification of diabetes by aetiology simply refers to types of diabetes. Classical juvenile onset diabetes is termed Type 1 diabetes. This wording is reserved for diabetes of

Table 1.2 A simplified classification and aetiology of diabetes mellitus

1. Type 1 ('insulin-dependent')
2. Type 2 ('non-insulin-dependent')
3. Secondary diabetes
    (a) Pancreatic disease
        Recurrent pancreatitis
        Malnutrition diabetes (calcific pancreatitis)
        Haemochomatosis
        Pancreatectomy
        Islet B-cell toxins
    (b) Hormonal/metabolic* disturbances
        Gestational diabetes
        Steroid excess (secretion or therapy)
        Acromegaly
        Glucagonoma
        Hepatic cirrhosis
        Catecholamine-induced diabetes
    (c) Drug-induced diabetes
        Thiazide diuretics
        Other
4. Genetic and other syndromes
    Insulin receptor abnormalities
    Insulin receptor antibodies
    Glycogen storage disease
    DIDMOAD syndrome (diabetes insipidus, diabetes mellitus, optic atrophy)
    Prader–Willi syndrome
    Lipodystrophy
    Ataxia telangiectasia
    Diabetes insipidus

*These conditions generally only result in hyperglycaemia if the patient already has insulin insensitivity or defective insulin secretion, but not sufficient to develop diabetes without further metabolic stress. The underlying metabolic condition is usually that of Type 2 diabetes, but may sometimes be Type 1 diabetes or other pancreatic disease.

auto-immune origin, progressing in the overwhelming majority of patients to complete failure of insulin production. It is generally accepted that, in the absence of a history of other pancreatic disease, an absence of endogeneous insulin production is indicative of such aetiology, thus allowing classification of the majority of insulin-dependent patients as having Type 1 diabetes without direct demonstration of the cause of their pathology. Nevertheless it will be necessary in many cases to make the classification on clinical grounds, particularly age of onset, proneness to ketoacidosis and body habitus.

Type 2 diabetes encompasses a very much broader and ill-defined group of patients, perhaps best delimited as those not likely to have Type 1 diabetes, diabetes induced by pregnancy or drugs, or a non-endocrine or pancreatic condition. Patients with Type 2 diabetes classically present in middle age or later, often with a history of being overweight, and by definition never progress to complete insulin deficiency. The diversity of age of onset and body habitus nevertheless convinces many physicians that Type 2 diabetes is aetiologically a group of conditions. However, it is more likely that the combination of insulin insensitivity and deficient insulin secretion necessary to produce overt Type 2 diabetes results in the heterogeneity of presentations.

Other forms of diabetes

Diabetes is otherwise classified by immediate causation, as in Table 1.2. The major groupings include diabetes secondary to pancreatic damage, with the subgroup of so-called tropical diabetes, and diabetes appearing during stress, endocrine disease, steroid and other drug treatment, and pregnancy.

A rare form of diabetes, but well characterized, is that of diabetes secondary to insulin receptor abnormalities, with which diabetes secondary to insulin receptor autoantibodies is sometimes grouped. There are also a number of rare syndromes in which diabetes occurs, as listed in Table 1.2, but the reason for these associations is generally unclear.

Aetiology of Diabetes

Type 1 Diabetes

Clues to the aetiology of Type 1 diabetes come from its association with the genes for the DR3 and DR4 molecules in the HLA immune response gene region on chromosome 6, the presence of islet cell antibodies in serum before and at the time of diagnosis, the finding of an aggressive round cell infiltrate in the islets of patients dying at diagnosis, and an association with other conditions more clearly recognized as being of autoimmune origin (Table 1.3).

Table 1.3 Factors associated with the occurrence of the two major types of diabetes

Type 1	Type 2
HLA susceptibility (DR3, DR4)	Insulin insensitivity
Islet cell complement fixing antibodies	Deficient insulin secretion (? islet amyloidosis)
Identical twin with diabetes (35% risk)	
Resident in northern Europe	Family history of Type 2 diabetes
Childhood	Some ethnic groups (e.g. Indian Asians)
? Stress	
? Exposure to islet B-cell toxins (nitrosamines)	High calorie intake (? obesity)
	Relative prosperity
? Viral infections	Reduced activity levels
	Drug therapy (e.g. thiazides)
	Old age
	Hypertension
	? Environmental factors

6   What is Diabetes Mellitus?

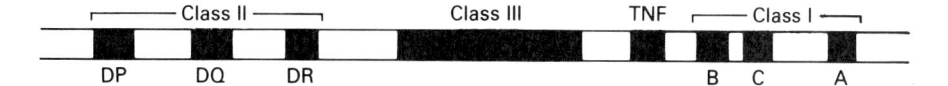

```
┌─────── Class II ───────┐        Class III        TNF   ┌── Class I ──┐
▕▇▇▇▏   ▕▇▇▇▏   ▕▇▇▇▏    ▕▇▇▇▇▇▇▇▇▇▇▇▇▇▇▏        ▕▇▇▏   ▕▇▏  ▕▇▏  ▕▇▏
  DP      DQ      DR                                      B    C    A
```

Fig. 1.1 Map of the HLA region of the short arm of human chromosome 6. The class I antigens were the first recognized to have an association with Type 1 diabetes, and with other auto-immune disease. However, although the HLA region contains many hundreds of genes (mostly unknown) very little recombination takes place at meiosis, so the relation between any allele in the class I region and any in the class III region is constant. The susceptibility to diabetes is now thought to lie mainly with the DQ genes (α and β), but there are many other genes close by, any of which might still be found to be involved.

The clinical observation of the association between Type 1 diabetes and other endocrine disease associated with circulating autoantibodies has been confirmed by cross-sectional survey, and is associated with an increased frequency of the B8 immune response gene. This association extends to other conditions with the same association (such as coeliac disease) and to non-endocrine conditions recognized as having an auto-immune basis (for example, alopecia areata, vitiligo). It is believed that these associations are particularly prevalent in a subgroup of Type 1 diabetes, termed Type 1b. These patients tend to be female, in early adulthood and have diabetes of clinically slow onset with long-term preservation of a degree of endogenous insulin production. In contrast to the large majority of people with Type 1 diabetes, circulating islet cell antibodies may persist for many years.

The HLA association with Type 1 diabetes was first recognized as an increased frequency of genes coding for B8 and B15 class I molecules, but this is now recognized as being due to linkage with the subregion coding for the class II molecules, the HLA D subregion (Fig. 1.1). These molecules may be classified as DP, DQ and DR, and while it is DR that is usually detected in typing, it seems that DQ is more closely linked to the genetic susceptability to Type 1 diabetes. Over 90% of individuals with Type 1 diabetes have the DR3 or DR4 allele, and if both are carried the relative risk of developing diabetes is increased four to five times. The HLA D molecules are expressed on B-lymphocytes, macrophages and other antigen-presenting cells, and their conformation is important in presenting foreign antigens to T-lymphocytes in the initiation of the immune response.

Genetically there is good evidence for quite a strong influence on Type 1 diabetes, with the lifetime incidence risk raised some 10 to 20 times by having a parent with the condition. Most of this effect probably lies in the genetics of the HLA D subregion genes, and the effect is considerably strengthened where there is HLA D identity between parents and children. Evidence also exists for a genetic influence from chromosome 11, which carries the insulin gene, suggesting that the susceptibility of the islet B-cell to auto-immune damage might lie in this region. Evidence for involvement of genes on chromosomes 2 and 14 is much weaker.

Genetics cannot be the only basis for the cause of Type 1 diabetes, however, since only around 35% of identical twins of patients with diabetes will also develop the disease. Some of the remaining 65% may, however, show minor metabolic abnormalities, short of impaired glucose tolerance.

The question as to whether viruses could be responsible for triggering an auto-destructive immune response remains unanswered. It is certainly the case that Type 1 diabetes is not simply due to viral isletitis, and that different viruses have been suggested as being associated with diabetes (for example, mumps, Coxsackie, influenza). This is a reflection of the weakness of the evidence. The case for a viral aetiology is generally regarded as being supported by the seasonal incidence of Type 1 diabetes, which increases in winter in both hemispheres of the world. However, the recognition (see below) that Type 1 diabetes is of slow onset, and might be precipitated clinically by infective stress, could account for this seasonal distribution. More recently, evidence of association with nitrosamine and rodenticide ingestion has suggested that a wide variety of environmental influences may be the necessary precipitating factors. Epidemiological evidence suggests that Type 1 diabetes should be regarded as a mainly environmental disease.

Sera from newly presenting cases of Type 1 diabetes nearly all contain antibodies of IgG specificity that react with pancreatic islet cells, including those secreting glucagon and somatostatin. More specific to islet B-cells are the complement-fixing islet cell antibodies. Islet cell surface antibodies are also often detectable. The aetiological role of these markers is uncertain, for it remains possible that they occur secondarily to damage to islet B-cells induced directly by other agents. It has been suggested that interleukin 1 might have such a direct toxic effect on B-cells. Nevertheless, studies of the siblings of children with Type 1 diabetes have shown that islet cell antibodies may be detected many years before clinical diabetes is precipitated, that complement-fixing antibodies are a particularly strong marker for this risk and that the ability to mount a maximal output of insulin declines when these antibodies are present.

Type 2 Diabetes

Any discussion of the aetiology of Type 2 diabetes begs the question as to whether we are dealing with a single condition or a multitude of conditions. This question is in itself not a simple one for there is clearly no single aetiology, as exemplified by the overweight patient whose diabetes remits on dieting. Furthermore, many patients who only have diabetes under conditions of stress (for example, steroid therapy, some gestational diabetic patients), but who would not normally be classified as having Type 2 diabetes, may have the same underlying aetiology.

Much of the argument that Type 2 diabetes is heterologous comes from simple clinical observation, in particular the contrast between the thin elderly non-insulin-requiring patient relatively sensitive to sulphonylurea therapy, and the obese patient with gross hyperinsulinaemia and insulin insensitivity. Although there are defined subgroups of non-insulin-requiring patients who appear more clearly to have a distinct aetiology (for example, maturity onset diabetes of the young), these syndromes are rare and should not detract from the main debate.

Clinical research, however, has not produced evidence that Type 2 diabetes is of multiple aetiology. Genetic and population studies suggest a single disease. Thus collections of identical twins with Type 2 diabetes, show, in contrast to Type 1 diabetes, that both siblings are nearly always affected. Although there are too few twin pairs brought up separately to be sure that this is a genetic influence, in order to postulate a double aetiology it would be necessary to suggest two or more separate conditions of genetic origin. The strong genetic influence on the aetiology of Type 2 diabetes is also seen in the positive family history that can be detected in about half of newly presenting patients in industrialized countries.

Some populations have a very high incidence of Type 2 diabetes. Two of these, the Pima Indians in the USA and the Micronesian inhabitants of the island of Nauru, are characterized by the recent and sudden acquisition of prosperity, a very high intake of refined carbohydrate and a very high prevalence of obesity. A similarly high prevalence of diabetes is seen in other populations where prosperity, high sugar intake and obesity occur together, notably in the higher economic classes of Latin America and Arabia. The geographical universality of this response suggests that environmental factors other than food and activity are not important in the aetiology of Type 2 diabetes, smoking and alcohol consumption *per se* not being directly implicated.

Studies of the Pimas and Nauruans show a bimodal distribution of fasting and 2-h post-glucose load blood glucose concentrations, suggestive of a single condition. It is noteworthy that an age effect only occurs in the subpopulation with the higher distribution of blood glucose concentrations, suggesting that age is not an independent causative factor. Although obesity is somewhat universal in these populations, there are thin individuals, and interestingly some of these are quite clearly in the diabetic population. Obesity alone, imposed on the genetic susceptibility, is thus not an absolute requirement for Type 2 diabetes, and it has not proved possible to show that these thin diabetic individuals have had a previous history of being overweight, or of high calorie intake.

Given that the environmental influences dictating the occurrence of Type 2 diabetes are not understood, it is not surprising that there is still much argument concerning the pathophysiological mechanisms initiating the biochemical disturbance. In essence the question is whether the primary abnormality is a defect of insulin secretion, which leads to secondary tissue resistance to insulin action, or whether a primary abnormality of hepatic or peripheral metabolism leads eventually to damage to the mechanisms of insulin production or secretion. It is evident that many patients with Type 2 diabetes have high serum insulin concentrations in the fasting and post-absorbtive states, thus strongly suggesting that hepatic tissues are less than normally sensitive to insulin. Equally, glucose clamp studies show abnormal insensitivity of skeletal muscle to administered insulin. Nevertheless, the raised fasting and postprandial insulin concentrations are abnormally low when compared to the insulin secretion rates of a non-diabetic subject if the blood glucose concentration is raised to the level of the diabetic patient. Furthermore, during the period immediately following a meal there is often absolute hypoinsulinaemia in these patients. On the basis of studies of insulin responses in younger offspring of people with Type 2 diabetes, and because insulin insensitivity can be demonstrated to improve with insulin replacement therapy, it is concluded by some that the primary abnormality is of insulin secretion, but such a view is opposed by many experts.

However, it should be recognized that the insulin insensitivity and insulin secretion theories are not exclusive. A more useful synthesis relies on the observation that many people who do not have diabetes have a similar spectrum of insulin insensitivity, dyslipidaemia, major vessel disease and

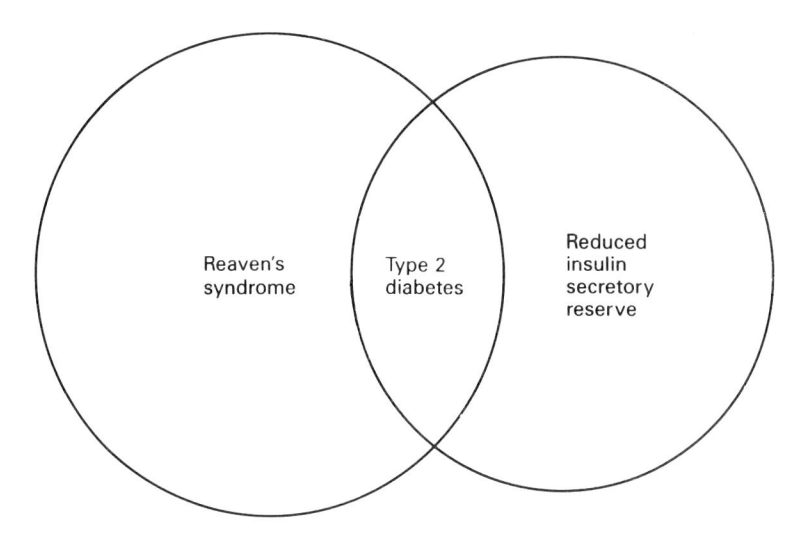

Reaven's syndrome:
Insulin insensitivity
Dyslipidaemia
Hypertension

Fig. 1.2 Schematic representation to show how insulin sensitivity and diminished insulin secretory reserve may interact to give Type 2 diabetes. The prevalence of Reaven's syndrome is likely to be influenced by factors related to high calorie intake, and will be much greater than that of reduced insulin secretory reserve in middle age. In old age the prevalence of insulin deficiency will increase, drawing into diabetes people whose degree of insulin insensitivity itself could hasten islet B-cell damage, through, for example, stimulation of the secretion of amyloid forming peptides.

hypertension, a combination becoming known as Reaven's syndrome. It is then possible that Type 2 diabetes only occurs in those patients with a propensity to develop B-cell failure in addition to having insulin insensitivity (Fig. 1.2). Indeed, it is possible that years of obesity or overeating are contributory to both Reaven's syndrome and islet B-cell failure.

Secondary Diabetes

Pancreatic damage

Diabetes secondary to pancreatic damage can occur with many forms of pancreatitis, pancreatic tumours or traumatic damage including pancreatectomy. The mechanism of diabetes will be that of insulin deficiency, although it must be recognized that some causes of pancreatitis or pancreatic infiltration, such as excessive alcohol consumption or haemochromatosis, may also lead to hepatic cirrhosis, which will exacerbate the tendency to diabetes by causing a profound insulin insensitivity. Any form of pancreatitis may lead to diabetes, and although the condition usually only develops with recurrent or chronic episodes, it may sometimes present with the first clinical event. Although diabetes occurs in association with calcific pancreatitis, radiological abnormalities on plain abdominal X-ray are uncommon, except in some tropical forms of the disease. Where the diabetes is noted in association with an acute episode of pancreatitis there may be remission with acute improvement in health, but once diabetes is established between episodes remission is rare.

Pancreatic diabetes, unlike other forms of diabetes, is associated with glucagon deficiency. These patients are often rather sensitive to insulin, and may be truely insulin-dependent on very small doses of insulin.

Endocrine disease

Diabetes is common in conditions where there is excessive secretion or delivery of the so-called counter-regulatory hormones, including Cushing's syndrome, acromegaly, glucagonoma and sometimes phaeochromocytoma. More common, in clinical practice is the association of diabetes with steroid administration, and problems may also arise through catecholamines used for inotropic cardiac support, or during stress reactions to major surgery, trauma or myocardial infarction.

In all these situations, however, many individuals do not develop more than minor degrees of glucose intolerance, and it seems clear that a patient already needs to have some degree of insulin insensitivity, or lack of pancreatic reserve, to develop diabetes or ketoacidosis under these circumstances. Problems of hyperglycaemia are more likely to occur with steroid therapy in people with a family history of non-insulin-dependent diabetes. It therefore seems likely that many patients who become diabetic under these circumstances have an underlying hormonal/biochemical abnormality related to the aetiology of Type 2 diabetes. People in the prodrome phase of Type 1 diabetes might be expected to react similarly.

Patients may become markedly diabetic on steroid therapy, requiring large doses of insulin. Unless they had undetected diabetes beforehand, it will remit on withdrawing the drug.

Gestational Diabetes

Diabetes appearing for the first time during pregnancy, and passing into remission afterwards, is separately classified as gestational diabetes. It has been suggested that what would be diagnosed as 'impaired glucose tolerance' in other circumstances (Table 1.4) should be classed as diabetes during pregnancy, although the evidence for this degree of glucose intolerance causing clinical problems is not strong.

The aetiology of gestational diabetes is not greatly different from endocrine diabetes, namely, the imposition of metabolic and hormonal changes on a biochemical milieu with little reserve. Human placental lactogen and prolactin both have anti-insulin metabolic effects. As many pregnant patients are young some of those who do go on to develop overt diabetes will have been in the prodromal phase of Type 1 diabetes, and will often require insulin therapy within a few months. However, if the patient is over 20 years of age and obese, particularly if she has a family history of diabetes, then there is a good chance of developing non-insulin-dependent diabetes very much later in life if dietary habits are not changed.

Other Forms of Diabetes

Other forms of diabetes have been reported from non-industrialized nations, but these probably only exist in pockets. Type 1 and Type 2 diabetes probably do occur in nations with low *per capita* incomes, but it appears that the diagnosis of insulin-dependent diabetes is often not made, and when it is prognosis is poor. Prevalence is thus very low. Dietary or other factors mean that Type 2 diabetes is rare in these countries. It may be that the condition sometimes described as J type diabetes (after Jamaica) is associated with malnutrition and secondary pancreatic damage. In these patients severe insulin insensitivity may be found, but ketosis is absent where adipose tissue mass is very low. Diabetes has also been described in association with cassava consumption and malnutrition, when pancreatic calcification is again common. A further possible source of pancreatic damage is locally brewed beers, presumably through a toxin in the plants used for flavouring.

Pathogenesis and Biochemistry of Diabetes

Clinically, diabetes has often been regarded as a single condition, because the biochemical disturbance is similar whatever the aetiology. Diabetes has generally been regarded by clinicians as a disease of glucose metabolism, because glucose is responsible for the commonest symptoms and is easily measured, but in reality it is a disturbance of the whole of intermediary metabolism as a result of relative or absolute insulin deficiency.

Metabolic Regulation and Acute Insulin Deficiency

Control of fasting metabolism

Insulin is secreted from the pancreas in a pulsatile fashion, probably with 'on' periods of 5 min in a cycle of 10–13 min. Although both proinsulin and C-peptide are also secreted (Fig. 1.3), only the first of these has any biological activity and this is too weak to be of biological significance. In the fasting state the major control of insulin secretion is determined by arterial plasma glucose concentration, although the islet B-cell is sensitive to other circulating compounds, including amino acids. In non-diabetic subjects control of plasma glucose concentrations is maintained very tightly, so that 80% of values in the course of a day will be within 10% of the mean concentration of around 4.3 mmol/l. In the fasting state this is achieved because insulin concentrations in the portal vein are high enough to restrain hepatic glucose production markedly. Any change in insulin delivery rate therefore modulates the input of glucose into the circulation, as the liver accounts for over 75% of glucose production (the rest being renal). Additionally the liver itself auto-regulates glucose production to some extent. Under basal conditions, by far the largest proportion of glucose disposal from the circulation is to the brain, and in the short-term this is purely a concentration-dependent phenomenon.

In the fasting state insulin will also have a restraining effect on triglyceride breakdown in the adipocyte, but this is not great enough to promote fat storage. There is therefore a significant output of non-esterified fatty acids (NEFA) from adipose tissue, and these provide the major fuel supply for skeletal muscle under fasting conditions. Non-esterified fatty acids and glycerol are also taken up by the liver, the former being oxidized to form 3-hydroxybutyrate and acetoacetate (ketone bodies) which again provide a useful fuel supply to peripheral tissues.

In skeletal muscle itself the major action of insulin in the fasting state will be to restrain protein breakdown, and hence loss of amino acids. The carbon backbone of amino acids, together with products of glycolysis, can be recycled to the liver to provide substrates for gluconeogenesis. Hepatic glycogen reserves will also be a major source of hepatic glucose production in the fasting (as opposed to the starved) state.

Insulin deficiency will therefore have predictable consequences (Fig. 1.4). Hepatic glucose output will rise with enhanced glycogen breakdown, and there will be diversion of the products of gluconeogenesis to glucose rather than to more glycogen. Triglyceride breakdown in adipose tissue will also be de-restrained, providing larger amounts of glycerol and NEFA, the latter en-

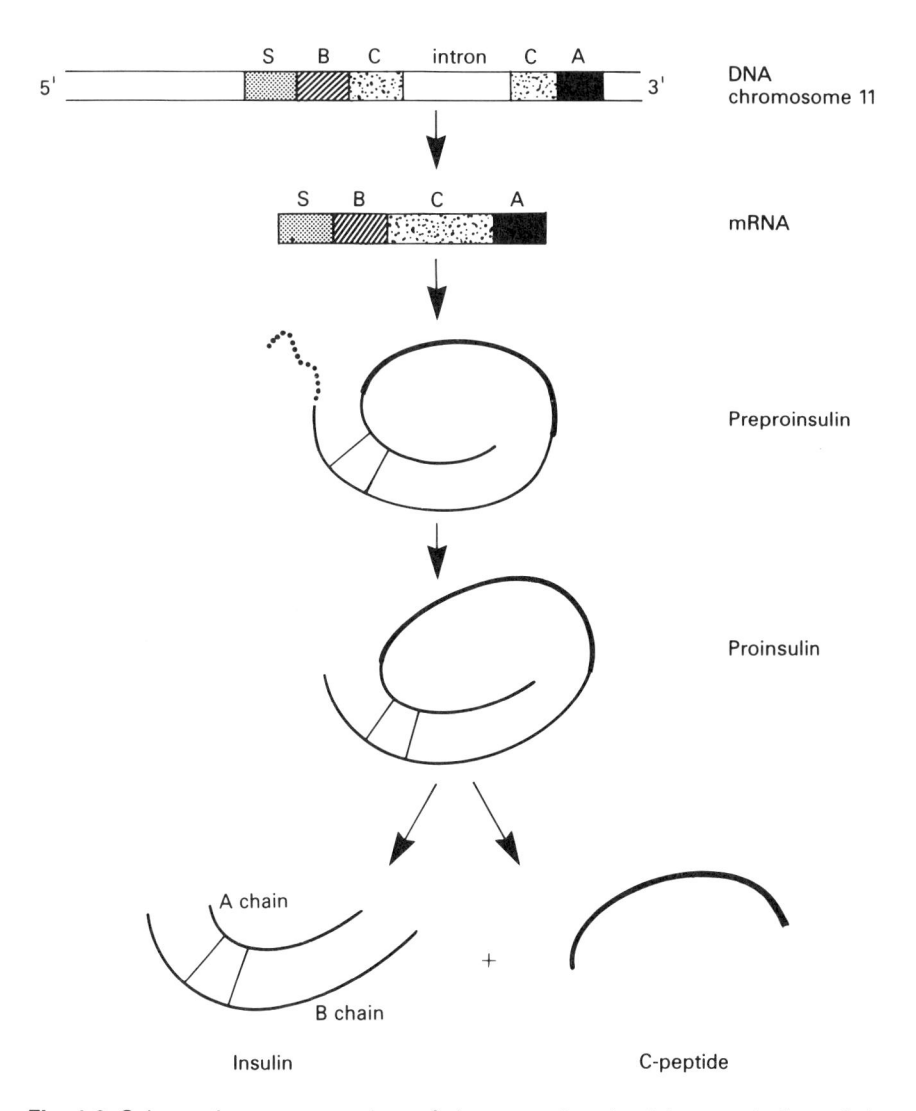

Fig. 1.3 Schematic representation of the steps involved in translation of the insulin gene on chromosome 11. One intron is spliced out in the formation of preproinsulin mRNA, which then guides the synthesis of the peptide. The signal peptide controls the destination of the molecule into granules, but is cleaved in doing so to leave proinsulin. Normally this is only secreted in small amounts, most being cleaved further before granule release to give equimolar amounts of insulin and C-peptide. Although the latter enters the circulation it has no metabolic actions.

14 What is Diabetes Mellitus?

hancing the output of hepatic ketone bodies. Plasma glucose, NEFA and ketone body concentrations will therefore rise, until their concentration-dependent removal comes into equilibrium with the rate of production. In the absence of enhanced counter-regulatory hormone secretion this will occur when glucose is around 12–15 mmol/l and plasma NEFA is 1–2 mmol/l. Ketone body concentrations will however rise from normal fasting concentrations (around 0.04 mmol/l) to levels where acidosis occurs (>5 mmol/l).

The role of the counter-regulatory hormones

The major hormone of physiological importance whose actions run counter to insulin is glucagon. Glucagon promotes hepatic breakdown of glycogen to glucose, and gluconeogenesis. It also promotes fatty acid oxidation by the liver and hence ketogenesis. There is a weak effect on peripheral lipolysis. Although its effects can be largely overcome by higher concentrations of insulin, in animals it does have a significant role in modulating hepatic metabolism in the fasting state. In diabetes, when insulin is relatively deficient, this action will be enhanced. Furthermore the restraining effect of blood glucose concentration on glucagon secretion is lost in insulin deficiency, and thus serum glucagon concentrations are raised in the diabetic individual.

Growth hormone concentrations are chronically raised in the poorly controlled diabetic patient, but only to a very small extent. Although growth hormone has significant effects on glucose metabolism in high concentrations, as in acromegaly, these are not important in diabetes, except in the disturbance of night-time blood glucose control.

Cortisol is also of little importance where insulin responses are adequate, but it is probably the most important deregulator of glucose metabolism in the stressed insulin-deficient patient. A major and clinically recognizable effect in these circumstances is on amino acid metabolism, where protein breakdown of muscle is enhanced, with consequent output of substrates for increased gluconeogenesis by the liver. The biochemical sites of action of cortisol are unclear, but effects are found both on regulation of hepatic glucose output and peripheral glucose disposal during chronic administration. Cortisol may be an important promotor of ketogenesis in the severely insulin-deficient patient.

Catecholamines may also be important in the promotion of ketogenesis, but this effect is assumed to be largely secondary to the increased supply of NEFA from adipose tissue as a result of the enhancement of lipolysis. These effects are further promoted by the dominant alpha-adrenergic effect of catecholamines on the islet B-cell, namely, to inhibit insulin secretion.

Fig. 1.4 Illustration of the effect of insulin deficiency on normal fasting metabolism. An arrow towards the tissue implies uptake. While the increased output of substrates from tissues are due to hormone deficiency, increased uptake (where indicated by *) may simply follow from the mass action effect of raised concentration. NEFA, non-esterified fatty acids. ↑ indicates increased levels of release of substrates into the bloodstream in insulin deficiency.

Tissue	Substrate	Normal uptake (←)/output (→) of substrate	Insulin-deficient uptake (←)/output (→) of substrate
Liver	Glucose	→	→→→
	Lactate	←	←←
	NEFA	←	←←
	Ketones	→	→→→
Muscle	Lactate	→	→→
	NEFA	←	←
	Ketones	←	←← *
Fat cell	NEFA	→	→→
Brain	Glucose	←	←← *
Blood	Glucose	←→	↑↑↑
	Lactate	←→	↑
	NEFA	←→	↑↑
	Ketones	←→	↑↑↑

The fed state

Although insulin is important in maintaining metabolic homeostasis after food intake, it is an error to consider insulin as a regulator only of ingested carbohydrate.

Anticipation of eating, and more particularly the presence of food in the gut, result in an increase in insulin secretion above basal rates, so that the metabolic status of the liver is already changing by the time absorption of food products begins to occur. Secretion of gut peptide hormones is thought to be a major mechanism of islet B-cell stimulation, but it is still unclear which major hormone(s) are concerned. Increased portal vein insulin concentrations will further restrain hepatic glucose output, so that gluconeogenic precursors (lactate) produced in the gut wall from the products of digestion are diverted to hepatic glycogen formation. *De novo* synthesis of fatty acids by the liver is also enhanced, while lipolysis in adipose tissue is further inhibited.

As glucose and amino acids are absorbed, and their arterial concentrations rise, insulin secretion will increase, reaching a maximum some 30–45 min after the start of the meal. These higher concentrations will, with some delay, enhance glucose incorporation into glycogen in skeletal muscle, and promote amino acid uptake in the same tissue. The larger part of carbohydrate in a meal appears as muscle glycogen. Insulin also promotes the synthesis of lipoprotein lipase in adipose tissue, and its expression on adjacent endothelial cells. This enzyme is responsible for the removal by digestion of triglyceride from chylomicrons, making the fatty acids available for esterification to triglyceride in the fat cell.

Acute insulin deficiency will impair all of these mechanisms. In particular the net nitrogen balance of skeletal muscle will remain negative, even in the fed state, and lipolysis and ketogenesis will continue unchecked. Any glucose load will only be removed from the circulation by non-insulin-dependent mechanisms, so that plasma concentrations of glucose will rise until the mass action effect can compensate for it. Renal loss of glucose in large quantities will inevitably give rise to an osmotic diuresis. Impaired clearance of lipoproteins from the circulation results in hyperlipidaemia.

Chronic Insulin Deficiency and Insulin Insensitivity

Prolonged deficiency of insulin will have metabolic effects predictable from its acute actions, as described above. The most evident of these will be the breakdown of skeletal muscle, whose products are turned into glucose through unrestrained gluconeogenesis in the liver. The glucose is then lost through the kidneys as a result of high plasma concentration. This calorie loss, coupled with failure to maintain fat stores, results in an inexorable reduction of body weight.

Where insulin deficiency is more modest, however, and where increased calorie intake matches the urinary calorie loss, the metabolic picture will be very different. Such patients can often maintain their fat stores and, to a lesser extent, retain muscle mass, while fueling gluconeogenesis with the products of peripheral glycolysis. While it may be that such patients have a relative insulin lack, many have an absolute elevation of plasma insulin concentrations in the fasting state, leading to the conclusion that they are relatively insensitive ('resistant') to the action of insulin. Furthermore, when exogenous insulin is given in larger amounts such patients prove to be insulin-insensitive even at the plasma concentrations found in the fed state.

The pathogenesis of insulin insensitivity in the chronically diabetic patient remains unclear. It appears to be a property of both hepatic and skeletal muscle metabolism. Insulin insensitivity is often found in non-diabetic obese subjects and the patterns of metabolic and other disturbances (for example, hypertension) suggest a similar cause. High levels of plasma NEFA may be a contributory factor, but they only account for a small part of the abnormality. Better defined as a cause of insulin insensitivity is insulin deficiency itself. Indeed it appears that restoration of insulin delivery to the insulin-insensitive Type 1 diabetic patient can largely return sensitivity to normal, while any effective treatment of the Type 2 patient (from diet to insulin) will improve this abnormality, although to far from normal values.

Metabolic Abnormalities in Non-Insulin-Dependent Tissues

It has recently been recognized that the chronic exposure of non-insulin-sensitive tissues to hyperglycaemia leads to a decreased capacity to take up and metabolize glucose. Consequently the mass action effect of higher plasma concentrations of glucose is reduced, so further lowering glucose disposal, and increasing hyperglycaemia. This will also mean that these tissues will take up less glucose at normal glucose concentrations, perhaps starving them of substrate supply and inducing intracellular metabolic abnormalities. Such mechanisms may also operate in tissues where glucose is important *per se* in the regulation of metabolic processes, in particular in the liver and the islet B-cell. As a result, hyperglycaemia may not effectively suppress hepatic glucose output, and the insulin secretory response to glucose will be blunted.

Abnormalities of insulin secretion

In the large majority of established Type 1 diabetic patients total insulin secretory failure is established one to three years from diagnosis. Patients with other forms of diabetes retain some insulin secretion, however, and indeed absolute plasma fasting and post-prandial insulin concentrations may be elevated. It is important to recognize that this may still be indicative of insulin deficiency, since the plasma glucose concentration will be elevated and the true yardstick for comparison should be the insulin concentration obtained in a non-diabetic subject if the plasma glucose level was raised accordingly.

The insulin secretory defect is more dramatically illustrated in the fed state, when plasma concentrations will rise much more slowly than in the normal

18 What is Diabetes Mellitus?

subject. Together with insulin insensitivity this results in ineffective glucose disposal and continuing elevation of plasma glucose concentrations (Fig. 1.5). These continue to stimulate insulin secretion, so plasma concentrations in the diabetic subject will again often be higher than in the non-diabetic subject in the period from 2 h after eating.

Studies with intravenous glucose administration have led to the division of insulin secretion into first and second phases, the former occurring in the first 6 min after plasma glucose concentrations are raised. Both first and second phase secretion are abnormal in diabetic patients, but the former is lost earlier in the disease and has acquired the reputation for being the underlying secretory defect. However, it is now clear that hyperglycaemia itself interferes with first phase release, and it is difficult to reconcile the significance of the observation with the continued abnormality of secretion throughout absorption of a meal.

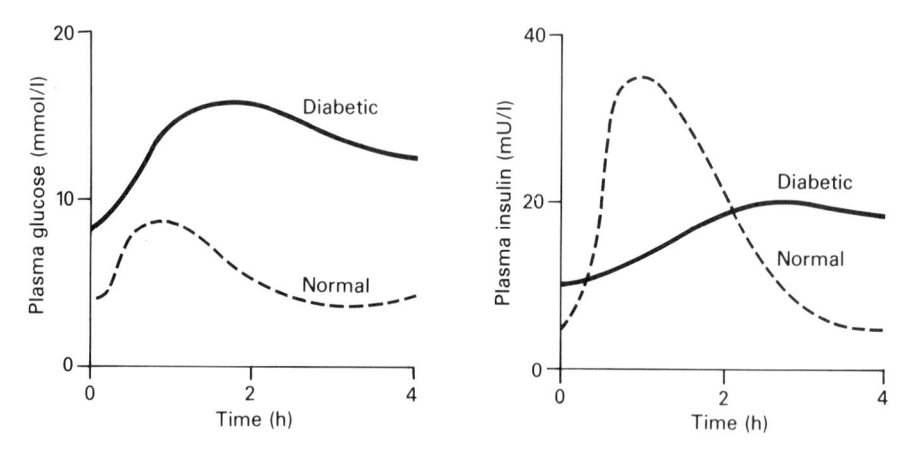

Fig. 1.5 Diagrams to show how the insulin response in non-insulin-dependent diabetes is influenced by the abnormal glucose profile after a meal. Raised fasting insulin levels are a response to fasting hyperglycaemia, but are inappropriately low for the abnormal blood glucose concentration. After the meal the insulin response is poor, so glucose concentrations go higher still, and continue to stimulate further insulin secretion long after physiological insulin and glucose profiles have returned to basal levels.

The metabolic abnormality underlying the insulin secretory defect is unclear, and investigations of the insulin gene have as yet proved unrewarding. It does appear, however, that the islet B-cell, as with other non-insulin-dependent tissues, becomes less sensitive to changes in glucose concentration as a result of prolonged exposure to hyperglycaemia. Any insulin secretory defect capable of causing hyperglycaemia is therefore likely to worsen the situation, particularly as target tissue insensitivity will develop as discussed above. It will be noted that effective treatment of any kind will thus have a doubly beneficial effect.

Definition of Diabetes Mellitus

It will be clear from the above that diabetes mellitus is not a single condition (disease or syndrome) in view of the heterogeneity of the aetiology and pathogenesis. Although heterogeneity is also to some extent a feature of treatment and natural history, the underlying common features of the biochemical disturbance and the specific late complications of diabetes make it worthwhile discussing the management, problems and outcome as if they were a single entity.

As discussed below confirmation of the diagnosis of diabetes is usually very simply obtained with a single blood test, and the severity of the metabolic disturbance is best assessed on treatment by self-monitoring in the patient's home environment, and confirmed by estimation of protein glycosylation. Nevertheless, it is useful to have a definition to which results of a patient's tests can be compared, if only for the reason that the diagnosis of diabetes may have significant consequences for the patient in terms of driving motor vehicles, piloting aircraft and shipping, life insurance, and in some forms of employment. Even here however the guiding principles are increasingly those of whether the presence of problems secondary to the diabetes (for example, angina, visual impairment) or to its treatment (for example, potential hypoglycaemia) are likely to give rise to risk to the patient or others.

The World Health Organization (WHO) has chosen a traditional measure of glucose handling for the purposes of defining diabetes, in the absence of evidence that any other metabolic measurement is of prognostic significance in the disease. The oral glucose tolerance test (OGTT) is now standardized as a 75 g glucose load (or 1.75 g/kg body weight if this is less) given in 250–300 ml of water, over the course of 5 min. Starch hydrolysates are an acceptable substitute. Diagnostic values are given in Table 1.4, and will vary according to whether blood or plasma glucose is measured (due to haemoglobin reducing effective water volume in the former) and whether the sample is taken from a site distal to glucose removing tissues (venous rather than capillary blood). A single blood sample should never be taken to be diagnostic of the condition in the absence of specific symptoms.

It will be noted that the WHO (1985) definition includes a category of 'impaired glucose tolerance'. People within this category are considered not to have normal glucose homeostasis, but to have a very low risk of specific diabetes-related late complications. They do however have an increased risk of major arterial disease, and should be given the same advice concerning diet and risk factor reduction as the Type 2 diabetic patient. It should not be assumed that the younger patient with impaired glucose tolerance will necessarily progress to diabetes, but a substantial proportion will do so over many years.

The WHO does not tackle the problem of whether a diabetic patient is still so defined if metabolism is returned to normal by treatment. Common sense dictates that this is not a problem when sulphonylurea or insulin treatment are used, but normal blood glucose levels are now increasingly found in patients

Table 1.4 Criteria for the diagnosis of diabetes mellitus

Criteria (alternatives):
1. Symptoms of diabetes + venous plasma glucose ≥11.1 mmol/l (or capillary glucose ≥11.1 mmol/l or venous blood glucose ≥10.0 mmol/l).
2. Venous plasma glucose ≥11.1 mmol/l on two separate occasions (or equivalent blood glucose).
3. Symptoms of diabetes + abnormal glucose tolerance test.
4. Two abnormalities (fasting and 2 h, or repeated 2 h) on glucose tolerance testing.

Criteria for abnormal glucose tolerance tests*:

	Fasting (mmol/l)	2 hour (mmol/l)
Diabetes		
Venous plasma	≥7.8	≥11.1
Venous whole blood	≥6.7	≥10.0
Capillary whole blood	≥6.7	≥11.1
Impaired glucose tolerance		
Venous plasma	<7.8	≥7.8–<11.1
Venous whole blood	<6.7	≥6.7–<10.0
Capillary whole blood	<6.7	≥7.8–<11.1

Applicability of criteria:
1. The patient is under no acute metabolic stress.
2. No metabolically active drugs are in use.
3. The assay of plasma or blood glucose is known to be reliable.
4. The physician is satisfied with the diagnosis.

*Criteria adapted from WHO Study Group (1985).
Glucose tolerance test: 75 g of anhydrous glucose in 250–300 ml water over 5 minutes.

following the same low sugar, high fibre diet recommended for their non-diabetic peers. However, even if normal glucose tolerance is achieved, it is possible for microvascular complications to develop for some years thereafter.

Presentation of Diabetes

Type 1 Diabetes

Although Type 1 diabetes most commonly presents between the ages of 4 and 30 years, with a peak in the 10–15 year age group, it may appear at any age. Nevertheless, it is uncommon in the elderly, and ketoacidosis presenting after the age of 40 years does not necessarily presage chronic insulin dependence. The peak season of presentation is during the winter in both hemispheres. Although the history of acute illness is usually short, often only a few days, pancreatic damage is known to proceed over years, marked by the presence of circulating complement fixing islet cell antibodies, while general ill health can often be recalled over a period of months.

The symptoms in the younger age group are generally those of polyuria, followed by polydipsia and weight loss. This often leads to a high consumption of soft drinks with high glucose content, thus exacerbating the symptoms. The history may, however, be too short for weight loss to have been evident. A history of infection of the skin or genito-urinary tract is also uncommon in the younger age group.

The progression into ketoacidosis will generally be announced by a complaint of feeling unwell, followed by loss of appetite, and then vomiting. Abdominal pain may accompany ketoacidosis and mimic an acute abdomen. Acidotic breathing, severe dehydration and loss of consciousness are severe events of grave prognostic significance if medical help is not sought immediately, or if diagnosis is delayed.

Over the age of 20 years symptoms may develop quite slowly, with weight loss despite increased appetite being a major marker. These patients may report problems with furunculosis, balantitis, vulval or vaginal candidiasis, and may have stigmata of other auto-immune disease. Below the age of 30 years patients presenting with diabetes are likely to require early insulin treatment, unless they are markedly overweight and have a family history of Type 2 diabetes.

Type 2 Diabetes

The presentation of Type 2 diabetes is much more heterogeneous, but the symptoms of polyuria, polydipsia and weight loss are still fairly common, often over a time course of only a few months. In the more elderly patient polyuria may result in initial urological or gynaecological referral. Other causes of polyuria and ill health are given in Table 1.5. Recurrent or chronic genito-urinary infections are common, and patients sometimes report furunculosis or intertrigo.

However, the metabolic disturbance is often so insidious that diagnosis is only made on presentation with a complication of the condition. The most common of these is due to major vessel disease, presenting through angina, myocardial infarction or a cerebrovascular accident. Less commonly the condition is picked up by routine urinalysis or screening in relation to employ-

Table 1.5 Causes of polyuria with ill health

Diabetes mellitus
Hypercalcaemia with or without malignancy
Renal failure
Psychological disturbance with habitual water drinking
Excessive beer intake
Diabetes insipidus
---

ment, and it is not unusual for relatives with diabetes to perform a diagnostic urine test when the patient is unwell for any reason. Presentation to an optician or ophthalmologist with diabetic retinopathy also occurs occasionally.

Although the patient with Type 2 diabetes is usually overweight, or has been for many years, this is not invariably the case particularly in the elderly. Even thin patients with marked weight loss may respond to dietary therapy.

Diagnosis and Differential Diagnosis of Diabetes

The diagnosis of diabetes presents little difficulty, and with the aid of blood glucose estimation at the time of consultation (using reagent strips) it is only rarely that there is any room for doubt. Any such estimation should, however, be confirmed in the laboratory. Glycosylated haemoglobin concentrations 2% of haemoglobin above the upper end of the normal range may also be regarded as diagnostic if the assay is known to be reliable. Doubt thus occurs only where casual blood glucose concentrations are below 10 mmol/l (whole venous blood, Table 1.4), and glycosylated haemoglobin is not markedly elevated. In these circumstances an oral glucose tolerance test may be useful.

A diagnosis must never be made on urinary glucose estimations alone, as a low renal threshold for glucose can, rarely, give misleading results.

Even where diabetes is diagnosed it is not unusual for there to be some need to consider whether polyuria may have an additional cause particularly in the elderly patient (Table 1.5). Furthermore, it is generally necessary to consider whether the diabetes is secondary to some other cause, such as drug therapy, pregnancy, or endocrine, hepatic or pancreatic disease.

Assessment of the Newly Presenting Diabetic Patient

The assessment of the newly presenting patient with diabetes is designed to establish the diagnosis, identify possible associated or causative conditions, establish the presence of risk factors for future ill health, and lay the basis for long-term management. It is often difficult to perform all these tasks at the initial consultation, particularly as it will be necessary at this time to lay the basis of knowledge about diabetes in a patient or parent who may be quite disturbed by the diagnosis.

Aside from the history of presenting symptoms of diabetes, it will be necessary in the putative Type 2 diabetic patient to find out by direct questioning whether there is any suggestion of pancreatic disease, liver disease or alcohol consumption. Smoking and eating habits need assessment before a programme for behavioural change can be planned. The presence of symptoms of coronary or peripheral vascular disease should be sought, together with those of peripheral or autonomic neuropathy. It is worth enquiring about visual disturbances so that appropriate advice can be given to avoid attending an optician until blood glucose levels are controlled, as the refractive properties of the lens change as it slowly looses water accumulated secondary to the osmotic effects of glucose. A drug history must be obtained, particularly to identify use of steroids, thiazides, or thiazides and beta-adrenergic blockers in combination. As diabetes is basically managed by the patient at home and at work, the circumstances of these need to be understood by the diabetes team.

The emphasis in general examination will be to ensure that other disease is not present, and that diabetic complications have not yet appeared. This can have a useful initial educational impact. Endocrine disease (for example, Cushing's syndrome, acromegaly) will usually be obvious, with the exception of the rare glucagonoma, but signs of haemochromatosis or pregnancy are sometimes easily missed. Optic atrophy, lipoatrophy or acanthosis nigricans will suggest the rarer syndromes of diabetes. Particular attention should be paid to foot condition, peripheral pulses, peripheral nerve function, blood pressure and to the condition of the retinae.

Investigations will also be directed towards the possibility of intercurrent infection or other illness, and to diabetes-related tissue damage. They will thus usually include assessment of circulating blood cells and erythrocyte sedimentation rate, liver function tests, urinalysis for protein and organisms, an electrocardiogram, renal function tests and serum lipids. A chest X-ray should be performed in those populations where tuberculosis is still endemic.

Further Reading

Allen, F.M., Stillman, E. and Fitz R. (1913). *Total Dietary Regulation in the Treatment of Diabetes*, pp. 1–78. Rockefellar Institute for Medical Research, New York.

Bliss, M. (1982). *The Discovery of Insulin.* Paul Harris, Edinburgh.

Bottazzo, G.F., Pujol-Borrell, R. and Gale, E.A.M. (1987). Auto-immunity and Type 1 diabetes: bringing the story up to date. In *Diabetes Annual 3*, pp. 15–38. Edited by Alberti, K.G.M.M. and Krall, L.P., Elsevier, Amsterdam.

Hitman, G.A. and Niven, M.J. (1989). Genes and diabetes mellitus. *British Medical Bulletin* **45**, 191.

Keen, H. and Ng Tang Fui, S. (1982). The definition and classification of diabetes mellitus. *Clinics in Endocrinology and Metabolism* **11**, 279.

Leslie, R.D.G., Lazarus, N.R. and Vergani, D. (1989). Aetiology of insulin-dependent diabetes. *British Medical Bulletin* **45**, 58.

Taylor, R. (1989). Aetiology of non-insulin dependent diabetes mellitus. *British Medical Bulletin* **45**, 73.

Taylor, R. and Agius, L. (1988). The biochemistry of diabetes. *Biochemical Journal* **250**, 625.

2
LATE TISSUE DAMAGE IN DIABETES MELLITUS

As discussed in Chapter 1, diabetes mellitus is well recognized to be a condition of multiple aetiology. It is unified as a single condition by two common features, found in all forms of the disease, although there are some varying features. Firstly, there is the characteristic metabolic disturbance, manifested by absolute or relative insulin deficiency, with consequent disturbance of hepatic glucose production, lipolysis, peripheral glucose disposal and protein metabolism. Secondly, there is a spectrum of tissue damage which occurs in many parts of the body, and often only becomes evident many years after diagnosis. Some aspects of the tissue damage that is associated with diabetes are very similar to the damage found in the absence of diabetes, in particular the atherosclerosis affecting many of the major arteries commonly diseased in modern people. Other aspects of this spectrum of tissue damage are, however, essentially unique to diabetes in terms of their natural history and pathological description (for example, retinopathy), even where individual features (for example, microaneurysms, mononeuropathy) may be found in other unrelated conditions.

It is the convention to use the phrase 'complications of diabetes' to describe specific tissue damage, particularly of the retina, kidneys and nerves, thus using the term 'diabetes' in its narrow metabolic sense. Pathological studies, however, reveal that in people in whom the metabolic state persists for decades, including therefore all Type 1 diabetic patients, tissue damage is eventually universal. It might therefore seem more correct to see this damage as part of the natural history of the disease, rather than as a complication of it.

Prevalence and Clinical Significance of Diabetic Tissue Damage

The importance of this tissue damage should not be underestimated, but it is difficult to obtain reliable figures for risk applicable to current diabetic populations. This arises because the damage is only manifested as a clinical problem many decades after diagnosis, and hence the current incidence of damage is a reflection of the cohorts of people who developed diabetes in the 1940s to

1960s, and of the techniques of management used during the intervening years. Management has certainly changed, and the increasing incidence of both the major types of diabetes might suggest that the population developing the disease will have different characteristics overall to past populations. An added difficulty is that deaths from diabetes are often recorded as being secondary to malfunction of the organ suffering the endstage damage (for example, myocardial infarction, renal failure, cerebrovascular accident), rather than the diabetes itself.

Morbidity is, however, probably an even greater problem for people with diabetes than mortality. In the USA and Scandinavia, countries for which there are adequate data, diabetes mellitus is the commonest cause of blindness before retirement age. In these countries renal transplantation is probably offered to the majority of people below the age of 70 years with progressive renal failure due to diabetes, and the disease then accounts for 20–30% of all such referrals. Nevertheless, it is not eye damage or kidney damage that accounts for the major part of in-patient bed occupancy by people with diabetes, and admission for metabolic problems *per se* is now comparatively uncommon. Foot problems, however, particularly foot ulcers secondary to neuropathy and arteriopathy, often requiring amputation, result in extended stays in hospital, and are a major cause of disablement.

When histological studies of kidneys in people with long-standing diabetes are made, it is found that the characteristic glomerular lesions are present in all specimens studied. Similarly, assessment of retinopathy over periods of years will reveal lesions in over 90% of eyes at one time or another, and use of fluorosciein angiography has confirmed the high penetration of the condition in diabetic patients. By contrast the malignant complications (for example, proliferative retinopathy, diabetic nephropathy) of this tissue damage only occur in a smaller proportion of patients, photocoagulation and management of renal failure only being needed in 10 to 30% of patient-lifetimes, depending mainly on age at diagnosis.

Classification of Late Tissue Damage of Diabetes

Classically late tissue damage of diabetes is divided into microvascular disease and macrovascular disease. The rationale for this division is that the so-called microvascular 'complications', including the classic triad of retinopathy, nephropathy and neuropathy, are nearly specific to diabetes, and have been assumed to be secondary to damage occurring in small vessels of the retina, glomerulus and nerves. It is, however, by no means clear that the metabolic damage in these tissues does have a single initiating cause, and indeed it has been suggested that, for example, vascular damage is not the major cause of neuropathy. By contrast, however, the spectrum of pathological features of the macrovascular disease (including peripheral vascular disease, ischaemic heart disease and hypertension) is very similar to that seen in people without diabetes. It is probably unsafe, however, to assume that the unknown metabolic disturbance underlying damage to small vessels is not capable of causing damage to arteries. In particular it is possible that leakage through the endothelium could be responsible for causing abnormal handling of lipids in the arterial wall. It is notable that retinopathy and systolic hypertension often develop together, and measurements of them correlate well, while diabetic nephropathy or glomerular leakage of albumin is associated with ischaemic heart disease.

The microvascular–macrovascular classification of tissue damage occurring in diabetes is also defective in not including other lesions of greater or lesser importance. The damage occurring to the fetus of the diabetic mother with poor control is the most significant of these, but chronic pyelonephritis can still cause renal failure, cataracts and glaucoma can lead to blindness; and some infections occurring secondary to poor lymphocyte and macrophage function are also potentially fatal.

The main sites and forms of microvascular and macrovascular disease are listed in Table 2.1, together with other forms of late tissue damage occurring in diabetes. Although all these types of damage occur in all forms of diabetes the spectrum of incidence can be very different, presumably reflecting the age groups in which the damage occurs, and the characteristics, duration and magnitude of the metabolic disturbance before diagnosis. Thus many people with Type 2 diabetes probably have a significant if mild metabolic disturbance for many years before diagnosis, either true diabetes or just impaired glucose

Table 2.1 Classification of late tissue damage in diabetes

Organ	Disease
Microangiopathy	
Eyes	Retinopathy
	Maculopathy
	Rubeosis iridis
Kidney	Nephropathy
Nerves	Neuropathy (see Table 2.6)
Heart	Cardiomyopathy
Musculo-skeletal	Soft tissue thickening
	Cheiroarthropathy
Skin	Dermopathy
Macroangiopathy	
Cardio-vascular system	Hypertension
	Ischaemic heart disease
	Cerebro-vascular disease
	Peripheral vascular disease
	Other arteries
Other	
Eyes	Cataract
	Glaucoma
Kidney	Chronic pyelonephritis

tolerance. The consequence is not only that such patients may present with retinopathy, but also that the various forms of major vessel disease have high incidence and prevalence, and are likely to provide the main management problems. By contrast the child with diabetes will only rarely suffer any of these problems, but grows up to face the possibility of eye and kidney problems in adulthood, with a major risk of large vessel disease if the patient survives until middle age.

Is Late Tissue Damage Caused by Metabolic Disturbance?

As the biochemical mechanism of late tissue damage is not known, it is important when considering the prognosis and management of diabetes to understand how the late manifestations of the disease are directly related to the characteristic metabolic disturbance, and to consider therefore whether they might be avoided by effective treatment. The pathogenesis of late tissue damage must inevitably have a biochemical basis of some kind, but it is quite possible to conceive that the metabolic disturbance recognized as 'diabetes' could co-exist with some independent tissue metabolic defects which could also be responsible for the tissue damage. Following from this there are five hypotheses which may be proposed:

1. There is a common genetic basis to the metabolic disturbance and the late complications, but that they are biochemically quite distinct. Thus a combination of genes could have different consequences in different tissues, leading to defects in insulin secretion when expressed in islets, and to capillary abnormalities when expressed in the pericytes of the retinal circulation.
2. There is a common environmental cause for the metabolic disturbance and the late complications, but that they are biochemically quite distinct. Thus a virus might be thought capable of causing islet B-cell damage, and damage in some other way (perhaps through immunological mechanisms) to vascular cells.
3. There is a common causative biochemical defect, which independently results in abnormalities of insulin secretion by the islet B-cells (or liver and muscle insulin insensitivity), and an abnormality causing late tissue damage. Thus hypothetically a membrane defect might initiate damage to the islet B-cell, and predispose to all the vascular manifestations.
4. Some aspect of the metabolic disturbance characteristic of diabetes is causative of damage in various tissues, through a common biochemical mechanism. Thus hyperglycaemia-induced accumulation of sorbitol might damage nerves, the lens and capillary function.
5. The metabolic disturbance of diabetes causes a number of different biochemical defects in different tissues, with resultant tissue damage. Thus glycosylation may damage lens crystallin, sorbitol may disturb neuronal function, and platelet changes cause arterial damage.

The first three of these hypotheses are indistinguishable at present and may be termed the co-causation theory. In the literature they are generally discussed in terms of a possible common genetic basis, the metabolic hypothesis being misleadingly termed the environmental hypothesis. Many specialists in the diabetes field would not distinguish between the fourth and fifth hypotheses, but would hold to the theory of the metabolic causation for the reasons discussed below. The fourth and fifth hypotheses may need to be distinguished if treatments become available which will interfere with one particular pathway previously demonstrated to cause one of the diabetic complications.

It is worth emphasizing that the concept of a genetic or a metabolic cause for late tissue damage is wholly misleading. Genes can only be expressed within the environment of the tissue they may govern. It may well be the case for example that there is a genetic influence on the development of complications, particularly the terminal events, but it is probable that this influence is only of significance when the tissue finds its biochemical homeostasis disturbed by diabetes. Thus even with the appropriate genes someone without diabetes would never develop retinopathy or nephropathy.

Evidence for the Metabolic Hypothesis (Table 2.2)

Cross-sectional and retrospective studies

A large number of cross-sectional and retrospective studies of the relationship between diabetic control and microvascular disease have been published. Cross-sectional studies suffer from the inevitable problem that they measure current control, while the relevant metabolic damage will have been accumu-

Table 2.2 Types of study supporting the metabolic hypothesis

Study	Conclusions
1. Animal diabetes	Microvascular lesions only after induction of diabetes
	Reversal/prevention with good control
2. Cross-sectional/retrospective studies in patients	Control related to development of complications
3. Prospective studies of patients	Microvascular lesions developing particularly in poorly controlled patients
	Proliferative retinopathy only if HbA_1 high
4. Intervention studies of established complications	Lesser progression of lesions with tight control
5. Epidemiological (population) studies	Microvascular complications only if marked glucose intolerance
6. Transplantation studies	Renal transplants develop microvascular lesions in diabetic patients
	Prevention of such changes can be achieved by good control of insulin levels
7. Genetic studies (identical twins)	Twin of a diabetic patient develops complications only if diabetes develops

lating over many years. Both cross-sectional and, to a greater extent, retrospective studies have suffered a further fundamental problem, however, for it has only been in the last decade that it has been possible to measure blood glucose control effectively. Even now the metabolic disturbance generally has been measured only as aspects of blood glucose concentration, body weight and serum lipids. Prior to the mid-1970s only urinalysis and clinic random blood glucose concentrations were available, and neither of these correlate well with diurnal blood glucose concentrations. Thus, assessment of control contained a large amount of random error, which would in turn be expected to remove the statistical significance of any relationship. It is not therefore surprising that many retrospective studies failed to find a relationship with control. However, some did find a relationship, and with improved assessment techniques (for example, glycosylated haemoglobin) there is now even semi-quantitative data on the degree of poor blood glucose control necessary for progression of early retinopathy.

Prospective and intervention studies

Only recently have the methods and understanding of insulin administration become sophisticated enough to modify control predictably and prospectively in any intervention study. Nevertheless, Pirart was able to show a relationship between microvascular complications and blood glucose levels in a large series of patients who were followed in ever decreasing number for 25 years.

More recently, the availability of continuous subcutaneous insulin infusion, glycosylated haemoglobin estimation and methods for measuring blood glucose profiles at home, has enabled a series of studies of control in patients with established microvascular disease. Studies have been directed towards retinopathy, nephropathy and neuropathy. It certainly appears that nerve conduction and neurological symptoms respond to tight control, but there has always been a suspicion that some of the disturbance of established neuropathy relates to current control, rather than being entirely due to long-term damage. Established retinopathy may worsen after an acute improvement in blood glucose control, possibly due to removal of the protective effect of hyperglycaemia, which itself promotes retinal blood flow. After a couple of years of tight control, however, it does seem that established retinopathy is improved, and progression as a whole halted. Similarly, two years of insulin infusion pump treatment may halt any deterioration in albumin excretion in patients with a subclinical leak ('microalbuminuria'), and the rise in blood pressure is arrested. Primary prevention studies are still desperately needed.

Epidemiological studies

Studies of diabetes in large populations have suggested that there is a relationship between the degree of abnormality of response to a glucose tolerance test, and the presence or development of retinopathy. It is on this basis that the blood glucose concentrations for the oral glucose tolerance test (OGTT) for the definition of diabetes by the World Health Organization (WHO) were determined (see Chapter 1). When populations as a whole change their habits, eating a Western style diet, taking less exercise and becoming generally obese, the incidence of diabetes rises. Although there will not be any genetic change in the short period involved, those people with diabetes now develop the complications, whereas previously they did not.

Animal studies

Experimentally it is possible to induce the development of characteristic microvascular damage, similar if not identical to that found in humans, in animals made diabetic in a variety of ways, including injection of drugs and pancreatectomy. This is possible in many species. Furthermore, in rats and dogs it has been possible to demonstrate a relationship between development of retinal lesions and blood glucose control. Glomerular lesions induced in diabetic rats can be reversed by transplanting the kidney concerned into a non-diabetic animal.

Transplantation studies in humans

Kidneys taken from donors killed in accidents nearly always develop the characteristic changes of diabetic glomerulosclerosis when transplanted into people with renal failure resulting from diabetic nephropathy. The exception is when concomitant pancreatic transplantation results in good blood glucose control.

Biochemical studies

Biochemical studies have succeeded only in demonstrating the enormous extent of the metabolic disturbance in diabetes, with many hundreds of abnormalities of blood and tissue concentrations of substrates, or enzyme activities, now on record. Whilst this draws attention to the large numbers of biochemical pathways that could be the initiating event in determining late tissue damage, it has been possible in some circumstances to imitate such damage by biochemical intervention. An example of this is galactose feeding to rats, resulting in characteristic cataracts. However, no similar evidence exists for classical microvascular damage. While the biochemical disturbances responsible for microvascular damage remain unclear, for many of the mechanisms that have been proposed (see below) it has been demonstrated that improved control in humans and animals leads to mitigation of the abnormality. This is the case for nerve polyol concentrations, serum growth hormone concentrations, platelet functional abnormalities and capillary fragility, for example.

Genetic arguments

As discussed in the sections on aetiology and pathogenesis (see Chapter 1), diabetes is not a single disease in the aetiological sense, as exemplified by clinical presentation, genetics and pathogenesis. As the specific late tissue damage of diabetes occurs in all forms of the syndrome, including diabetes secondary to various forms of pancreatic damage, but not in euglycaemic people, it becomes difficult, if not impossible, to hold to the theories of co-causation. Thus specific complications are found in patients with tropical diabetes, diabetes after pancreatitis and pancreatectomy, diabetes in acromegaly, and diabetes secondary to haemochromatosis, as well as in the major types of diabetes.

Where only one of a pair of identical twins develops diabetes, as happens in the majority of pairs in Type 1 diabetes, then the normal twin never develops microvascular damage. This is true even though most twin pairs share childhood environments, as well as genes.

Evidence for the Co-causation Hypothesis

Basement membrane studies

A feature of many tissues in people with diabetes is thickening of the basement membrane which occupies the space between the endothelial cells lining the capillaries and the cells of the tissues. It is an early feature in the retina and the renal glomerulus. It has been suggested that such thickening is universal in diabetes, and is an important factor in the development of microvascular disease. This may or may not be the case, but the argument then put is that basement membrane thickening is sometimes demonstrable before the onset of diabetes (the metabolic disturbance). There are major methodological difficulties in measuring basement membrane thickness, however, and it now seems to be generally accepted that this is not the case. In performing these kinds of studies it is important to recognize that diabetes is a disease of slow onset, with the exception of some forms of pancreatic damage, and that the metabolic disturbance may have been present for a good while before diagnosis.

Sparing from microvascular disease

It is often pointed out that many patients do not suffer the microvascular complications, even though they all, by definition, have the metabolic disturbance. This is then taken to mean that the metabolic disturbance cannot be the cause of microvascular disease, in those who do suffer the problems. In practice this is based on a false assessment of the incidence of microvascular disease, since careful searches in patients with diabetes of sufficient duration will reveal retinopathy in over 90% of cases, and nearly universal renal glomerular changes. It is true that there is incomplete penetration of the malignant aspects of the complications, proliferative retinopathy or progressive nephropathy, but these only occur in the presence of background changes. However, proliferative retinopathy not only shows incomplete penetration between patients, but also within single patients from year to year, so it is difficult to attribute this phenomenon to genetic differences alone.

Clearly there are other metabolic factors which determine the natural history of tissue damage in any particular individual. It may well be the case that some are even protective against microvascular complications (the high tissue blood flow induced by hyperglycaemia, for example), and that it is a balance of factors which determines the spectrum of problems.

Clinical impressions

'Some patients with poor control have no complications, and some patients with good control do badly'. This is undoubtedly true, but the argument that it supports a co-causation hypothesis is flawed. Many patients with poor control are young and have a short duration of diabetes, while many patients regarded as having relatively good control have not in fact had documented glycosylated haemoglobin concentrations close to normal throughout their diabetic lifetime, and many are well into adulthood and past the age when control was at its poorest.

Control and Complications: Conclusions

It now seems clear that the evidence shows that the microvascular complications of diabetes do not occur in the absence of metabolic disturbance, and hence that its appropriate correction should result in the prevention of these complications. It is at present unclear, however, whether the appropriate correction of the metabolic disturbance will merely mean the delivery of insulin to obtain glycosylated haemoglobin concentrations below some set figure close to the top end of the normal range, or whether more specific and careful control of some other metabolic variable will be necessary.

Meanwhile it would seem unwise for any physician not to advise the majority of adult patients of the relationship between control and complications, since not to do so could be regarded as a breach of duty of care. Nevertheless, it remains the case that at present we do not have the means to guarantee a high proportion of patients freedom from complications, while meanwhile allowing them a satisfactory lifestyle.

Pathological Mechanisms of Microangiopathy (Table 2.3)

The pathological mechanisms resulting in damage to various tissues in diabetes have not been defined, and the underlying biochemistry is not understood. It even remains unclear, for example, whether there is a common initiating

Table 2.3 Postulated mechanisms for development of microvascular lesions

Cell membrane damage
  Vascular leakage
  Basement membrane thickening
  Sodium/Lithium counter-transport abnormalities
  Free radical damage
  Gamma-linolenic acid deficiency

The polyol hypothesis
  Sorbitol accumulation
  Myo-inositol depletion

Glycosylation
  Glycosylated proteins (structural, enzymatic)
  Advanced glycosylation end products

Rheological and clotting abnormalities
  Microthrombosis (abnormal platelet function)
  Clot lysis abnormalities
  Abnormal erythrocytes

These mechanisms are not necessarily exclusive. Thus membrane damage might be the basis for platelet dysfunction.

pathway for retinopathy, neuropathy and nephropathy, or whether their development is essentially biochemically independent. Although a number of potential pathological mechanisms have been suggested, and some of the more promising are described below, evidence of a definite role for any of them, and therefore for a definite site for clinical intervention, is lacking.

Altered Capillary Permeability

Leakage from capillaries is an early feature of diabetes in the eye. This can be demonstrated by fluoroscein angiography well before any structural vascular changes are discernible. Similarly, transcapillary albumin escape is demonstrable early on in the development of diabetic nephropathy. Early permeability changes are presumably a reflection of abnormal function of the intercellular junctions between endothelial cells. The characteristics of these junctions can be altered by biochemical changes occurring within the endothelial cells. The biochemical mechanism of the leakage, and how it might lead to later structural changes of the capillaries, is unclear. Leakage may be an important factor in the early changes seen in the basement membrane (see below), and could account for stiffening of arterial walls (and hence hypertension) and arterial wall lipid deposition.

It has recently been suggested that those diabetic patients who go on to develop diabetic nephropathy can be distinguished by the properties of their sodium/lithium counter-transport across cell membranes, inherited properties that may be linked to hypertension alone in non-diabetic people. It may well be, however, that sodium/lithium pump activity is simply a marker for some more fundamental membrane defect, itself related to increased membrane permeability under conditions of hyperglycaemia.

Basement Membrane Thickening

Thickening of the capillary basement membrane and basement lamina is evident in many tissues in people with uncontrolled diabetes, including the retina, renal glomerulus and even skeletal muscle. In animals made diabetic with drugs, basement membrane thickening develops quite quickly. The biochemical nature of this abnormal basement membrane remains to be established, although abnormalities of its carbohydrate content and glycoprotein constituents are well documented. The increased amounts of hydroxyproline present in the diabetic retina do, however, suggest that either synthesis of the Type IV collagen skeleton is abnormally rapid, or that scavenging, a pericyte function, is deficient. Capillary leakage of large molecules, as manifested by transcapillary albumin escape and retinal leakage of lipoproteins, may be a function of the abnormal basement membrane. Albumin leakage probably occurs because of loss of the normal charge of the basement membrane, a charge conferred by its content of glycosaminoglycans, such as heparan sulphate. The presence of immunoglobulins and other blood constituents in the thickened basement membrane is probably only a reflection of this leakage from plasma, rather than their presence making a significant contribution to thickening as such.

It remains unclear, however, what role, if any, thickening and abnormalities of the basement membrane might have in the development of capillary closure and later microvascular damage.

The Polyol Hypotheses

Sorbitol accumulation

Many cells contain an enzyme, aldose reductase, which at high glucose concentrations will convert glucose to the polyol, sorbitol (Fig. 2.1). This is removed by a second enzyme, alcohol dehydrogenase, but only when sorbitol is present at high concentrations. Sorbitol therefore accumulates in many tissues when the cells are exposed to high glucose concentrations, although it is unclear whether, and if so how, sorbitol accumulation does any damage. Two possibilities are an osmotic effect or a direct toxic effect, with possible sites of damage being the pericytes of the retinal capillaries and the Schwann cells of nerves. Although use of aldose reductase inhibitors in experimental models can prevent cataracts, the clinical use of these drugs has as yet proved unexciting. Formation of sorbitol requires the use of reducing equivalents, and it is possible that a resulting alteration of cytoplasmic redox state could itself be an initiating pathway for a significant biochemical disturbance.

```
Glucose                    Sorbitol                    Fructose
    \                      /      \                      /
     \                    /        \                    /
      \                  /          \                  /
NADPH   ───────────────▶ NADP  NAD   ───────────────▶ NADH
          Aldose reductase         Alcohol dehydrogenase
```

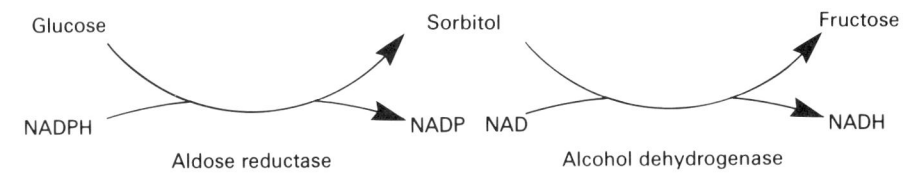

Fig. 2.1 Diagram of the mechanism of accumulation and removal of sorbitol in cells. Aldose reductase has a high capacity for glucose, so that sorbitol formation increases proportionately to glucose concentration. However, alcohol dehydrogenase is a low capacity enzyme, and clearance of sorbitol can rise very little. The result is marked increases in intracellular sorbitol concentrations.

Myo-inositol depletion

Myo-inositol is a cyclic polyol, found throughout the animal and plant kingdoms. It is of particular interest because of its concentration in nervous tissue, but which is relatively low in diabetes. For reasons that remain unclear myo-inositol depletion is related to sorbitol accumulation, and reversed by aldose reductase inhibitors in experimental diabetes. Myo-inositol is a precursor of phosphoinositides. They are an important part of phospholipids, and are now known to be intimately involved in extensive intracellular and intercellular signalling systems, and modulation of enzyme activities through the regulation of protein kinase C. It has been suggested that myo-inositol depletion may affect nerve conduction through effects on membrane sodium/potassium ATPase, but other alterations of membrane metabolism may well occur through disturbed inositol phospholipid metabolism. As yet no direct link with intercellular junction function has been demonstrated.

Glycosylation

Increased non-enzymatic glycosylation will occur on all susceptible proteins exposed to high glucose concentrations. This non-catalysed reaction is, however, slow and will be of little consequence for proteins whose turnover is quite fast. Thus very high concentrations of glucose are required to obtain glycosylation of a significant fraction of apolipoproteins, and it would be surprising if this could account for lipid turnover abnormalities. Some proteins do, however, turn over at rather slower rates, particularly structural proteins including those of the basement membrane. Glycosylation of these might lead to a change of biochemical characteristics. Possible sites for detrimental effects of tissue glycosylation would be lens crystallin, Type IV collagen in basement membrane, collagen in skin and connective tissue, and nerve myelin. All these proteins are known to show increased glycosylation in human or animal diabetes.

Platelets, Prostaglandins and Clotting Factors

Many aspects of thrombotic and clotting mechanisms have been shown to be disturbed in diabetes, and it is hypothesized that these might predispose to capillary endothelial cell damage. Thus there is some evidence of decreased endothelial cell prostacyclin synthesis in experimental diabetes, and with it increased platelet stickiness. Similarly there is evidence of reduced fibrinolytic activity in plasma, and a combination of these might be expected to lead to an increased rate of vascular occlusion at the microscopic level. Similarly, erythrocytes show decreased deformability in diabetes, possibly through haemoglobin glycosylation.

Diabetic Eye Disease

Natural History and Retinal Appearance (Table 2.4)

The initial changes in the diabetic retina are not visible on ophthalmoscopy, but consist of leakage through the blood–retina barrier between endothelial cells and thickening of retinal capillary basement membranes. Abnormalities of the retinal capillaries then follow, with subsequent loss of the pericytes. Damage to the small vessels eventually leads to capillary closure. This, and capillary leakage, may be demonstrated by fluoroscein angiography. These changes in the walls of the smallest vessels eventually lead to distortion and dilatation, giving rise to the earliest observable changes, the characteristic microaneurysms. Microaneurysm counts may vary from very few up to hundreds per eye. They may be of variable size and individual microaneuryms often thrombose and therefore disappear.

The next lesion to appear is usually the intraretinal haemorrhage (Fig. 2.2).

Table 2.4 Classification of the lesions of diabetic retinopathy

Background retinopathy	Proliferative retinopathy	Maculopathy

Early lesions
  Microaneurysms
  Small intraretinal
    haemorrhages
  Hard exudates
Pre-proliferative lesions
  Multiple large blot
    haemorrhages
  Cotton wool spots
  Venous tortuosity
  Venous beading
  Intraretinal
    microvascular
    abnormalities
	New vessel formation
	Fibrosis and traction
	Vitreous haemorrhage
		Exudative maculopathy
		Macular oedema
		Ischaemic maculopathy

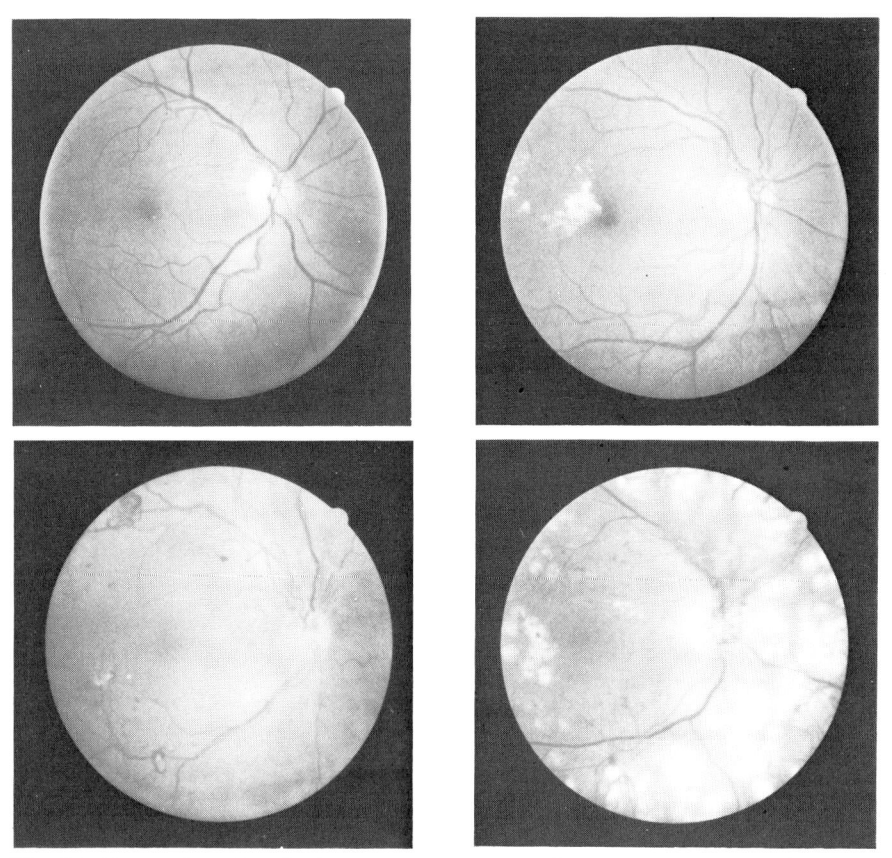

Fig. 2.2 Examples of diabetic retinopathy. **Top left**: Maculopathy with minimal retinopathy. Most of the retina appears normal. Careful inspection of the macula reveals a microaneurysm and a small hard exudate. Another microaneurysm is present above and to the right of the macula. Visual acuity had dropped one line over the last year. **Top right**: Hard exudates in a typically circinate pattern, temporal to the macula, and threatening it. Plasma will be leaking from a single point in the centre of the ring. Visual acuity is as yet still normal. **Bottom left**: Proliferative retinopathy. New vessels are visible growing both upwards from the disk, and in the periphery (top left). Two areas of infarction surrounded by haemorrhage are seen bottom left, together with scattered microaneurysms and retinal haemorrhages. **Bottom right**: Laser photocoagulation scars are seen throughout the peripheral retina. Venous abnormalities are extensive, particularly microaneursyms, retinal haemorrhages, and new vessels. A leash of new vessels is growing upwards and forwards from the optic disk, and is hence out of focus. *See* colour plates between pages 166–167.

Bleeding is confined by the retinal membrane. The shape of the haemorrhage is determined by the orientation of the nerve fibres at the point of haemorrhage. Many haemorrhages are seen end on, and will usually be interpreted as microaneuryms. Such haemorrhage occurs after rupture of a small venule or microaneurysm, possibly secondary to more distal obstruction. Although these two lesions do not in themselves threaten vision, or necessarily suggest the immediate further evolution of the retinopathy, they should be regarded as indicating that quite significant damage to the retinal circulation has already occurred. Multiple large blot haemorrhages suggest a more sinister prognosis, however.

Hard exudates, composed mainly of lipid and macrophages, probably form because of small vessel leakage in poorly controlled diabetes, to an extent that overcomes the scavenging mechanisms. Like many of the lesions of diabetic retinopathy they are commonest in the part of the retina lateral to the macula. Hard exudates are associated with high serum cholesterol levels, and their presence correlates with hypertension. They may enlarge and coalesce, but they can also shrink and even disappear altogether over periods of months. Hard exudates in themselves are generally benign, unless they are near the fovea.

Cotton wool spots are of more concern. Once termed soft exudates these are extensive areas of axonal swelling due to local retinal ischaemia. These are common lesions, but individual areas resolve quite quickly, so that only small numbers are usually seen at one time. When more than a handful are present at once they generally presage new vessel formation.

Less obvious on ophthalmoscopy, but very common, are arterial abnormalities, observed as sheathing and irregularity. Venous abnormalities are more readily observed, and are usually a sign of severe damage to the retinal vasculature, often being followed by new vessel formation. Venous tortuosity and venous beading are typically seen, but venous loops and other bizarre appearances are not uncommon. New vessels may first form within the retina, where they are not very striking, and are termed intraretinal microvascular abnormalities (IRMA). They do not in themselves carry the dangers of pre-retinal neovascularization.

Proliferative retinopathy occurs when new vessels grow out from the venules into the area in front of the retina. As vitreous detachment usually occurs with new vessel formation in diabetic retinopathy, pre-retinal neovascularization is not generally within the vitreous itself, but along the posterior vitreous membrane. These vessels present two acute risks to vision. Firstly, they may bleed into the pre-retinal space (pre-retinal or vitreous haemorrhage) to an extent that causes temporary or permanent visual loss. Recurrent bleeds into the vitreous often clear more and more slowly and incompletely, hence having a poor prognosis for vision. Secondly, the growth and regression of new vessels is associated with fibrosis, and contraction of this fibrous tissue can cause traction retinal detachment. Fluoroscein angiography will generally show new vessel formation to be much more widespread than observed on ophthalmoscopy. New vessels developing from the optic disc tend to grow faster, and have a poorer prognosis, than peripheral new vessels.

Visual loss can also occur through local macular problems, all of which are common, and hence a particular problem, in the more elderly Type 2 diabetic patient. This age group has the usual significant risk of ordinary senile macular degeneration. In the diabetic patient with background retinopathy hard exudates often appear to form particularly around the macula (exudative maculopathy), and will cause blindness if they extend across it. Much more difficult to recognize by ophthalmoscopy is macular oedema, but this can be detected as a significant deterioration in visual acuity. Ischaemic maculopathy is also difficult to recognize by ophthalmoscopy, and carries a poor prognosis.

Clinical Examination of the Diabetic Eye

Screening for diabetic eye disease should be performed yearly in all patients, but more frequently once abnormalities are detected or during pregnancy, after the onset of albuminuria or after major changes in metabolic control. Screening consists of comparing corrected visual acuity with the results from previous years, examining the iris and lens, and then examining the retina by ophthalmoscopy with mydriasis. Tropicamide eye drops (0.5 or 1.0%) are recommended for their rapid and short-lived effects. Occasionally patients suffer blurring of vision for two to three hours. These eye drops should not be used if glaucoma has previously been diagnosed. Opticians have been used with success to perform yearly screening checks if some form of appointment and default identification system can be instituted. In the presence of glaucoma, or diffuse cataracts, screening will need be done by an ophthalmologist.

Non-mydriatic retinal cameras have recently become available. These can give adequate pictures of the central retina, but it remains to be established whether they are suitable for patients with minor degrees of lens opacity, and whether peripheral lesions of significance will be missed. Present experience suggests, however, that they miss fewer problems than all but the most competant ophthalmoscopists.

Prevalence and Clinical Aspects

Retinopathy will not be evident at diagnosis in the younger patient, nor indeed will there usually be any evidence of retinal damage throughout childhood. However, people with onset of diabetes later in life may have had hyperglycaemia for many years, even decades, before diagnosis and it is not uncommon for them to have significant, even proliferative, retinal disease. The presence of retinal lesions is otherwise related very strongly to the duration of the disease in all age groups; microaneurysms often appearing after about 10 years of insulin-dependent diabetes. In many patients these will be the only lesions visible at any one time. They may be found in anything from 10 to 50% of the clinic population, dependent on its age structure.

In many patients background retinopathy will be stable for many years, with occasional intraretinal haemorrhages coming and going over that time. It is unclear why some patients rapidly progress to the lesions suggestive of a more serious ischaemic process (for example, multiple cotton wool spots, venous abnormalities, IRMA, multiple haemorrhages), but such change will often be followed by new vessel formation. Factors which are thought to be associated with the rapid evolution of diabetic retinopathy are the development of diabetic nephropathy, pregnancy and acute improvement of previously disturbed metabolic control. Angiogenesis is believed to be sensitive to serum growth hormone or somatomedin concentrations, but this relationship is probably not specific to the diabetic retina.

Without treatment new vessels carry a 30% risk of blindness within five years. Photocoagulation will prevent progression to blindness in around 70% of these eyes, but it is not yet possible to say that photocoagulation remains beneficial over more than one decade. It is not clear what proportion of patients with diabetes will need photocoagulation in time, but in the younger insulin-dependent patient it seems likely to be at least 30% at 40 years from diagnosis.

Management of Diabetic Retinopathy

Diabetic control

For the reasons given above the main aim of the treatment of diabetes must be to maintain metabolic control as close to normal as is possible in any individual. It is not yet possible to say how tight control needs to be to avoid development of retinopathy, but there are indications that a glycosylated haemoglobin concentration below mean +4 standard deviations of normal people will suffice. The appearance of diabetic retinopathy in any patient must therefore be recognized as a failure of preventative management. Once retinopathy is present it appears that only the best possible control, achieved with intensive supervision and infusion pumps, can offer any hope of reversing retinopathy in a population of patients. Many would argue that clinic resources are better devoted to maintaining good control from diagnosis. Even with very tight control many patients with established background retinopathy will still go on to develop proliferative retinopathy, which may indeed be precipitated by rapid correction of hyperglycaemia.

Photocoagulation

Patients with new vessel formation, or the more severe background lesions (see above), need urgent assessment by an ophthalmologist, who may want to employ fluoroscein angiography to detect all possible areas of neovascularization. Photocoagulation is generally delivered over large areas of the retina (pan-retinal), with many hundreds of burns. It is then usually successful in preventing or causing regression of neovascularization, even where this cannot be tackled directly. New vessels originating on the optic disc generally carry a worse prognosis, and require more urgent attention, than peripheral new vessels. Pan-retinal photocoagulation often results in no apparent visual disturbance to the patient, but photocoagulation near to the macula may cause noticeable loss of the field of vision.

When new vessels present a risk of bleeding, this risk appears to be increased by hypoglycaemia. A further problem arises with anticoagulation, and retinopathy must be particularly carefully assessed before open heart surgery or any vascular operation. Antiplatelet therapy (aspirin) might be expected to reduce progression of retinopathy in patients with poor blood glucose control, but again may be contraindicated in the presence of new vessels and recurrent vitreous haemorrhage.

Vitrectomy

Where advanced proliferative retinopathy with fibrosis threatens or has caused a fairly recent detachment in the foveal region, and where this is otherwise healthy, then it may be worthwhile removing the vitreous (vitrectomy) and dividing the fibrous bands along the posterior vitreous membrane pulling the retina forwards. This operation is only successful in a proportion of patients, generally those already retaining some vision.

Vitreous haemorrhage

Management of vitreous haemorrhage is an emergency, requiring sealing of the bleeding point if this is still visible. If not, blood within the retro-hyaloid space (behind the detached vitreous) will settle under the influence of gravity quite quickly if the patient is nursed sitting up and keeping still, but will settle in front of the macula if the patient is supine. Bleeding into the vitreous itself clears much more slowly, and in time leads to vitreous degeneration, thus obscuring vision, and is then only treatable by vitrectomy.

Maculopathy

A drop in visual acuity of more than one line on the Snellen chart, or evident perimacular abnormalities, also require early specialist assessment. Recent studies have shown that photocoagulation may help patients with maculopathy, although less reliably than with new vessels. Photocoagulation near the macula may require a general anaesthetic. The role of the newer lipid lowering drugs (bezafibrate or gemfibrozil) when hard exudates threaten the fovea has yet to be assessed, but they would appear to be a logical therapy, as would attention to dietary fat intake.

Other Eye Problems in Diabetes

Rubeosis iridis

Rubeosis iridis is essentially new vessel formation occurring on the iris. It is usually an accompaniment of proliferative retinopathy or a complication of vitrectomy. Repeated haemorrhage into the anterior chamber generally leads to eyesight-threatening glaucoma.

Cataracts

Cataracts are very common in diabetic patients past middle age. Apart from the increased incidence the large majority behave in the same way as senile cataract in the patient without diabetes. Thus the progression of the cataract is slow in the majority of patients, and the indications for surgical management are essentially the same. Cataracts may, however, pose a problem to the diabetologist screening for retinopathy, and it may be necessary to seek specialist assistance before the patient notices significant visual impairment. Nevertheless, it will inevitably occasionally be the case that cataract extraction reveals a retina in which vision has been lost through unobserved retinopathy or maculopathy. Photocoagulation requires a clear light path, and may also be impossible in the presence of cataract.

The classic metabolic cataract, termed a snowflake cataract, is now rare. It is associated with very poor metabolic control in the young insulin-dependent patient, and might appear quite suddenly at any time from diagnosis through to many years later. Some resolution may be expected with acute tightening of control, but extraction may be necessary. More minor forms of lens opacity may be noted on occasion, and again will often regress with effective treatment.

Glaucoma

Classical open angle glaucoma is more common in people with diabetes than the general population. It is not clear why this might be. Retinal changes and changes in visual acuity are the same as those found in non-diabetic patients, and may be picked up on routine annual screening. Glaucoma in people with diabetes is managed conventionally. Use of miotic eye drops renders fundoscopy difficult for the non-specialist, and diabetic patients with glaucoma will need to have their retinae checked regularly for retinopathy by an ophthalmologist. Theoretically, closed angle glaucoma may occasionally be precipitated in susceptible patients with the mydriatic eye drops used to facilitate ophthalmoscopy.

Blurring of vision

Blurring of vision, occuring as a symptom in people with diabetes, is usually a benign occurrence associated with rapid changes in blood glucose control. It is most commonly reported in the newly diagnosed and therefore in newly treated patients with insulin-dependent diabetes in whom a rapid reduction in blood glucose levels occurs with insulin therapy. It is believed to be due to osmotic distortion of the lens as a result of the relatively slow loss of glucose and its metabolites from within the lens structure. It is important to warn patients that this might occur, and in particular to explain that it is temporary, and that visits to the optician should be delayed until blood glucose levels are relatively stable.

Sudden changes of visual acuity should suggest haemorrhage into the vitreous (see above), or retinal detachment affecting the macula. Fairly fast changes in vision may also be found with some forms of cataract.

Diabetic Renal Damage

Prevalence and Natural History

Post-mortem and renal biopsy studies have shown that glomerulosclerosis will affect the kidneys of nearly all insulin-dependent patients two to three decades from diagnosis. However, only a proportion of diabetic patients eventually develop progressive urinary protein loss followed by a fall in glomerular filtration rate leading to end-stage renal failure. Precise incidence figures cannot be given because severe cardiovascular disease often develops in concert with the renal failure, but perhaps 20 to 40% of patients may be so affected. The peak incidence of renal problems is between 20 and 30 years from diagnosis, and those patients not showing proteinuria at 30 years are likely never to develop diabetic nephropathy. The condition is less of a problem in non-insulin-dependent diabetes, but this is probably partly due to the development of diabetes late in life in many of these patients, and the high mortality from cerebrocardiovascular disease.

Poor control of diabetes is associated with an enlargement of the kidneys and a high glomerular filtration rate, 10–20% above normal. Both these features are generally present at diagnosis, and will resolve if and when metabolic control is restored to near normal. In many patients, however, this glomerular hyperfiltration will persist up to the time when a significant loss of nephrons occurs. The significance of hyperfiltration in the development of diabetic nephropathy remains a subject of investigation.

Urinary albumin losses in a non-diabetic individual are very small, the tubules recovering any that is filtered, so that daily urinary output is rarely above 10 mg in the healthy subject. Most diabetic patients lose rather more than this, and if provoked, for example, by exercise, urinary albumin losses may rise quite markedly. After only a few years of diabetes albumin excretion in some patients rises to over 20 µg/min even in a resting overnight sample. It is these patients (with so-called microalbuminuria) who are thought to be at risk of development of frank albuminuria and renal failure many years later. Microalbuminuria is only detectable with immunological assays, as yet only available in specialist centres, but on present evidence the test should be applied to all patients every one to two years.

Screening for microalbuminuria is most easily performed on an early morning urine sample. An albumin:creatinine ratio of >3.5 mg/mmol should suggest the need for measurement of albumin excretion with a timed overnight sample.

The development of intermittent abuminuria, detectable with reagent strips, is a sign of advanced renal damage. Commercial reagent strips require about 0.30 g/l of albumin before a colour change occurs. While on average patients will progress from intermittent albuminuria to renal failure in about five years, with serum creatinine rising from three years, this is very variable and some patients have a much slower course. Once above normal, serum creatinine usually rises linearly if a reciprocal plot against time is constructed.

The development of diabetic nephropathy is usually accompanied by a rise in systolic and diastolic blood pressure, beginning before albuminuria is detectable. At the stage of frank albuminuria and rising serum creatinine concentrations worsening (or appearance) of retinopathy is nearly invariable, and pre-retinal new vessel formation is common. Nephrotic syndrome with protein losses of around 2–6 g/day is common at this stage. At the same time insulin dose requirement usually begins to fall, often to half or less of the original dose, and there is an increase in the rate of damage to the major arteries, often with severe medial calcification. Blood pressure control may become problematic, particularly if autonomic neuropathy develops at the same time.

Diagnosis of Diabetic Nephropathy

When proteinuria develops in the diabetic patient 15 to 30 years from diagnosis in the absence of factors suggestive of other forms of renal disease, then the diagnosis of diabetic nephropathy can generally be made without resorting to renal biopsy. If, however, there is no evidence of retinopathy, or if serum creatinine levels are rising in the absence of proteinuria, then the diagnosis must be questioned, even if still likely. The presence of haematuria, an abnormal erythrocyte sedimentation rate (ESR), pre-existing hypertension, or a history of recurrent urinary tract infection, would also suggest the need for further investigation. Diabetic renal disease is characterized by glomerular damage, the characteristic lesion being marked thickening of the basement membrane of the glomerular endothelium, together with a gross expansion of the mesangium, probably due to deposition of the same material. The classic nodular Kimmelstiel–Wilson lesions are seen less often. Hyalinization of the afferent and efferent arterioles may be found, and sometimes a non-specific fibrinoid cap may be seen within Bowman's space. Basement membrane thickening also occurs around the renal tubules.

Management of Diabetic Renal Disease (Table 2.5)

Prevention

As with diabetic retinopathy, very good metabolic control from the time of diagnosis is probably the most important measure in the management of diabetic renal disease. Early detection of Type 2 diabetes will therefore be important.

Stage of microalbuminuria

For patients with microalbuminuria the position is as yet unclear, but it now seems likely that very good control of both blood glucose concentration and hypertension may prevent progression to diabetic nephropathy. Blood press-

Table 2.5 Principles of the management of diabetic renal disease

Screening
Proteinuria (for urinary tract infection) if control poor
Microalbuminuria
   yearly albumin/creatinine ratio
   confirm with overnight albumin excretion rate if abnormal

Patients with microalbuminuria
Maintain blood pressure below 90th centile for age
Maintain HbA_1 within normal range if possible
Avoid high protein intake
Treat hyperlipidaemia if present
Monitor serum creatinine

Patients with frank proteinuria
As microproteinuria
Monitor retinopathy frequently
CAPD when necessary
Early renal transplantation

ure in particular should be maintained below the 90th centile for age and sex, using ACE inhibitors or calcium antagonists. As the inevitable consequences of this progression have profound resource and health costs, intensification of therapy must be considered worthwhile. The role of low protein diets has yet to be defined, since although they reduce the output of urinary albumin, it has not been established yet that they prevent progression of nephron loss.

Patients who progress to nephropathy very often die of cardiac disease, and those with microalbuminuira tend to have abnormal serum lipid levels. These too should be actively managed.

Stage of intermittent proteinuria

By the time that intermittent proteinuria has appeared structural renal damage is too far advanced for progression to be influenced by a tightening of metabolic control. More promising at present is the treatment of hypertension, which may slow progression of the disease. Very good control may, however, be necessary, keeping lying diastolic pressure below 85 mmHg, and usually requiring multiple drug therapy.

Renal failure

When renal failure develops stardard therapy may be used to cope with any troublesome symptoms. If a very high carbohydrate, low protein diet is instituted blood glucose control may change, at a time when insulin doses tend to be dropping rapidly as creatinine rises. Intermittent haemodialysis may be used to good effect in people with diabetes, although there can be problems with vascular access. Continuous ambulatory peritoneal dialysis (CAPD) does not have this problem, is cheaper and offers a more flexible lifestyle to the patient. The use of CAPD carries a significant risk of peritonitis, with loss of the effective exchange surface occurring in about 20% of patients in the first year. Diabetic control must therefore be monitored and controlled carefully. On CAPD it is possible to give the insulin in the peritoneal infusate, and this may provide some match to the high carbohydrate loads involved.

Renal transplantation

People with diabetes may be judged as suitable for renal transplantation by the same criteria used for the non-diabetic patient. Because of the rapid evolution of major vessel disease and retinopathy in these patients there is an argument for transplantation at relatively low creatinine levels (below 500 µmol/l), since distal arterial disease and myocardial infarction may complicate the late post-operative course. Cyclosporin is a particularly useful agent for immuno-suppression in diabetic patients, as it may largely obviate the need for predniso-lone therapy, and hence the problems of disturbance of metabolic control caused by this drug.

Control of diabetes is important in immunosupressed patients, particularly during adjustments of prednisolone dosage if that drug is used. For the long-term it must be remembered that the transplanted kidney is itself at risk of diabetic renal damage, and indeed will show characteristic histological damage within a few years.

Other Urinary Tract Problems in Diabetes

Renal and urinary tract infection

Urinary tract infection is still very common in people with diabetes, particularly where diabetic control is not good. It should not be assumed that urinary frequency is due to poor control, or that albuminuria is due to glomerular damage, without investigating the possibility of infection. Management is identical to the non-diabetic patient, except that infection is often recurrent, so providing another reason for checking a urine specimen for albumin at each clinic visit. Documented recurrent infection should be monitored by repeated urine microscopy and culture. It is unclear whether the use of prophylactic antibiotics prevents chronic renal damage when repeated infections occur in this group of patients, but, where their use is effective in controlling recurrent infection, it would seem sensible to continue this potential protection.

Chronic pyelonephritis would now seem to be less common since the advent of effective antibiotic therapy, although it is possible that it is underdiagnosed in the failing diabetic kidney. Renal carbuncle is an occasional occurrence in the poorly controlled diabetic patient. Renal tuberculosis is still an occasional problem in people with diabetes, particularly in less developed countries.

Urinary frequency

Polyuria and nocturia are common in people with diabetes, and may present a problem of differential diagnosis especially in elderly men. Once diabetes is even modestly controlled, however, it is unusual for glycosuria to be heavy enough to cause urinary frequency. Where this is suspected it is easy to arrange for urine specimens to be checked for 2% glycosuria at the times frequency is complained about.

Diabetic Neuropathy

Diabetic nerve damage may affect visceral, somatic and cranial nerves, as well as spinal nerve roots, but signs of damage are generally present in more than one branch of the peripheral nervous system. Possible biochemical abnormalities underlying conduction disturbance have been discussed above. Histologically the most prominent changes in diabetic nerves are to their vasculature, with closure and thrombosis of a high percentage of small vessels when neuropathy is evident.

A classification of diabetic neuropathies is given in Table 2.6.

Characteristics and Management of Somatic Neuropathy

Distal sensory neuropathy

This is the commonest of all the diabetic neuropathies, but the majority of patients with the problem are asymptomatic. It is generally symmetrical, affects mainly the small fibres and is manifested particularly in the feet. It is particularly prevalent in the elderly, non-insulin-dependent patient, but may be found with any type of diabetes. It has a prevalence of 10–20% in insulin-dependent patients. In those who become symptomatic the complaint is usually

Table 2.6 Classification and syndromes of diabetic neuropathies

Somatic neuropathy	Autonomic neuropathy
Distal sensory neuropathy	Sympathetic efferent neuropathy
Asymptomatic	Postural hypotension
Symptomatic	Loss of adrenal medullary activation
Painful	Gut motility disorders
Mixed peripheral neuropathy	Gastroparesis
Proximal motor neuropathy	Diarrhoea
Mononeuropathy	Genitourinary disorders
Pressure point, nerve entrapment neuropathies	Bladder dysfunction
	Impotence
Acute mononeuropathy	Neuropathy of cardio-respiratory reflexes
Mononeuritis multiplex	
Radiculopathy	Sweating disorders

of numbness or heaviness affecting the soles of the feet, although mild paraesthesiae in toes and fingers may also be commonly reported.

Distal sensory neuropathy is a major risk factor for foot problems (see below), and should be documented yearly in every patient. At present the only instrument widely used for quantification is the Biothesiometer, which measures vibration threshold, a large fibre function. Hallux thresholds of over 30 have, however, been shown to be associated with a risk of foot ulceration. Semi-quantitative versions of the traditional tuning fork are also available as well as expensive apparatus for quantifiying temperature sensation. However, these have not yet been calibrated against foot ulcer risk. Management of the diabetic foot is discussed below.

Distal sensory neuropathy carries a small risk for the development of Charcot's arthropathy. Although usually affecting the ankle, other joints of the feet, or even the hands and arms, may become disorganized. Joint destruction sometimes follows what otherwise seems to be a very mild injury.

Mixed distal neuropathy

In some patients with a distal sensory neuropathy there is also a distal motor neuropathy. This may be of clinical significance where loss of tone in the intrinsic muscles of the feet leads to clawing of the toes, and hence increased pressure on the metatarsal heads.

Motor neuropathies

Isolated, diffuse, motor neuropathy is rare. More notable amongst the motor neuropathies is **diabetic proximal motor neuropathy**, previously termed diabetic amyotrophy, or femoral neuropathy. In this condition there is often a rapid onset of weakness and wasting affecting principally the thigh muscles, often asymmetrically. Knee jerks are absent. The condition may progress until the patient cannot walk. The degree of weight loss and ill health associated with this condition often leads to unnecessary investigation for malignancy. Nerve conduction studies, and electrophysiological muscle studies, may be useful for defining the site of the lesion, and confirming the nature of the problem.

Muscle pain is common and often severe enough to need opiate analgesia. As the patients are usually non-insulin treated it is general practice to transfer them to insulin therapy, and obtain the best possible control, but it is unclear if this aids resolution, which occurs in 6 to 24 months. Meanwhile reassurance and psychological support are usually necessary, while physiotherapy can help retention and recovery of muscle power.

Painful diabetic neuropathy

Painful neuropathy occurs unpredictably and often apparently randomly amongst patients with different degrees and patterns of sensory neuropathy.

Again it is more common amongst non-insulin-dependent patients, and may be the presenting symptom. There is a suggestion that it may occur with improvement of diabetic control, perhaps indicating a return of nerve function. The sensations are variable in character, and may be so severe that they may be nearly intolerable to the patient. Painful neuropathy is usually symmetrical, affects mainly the feet, and tends to remit over a period of several months.

Mild symptoms may respond to simple analgesic therapy with aspirin or paracetamol, which should be given prophylactically in patients with predominantly night-time symptoms. A bed cradle to remove pressure of bed clothes may give great relief. More painful neuropathy responds well to full doses of tricyclic antidepressants, but it is worth explaining to the patient that these are not given for treatment of depression. Carbamazepine and phenytoin are usually disappointing, and the dose needs to be worked up to the maximum tolerated recommended level. Transcutaneous electrical stimulation may help, but any response is often short lived.

It is usual to tighten metabolic control with intensive insulin regimens in any patient suffering problems from diabetic neuropathy. Clinical impressions are that this is worthwhile, but it is unclear whether remission is definitely promoted.

Diabetic mononeuropathies

Diabetic nerves are very sensitive to traumatic damage, at all the usual pressure points, giving rise to both motor and sensory problems. Carpal tunnel syndrome is common, and responds to decompression, while ulnar nerve damage, although also common, is usually asymptomatic. A rare but characteristic mononeuropathy is a sudden and isolated loss of function of one of the nerves to the external occular muscles, often the sixth. Although recovery, sometimes incomplete, occurs in one to six months, it is useful to refer the patients to an eye department for eye exercises.

Diabetic radioculopathy

Painful radiculopathy is not uncommon in people with diabetes, but usually resolves in three to six months. Analgesia and reassurance are all that is required, once disc or other lesions have been excluded.

Characteristics and Management of Autonomic Neuropathy

Autonomic neuropathy may affect any part of the sympathetic and parasympathetic nervous systems (Table 2.6), including the nerve plexuses of the gut. In any individual patient, however, one symptom usually predominates. While patients with autonomic neuropathy will generally have a demonstrable somatic neuropathy, this is not invariable. Indeed the sympathetic and parasympathetic nerves often seem to be affected independently.

Erectile impotence

In diabetic men impotence appears to be the most commonly recognized symptom, affecting from 10% of men at age 30 years to 50% by age 50 years. Diabetic impotence is difficult to distinguish from psychogenic impotence, particularly when the problem is partial and variable in time, which is often when the patients most need help. Even where the problem is organic (neurogenic or vascular), secondary psychogenic disturbance may occur. Once organic impotence is established and complete, however, erections will not occur at any time including during sleep, and at this stage a return of function is very unlikely.

Intrapenile papaverine injection will allow differentiation of vascular problems from neurogenic or psychological impotence. The presence of other vascular disease, or neuropathy, may also help, and retinopathy also suggests an organic problem. Sensitive counselling is necessary to discover whether the patient wishes to obtain help through psychosexual counselling, prosthetic implantation, vacuum aids, or papaverine self-injection. Surgical implants are expensive and sometimes painful at first, but may give great satisfaction to some patients. Papaverine injections are not known to be safe in the long-term, and are associated with a significant incidence of priapism, needing urgent treatment.

Bladder dysfunction

Bladder dysfunction usually takes the form of loss of tone with a large increase in volume. It is therefore usually asymptomatic. Urinary tract infection may become recurrent, and eventually retention may occur. Ultrasonography may help establish the diagnosis. Cholinergic agents (for example, carbachol) are usually disappointing. Bladder neck incision or reconstruction may help, at the risk of giving rise to other urinary symptoms.

Diabetic diarrhoea

This is also uncommon, but can be very troublesome. Large volumes of watery stool may be produced, often with urgency or even incontinence, and with a tendency to occur at night. The condition is usually chronic, but with long periods of remission. Bacterial overgrowth and exocrine pancreatic disease need to be considered in the differential diagnosis, but these will usually give steatorrhoea rather than diarrhoea. Bacterial overgrowth is itself possibly a manifestation of disordered gut motility.

Management will initially be with opiate derivatives (for example, codeine phosphate, loperamide), but ephedrine, tetracycline and metronidazole have also been recommended.

Gastroparesis

Diabetic gastroparesis can be extremely problematic when it leads to intestinal hold up or to vomiting, particularly where this interferes with food absorption in the insulin-treated patient. It can be very debilitating, and is associated with a very poor prognosis. Diagnosis is by barium meal with screening, when the effect of metaclopramide can be monitored. The drug, domperidone, and the newer agent cisapride, may be effective if given in large doses.

Postural hypotension

Postural hypotension due to autonomic neuropathy is uncommon in diabetes, anti-hypertensive therapy being a much more likely cause. Management is by attention to drug therapy (including antidepressants and tranquillizers), a high salt intake and increasing fludrocortisone from 0.1 to 0.4 mg/day. Indomethecin or chlorpropamide may be worth trying, but overall the results are disappointing and oedema may be troublesome. Suitable explanation and instruction on rising slowly helps many patients.

Cardiorespiratory arrest

Disorders of the efferent and afferent nerves controlling cardiac and respiratory performance are more common, but are not usually symptomatic. Tachycardia can be quite marked, however, and this form of autonomic neuropathy may predispose to cardiorespiratory arrest during and after anaesthetic procedures. Assessment of beat-to-beat interval with deep breathing, or 15 and 30 s after standing, are commonly used as tests of autonomic neuropathy.

Sympathetic efferent nerve damage

Loss of the fight-or-flight reflex controlling secretion of adrenaline from the adrenal medulla can be troublesome in the insulin-dependent patient, as it will remove some of the main warning symptoms of hypoglycaemia.

Sweating disorders

Gustatory sweating may also be a troublesome condition, and occasionally sweating may become entirely unpredictable, often occurring asymmetrically. Disorders of sweating may give rise to concern by the patient that he/she is hypoglycaemic. Anticholinergic agents such as poldine may be helpful.

Musculo-skeletal Problems in Diabetes

Diabetes quite commonly causes joint and connective tissue problems which can be revealed by careful examination of the hands of any cohort of patients.

The aetiology of this damage is unclear, but it has been suggested to be due to abnormal forms of collagen, perhaps as a result of advanced glycosylation end products. The commonest lesion is probably simple palmar thickening, but this is not generally a significant problem to the patient. It may progress to Dupuytren's contracture, however, which is significantly more common in diabetic patients than in the general population. Thickening of the fascia over the joints of the fingers is also common, and leads to limited joint mobility in many patients. Such cheiroarthropathy is easily demonstrated with the 'prayer sign', where the fingers cannot be approximated when the palmar surfaces of the hands are placed against each other. Limitations of shoulder movement, indistinguishable from a classical 'frozen shoulder', and with the same management and outlook, are also not uncommon.

Diabetic Dermopathy

Rarely patients with other evidence of microangiopathy develop a specific dermatosis usually affecting the lower leg. Oval dull red papules form and evolve in time to blisters and then scars.

Diabetic Specific Heart Disease

People with diabetes have a higher prevalence of congestive cardiac failure, and do less well after myocardial infarction, than would be predicted from overt ischaemic heart disease. However, in the majority of patients more detailed investigations will show diffuse disease of the coronary arteries to be the underlying problem. A small percentage of patients with ventricular dysfunction, not explainable by coronary artery disease, are believed to have a specific diabetic cardiopathy, but the condition is not well understood, and the outlook for such patients is generally poor.

Cardiac and Major Vessel Disease in Diabetes

Prevalence and Natural History

Ischaemic heart disease is very common in people with diabetes, the relative risk of myocardial infarction being perhaps four in the middle-aged man, and rather higher in women. Around 15 to 20% of admissions to coronary care units are of people with pre-existing diabetes. Myocardial infarction in people with diabetes has a poorer prognosis than in the population as a whole, and probably accounts for more deaths than any other diabetes-associated health problem. Indeed myocardial infarction may be the largest killer of patients with insulin-dependent diabetes, although some of these will have had diabetic nephropathy for some time. Peripheral vascular disease is also very common in people with diabetes, although its true prevalence has never been properly assessed. It is of particular concern in people with diabetes, since ischaemia accounts for much of the morbidity associated with foot problems. Cerebrovascular events also occur at increased frequency; in some series these account for as much as 30% of acute cerebral infarction. Other less common problems due to major vessel disease (for example, mesenteric ischaemia, subclavian steal, ophthalmic artery thrombosis) are probably seen more often than in the general population.

Hypertension is extremely common in people with diabetes, in association with both macrovascular and microvascular disease (for example, retinopathy, early nephropathy). In some populations of non-insulin-dependent patients the prevalence of blood pressure greater than 160/90 may be as high as 50% of all those attending a clinic. For younger patients with early nephropathy a tighter definition of hypertension is needed (see above), usually above the 90th centile for their age group.

Pathogenesis of Macrovascular Disease

There appears to be no single reason for the marked increase in the incidence of major vessel disease in diabetic patients. In a number of respects, however, diabetes is associated with factors known to be related to atherogenesis in non-diabetic people (Table 2.7). These are enumerated below, but it should be noted that many of these factors influence and interact with each other (for example, diet and diabetic control; control and coagulation disturbance).

Poor dietary habits

While it is uncertain what aspect of dietary behaviour predisposes to (or causes) non-insulin-dependent diabetes, it does seem to be related to the high sugar, low fibre, high fat diets eaten in industrialized nations. These diets are also high in cholesterol and saturated fats, which are in turn associated with high serum lipid concentrations, and an increased risk of arterial disease. The risk of major arterial disease is steeply related to cholesterol concentration throughout the range found in the general population, or at least from above 4.0 mmol/l, and it must be assumed this applies to people with diabetes.

Table 2.7 Possible mechanisms for excess major vessel disease in diabetes

Poor dietary habits
Concurrent Reaven's syndrome
Secondary dyslipidaemia
Exacerbation of primary dyslipidaemia
Hyperinsulinaemia
Endothelial damage
   Membrane defects (see Table 2.3)
   Platelet clotting abnormalities (see Table 2.3)

Poor diabetic control

Poorly controlled diabetes itself causes a rise in serum cholesterol and triglyceride concentrations, including a rise in the higher risk low density lipoprotein (LDL) cholesterol concentration. Abnormalities of lipid and lipoprotein turnover are demonstrable in experimental diabetes. It is possible that high blood glucose levels may cause abnormal apolipoprotein function through non-enzymatic glycosylation.

Microvascular disease

It is difficult to ignore the possibility that the mechanisms responsible for microvascular disease might also be responsible for metabolic damage to the walls of major vessels. There are strong associations between retinopathy and hypertension and between diabetic renal disease and accelerated major vessel disease. As discussed above endothelial cell abnormalities are an important feature of microvascular disease, and it cannot be ruled out that arterial endothelial cell damage, and leakage into the arterial wall, might play a role in the development of macroangiopathy. A further possibility in the larger arteries is that the vasa vasorum of the arterial wall itself may become damaged by microangiopathy.

Hyperinsulinaemia

Epidemiologically, high plasma insulin concentrations are associated with a risk of arterial disease in people with diabetes, with impaired glucose tolerance and even with normal glucose tolerance. Poor and even moderate control of diabetes is associated with tissue resistance to the action of insulin, and basal plasma insulin concentrations are elevated in both the treated insulin-dependent patient, and most non-insulin-dependent patients. Experimentally insulin influences many aspects of arterial wall smooth muscle cells, including endogenous sterol synthesis, LDL uptake and proliferation. These effects are demonstrable at physiological insulin concentrations, and their normal role may be in the repair of thrombus associated arterial wall damage.

Coagulation and thrombotic disorder

Poorly controlled diabetes is associated with abnormalities of platelet function, prostacyclin activity, clotting mechanisms and erythrocyte deformability. Though it is not clear that these contribute to the pathogenesis of major vessel disease, they should make it more likely that atherosclerotic damage predisposes to arterial thrombosis.

Prevention of Major Vessel Disease

On biochemical grounds good control of diabetes should be important in preventing the gradual development of arterial disease. Thus improvement in blood glucose control is associated with normalization of serum cholesterol and triglyceride concentrations, as well as all measurements related to platelet and clotting mechanisms. There is no evidence that improvement in control leads to higher insulin concentrations overall, probably because tissue insulin sensitivity improves in parallel with improved insulin delivery. Dietary attention should be directed to a reduction in total fat intake, particularly of saturated fats and cholesterol. Risk factors, in particular smoking, deserve regular educational follow-up. Diabetic records should be constructed to give attention to regular measurement of blood pressure and examination of peripheral vessels.

Ischaemic Heart Disease in Diabetes

Many of the features and management of ischaemic heart disease in people with diabetes are identical to those of the non-diabetic patient. Myocardial infarction is apparently more often silent in the diabetic patient, however, and may present as ketoacidosis. Care must be taken in the interpretation of electrocardiograms during severe metabolic disturbance. Diabetic patients appear to suffer more diffuse disease of the coronary arteries, and probably as a result do less well after infarction, with a much higher frequency of left ventricular failure and cardiogenic shock. Although occasionally cardiopathy may be specifically related to diabetes (see above), in general it may be presumed to be due to diffuse coronary artery disease.

The stress of myocardial infarction may cause hyperglycaemia, and is best managed with intravenous insulin therapy, beginning at 3 units/h in the absence of acidosis, and transferring to a glucose/insulin infusion (see surgical management) when the blood glucose concentration drops below 13 mmol/l. Transfer to subcutaneous insulin therapy may follow when hyperglycaemia is controlled and skin perfusion is good. People with hyperglycaemia after myocardial infarction, but not previously known to have diabetes, often turn out to be diabetic on formal testing a couple of months later. Glycosylated haemoglobin estimation at the time of infarction may be a useful indicator in this respect.

Hypertension

Hypertension is a risk factor for major arterial catastrophes in diabetes as in non-diabetic patients. In many people with diabetes the blood pressure elevation is mainly systolic, and can be difficult to treat successfully. Many of the drugs available for the treatment of hypertension have some diabetogenic effects, or are believed to elevate serum lipid concentrations. Thiazides are effective drugs in most age groups, but they are likely to worsen glucose tolerance, particularly if used in conjunction with beta-adrenergic blockers. Beta-blockers may themselves cause problems in patients with peripheral arterial disease and it is important to ensure that blood supply to the feet is not impaired before they are prescribed. Beta-blockers can disguise and inhibit the catecholamine response to hypoglycaemia, so that the cardioselective beta-blockers, atenolol and metoprolol, are to be preferred. They may also raise serum lipid levels, particularly when used together with thiazides, and care must be taken not to precipitate cardiac failure if left ventricular function is poor. Some calcium antagonists appear to be effective agents in diabetic patients, without major metabolic effects. Other vasodilators (for example hydrallazine, prazosin), and centrally acting alpha-adrenergic-antagonists (for example clonidine), are effective second or third line drugs, without special problems in diabetic patients. Angiotensin converting enzyme (ACE) inhibitors are also effective, and accumulating experience suggests that they are useful drugs in people with diabetes, with no metabolic effects and little likelihood of exacerbation of problems such as erectile impotence or postural hypotension. The evidence that ACE inhibitors may have specific advantages in diabetic patients through alteration of glomerular haemodynamics is as yet unconvincing.

Peripheral Vascular Disease

Peripheral vascular disease in diabetic patients is often more diffuse and distal than in the non-diabetic patient, but some patients do have lesions which can be by-passed surgically. Iliac and femoral disease should therefore be sought if feet are threatened by ischaemia, or if claudication is troublesome. Unrecognized claudication should be sought annually by direct questioning, so that suitable reinforcement can be given to advice about smoking, regular exercise and foot care (see below). Out-patient drug therapy is not indicated, but standard infusion regimens of naftidrofuryl or dextrans may be tried in patients admitted to hospital because of incipient gangrene.

The Diabetic Foot

Foot problems in diabetic patients cause more in-patient bed occupancy than all their other medical problems put together. Amputation causes major disability, and quite often needs to be performed bilaterally. Skin condition is poor in diabetic patients and, apart from stump healing problems, there seems to be an increased risk of pressure sores. These operations carry a significant mortality in this group of patients.

Many studies have demonstrated that foot problems are largely preventable by suitable and repeated education. The importance attached to the problem is best emphasized to the patient by regular and detailed examination (Table 2.8) of the feet, at least once a year, while talking about the risks. At this examination skin and sole condition are inspected, and deformities putting the feet at risk noted. Assessment is made of arterial supply to the feet, and examination made to detect neuropathy. A relative threshold above 30 on the Biothesiometer has been shown to be associated with a risk of future ulcer-

Table 2.8 Examination of the feet in diabetes

Frequency
Every visit if Poor skin
　　　　　　　Deformity
　　　　　　　Neuropathy
　　　　　　　Peripheral vascular disease
Otherwise annually

Education
Examination should always be accompanied by an explanation

Procedure
Remove all shoes, socks, stockings, dressing, plasters
Inspect shoes including contents
Shape of feet (deformities)
　　　　　　Over-riding toes
　　　　　　Clawed toes
　　　　　　Hallus valgus
　　　　　　Amputation
　　　　　　Loss of arch
　　　　　　Charcot joints
Skin condition (especially soles) including
　　　　　　Thinning and rubbing
　　　　　　Callosities
　　　　　　Fungal infection (between toes)
　　　　　　Dirt
　　　　　　Foreign bodies (in soles)
　　　　　　Ischaemia
　　　　　　Ulceration
Nails
　　　　　　Length
　　　　　　Shape (local skin trauma)
　　　　　　Shape of cut
Nerves
　　　　　　Pin prick
　　　　　　Vibration sense (quantitative)
　　　　　　Temperature sense
Vasculature
　　　　　　Dilated veins
　　　　　　Peripheral pulses absent
　　　　　　Leg hair loss

ation. Shoes should be examined at the same time, with advice given to buy well-fitting shoes which accommodate the feet without distortion. Patients should be advised to examine their feet daily for sores, thinning, or reddening of the skin, to cut nails proud (or preferably have a chiropodist do them), not to walk about without shoes, and to report any change to a doctor within 24 h. Patients or their relatives should not themselves attempt minor surgery to the feet, or use corn plasters; these matters should be left to a chiropodist.

The ischaemic foot will be cold, with altered skin colouration, absent peripheral pulses, and have hair loss over the outer aspects of the shins. By

58 Late Tissue Damage in Diabetes Mellitus

contrast, the purely neuropathic foot will feel warm, often with bounding pulses, and dilated veins over the dorsum which will not empty until the foot is raised. This appearance is deceptive, however, for it arises through the opening up of arteriovenous connexions, and the tissues will be relatively hypoxic.

Foot Ulcers

Neuropathic foot ulcers

These occur particularly on the sole of the foot, generally under an area of callus, often at an area of high pressure, and are usually surprisingly deep due to the callus being forced into the ulcer on walking (Fig. 2.3a). They are always painless. Neuropathy leds to clawing of the toes, with transfer of foot pressure to the metatarsal heads, so that these are the commonest site of callus

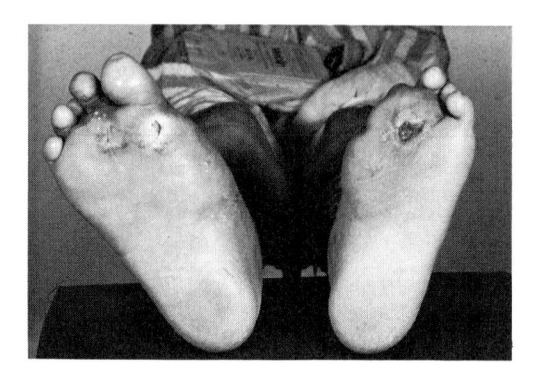

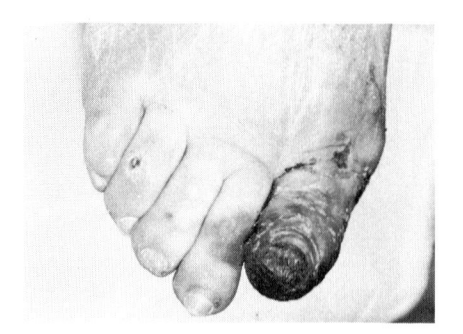

Fig. 2.3 Examples of neuropathic (a) and vascular ulceration (b). *See* colour plates between pages 166–167. Neuropathic ulcers are typically on the plantar surface of the foot, in a site of high pressure on standing or walking, and thus often covered by callus. Removal of the pressure will usually result in quite rapid healing. Vascular ulceration typically occurs distally at the toes, and proceeds to ischaemia and mummification. Ulceration in areas of thin skin over the dorsal aspects of the toes or the sides of the feet is often mixed in aetiology, but will generally heal slowly provided infection is superficial.

formation, and hence ulceration. The best form of treatment is to put the foot in a plaster cast boot, with the ulcer exposed through a window, and healing is then often surprisingly rapid. Callus should be removed, and reulceration prevented by attention to any new areas of skin hardening. Shoes should be provided with the soles moulded to spread foot pressure evenly. Neuropathic ulcers are never an indication for amputation.

Ischaemic ulcers

These are classically painful, often usually on the distal ends of the toes (Fig. 2.3b), and are associated with the usual signs of peripheral vascular disease and ischaemia. Ischaemic feet must be kept warm (but not hot) if the ulcers are to have a chance of healing. Infusions of plasma expanders and peripheral vasodilators are generally disappointing in incipient ischaemia. Where distal tissue death occurs in the absence of infection the best course of action is to wait until the dead tissues separate. Strong analgesia may be required, and its failure to control pain is an indication for surgery.

Even the more superficial ulcers will not heal if arterial supply to the leg is compromised. In these circumstances, and before consideration of amputation, the possibility of angioplasty, or proximal vascular reconstruction or by-pass should be entertained. Where amputation is contemplated a definitive procedure is often more successful in the long-term than repeated local nibbling.

Infected foot ulcers

Superficial infected foot ulcers are more common than either of the above classical lesions. Infected ulcers may range from small superficial lesions in areas of skin damage due to rubbing of shoes or pressure of one toe on another, through to paronychia and nail bed infections, and to deep traumatic lesions. It may often be difficult to decide whether vascular disease, neuropathy or simply poor hygiene and poorly controlled diabetes are the most important contributory causes. The deeper lesions are often the worse for being detected late as a result of neuropathy, but if ischaemia is not a problem they may heal quite rapidly.

Superficial lesions are best treated by daily surgical toilet with antiseptic solutions (such as dilute hypochlorite) and non-adherent dressings until clean, and dry dressings only thereafter. Healing is usually very slow, particularly if there is an ischaemic element. When considerable slough is present in the ulcer, absorbant materials may promote healing. If local cellulitis is present in the surrounding tissue then antibiotic therapy may be useful antistaphylococcal drugs such as flucloxacillin being the agents of first choice, with the addition of antistreptococcal therapy for cellulitis beyond the immediate surrounds of the ulcer.

Diabetic control should be managed intensively in order to ensure that leucocyte function is promoted and local tissue responses optimized. Blood glucose concentrations should be kept as close to normal as possible, and certainly below 11 mmol/l, usually with insulin therapy.

The Infected Foot

Any of the above types of ulcer may lead to an infected foot, particularly where diabetic control is poor. Spread of infection occurs along the tissue planes and the foot feels warm and boggy, while the patient is pyrexial. Surgical treatment then needs to be fairly radical, with excision of affected tissue deep into the foot. The wound is often best left open. Antibiotic therapy is again indicated, and may be guided by cultures, but again optimal diabetic control is probably at least as important if the foot is to be saved.

Osteomyelitis is not uncommon as a complication of diabetic foot ulcers, particularly where blood glucose control is poor, and is often not amenable to treatment with antibiotics in the foot compromised by metabolic problems and large or small vessel disease. Osteomyelitis is therefore an indication for surgical removal of the affected bone.

Further Reading

Betteridge, D.J. (1989). Diabetes, lipoprotein metabolism and atherosclerosis. *British Medical Bulletin* **45**, 285.

Boulton, A.J. M. and Ward, J.D. (1986). Diabetic neuropathies and pain. *Clinics in Endocrinology and Metabolism* **15**, 917.

Colwell, J.A. (1987). Atherosclerosis in diabetes mellitus. *Diabetes Annual 3*, pp. 325–53. Edited by Alberti, K.G.M.M. and Krall, L.P. Elsevier, Amsterdam.

Drury, P.L., Watkins, P.J., Viberti, G.C. and Walker, J.D. (1989). Diabetic nephropathy. *British Medical Bulletin* **45**, 127.

Edmonds, M.E. (1986). The diabetic foot: pathophysiology and treatment. *Clinics in Endocrinology and Metabolism* **15**, 889.

Ewing, D.J. and Clarke, B.F. (1986). Autonomic neuropathy: its diagnosis and prognosis. *Clinics in Endocrinology and Metabolism* **15**, 855.

Keen, H. and Jarrett, J. (1982). Complications of diabetes. Edward Arnold, Sevenoaks.

3

DELIVERING OPTIMAL CARE TO THE PATIENT WITH DIABETES

Management of diabetes differs to a considerable degree from the management of many other medical illnesses. This arises through the combination of the following:

1. Most of the day-to-day management of the condition is organized and put into effect by the patient him/herself;
2. Management of the condition rather than the condition itself interferes with and modifies the patient's lifestyle;
3. Most of this management is not directed towards improving the symptoms (the patient being asymptomatic), but to prevention of the consequences of late tissue damage as described in Chapter 2.

The combination of these factors, together with the high prevalence of diabetes in the older and less well population, means that organization and delivery of care for people with diabetes is an important subject in its own right. While these aspects are discussed in the current chapter, more conventional aspects of care (for example, diet, oral agents, insulin) are discussed in Chapter 4.

Concepts Underlying the Organization of Care

Remedial and Preventative Medicine

Much of medical and surgical practice is remedial in nature, either in the sense of coping with acute events such as chest infection or haematemesis, or in the sense of avoiding acute complications such as heart failure after myocardial infarction. Although some procedures might be seen as having a preventative aspect (for example, coronary artery by-pass grafting) this occurs in the context of an already damaged organ in order to prevent further deterioration. Some aspects of the treatment of diabetes are also clearly remedial, for example, the continuing prevention of ketoacidosis in the insulin-dependent patient, while other aspects help prevent the occurrence of acute complications of the condition, such as candidal infections.

Table 3.1 The preventative emphasis of diabetes care

Feature managed	Example	Comment
Classical remedial medicine		
Acute symptoms	Polyuria	Easily controlled
Acute deterioration	Ketoacidosis	Uncommon
Acute complications	Infections	Uncommon if control is good
Treatment of side-effects	Hypoglycaemia	Complication of preventative care
Preventative medicine		
Treatment of side-effects	Hypoglycaemia	Avoid with good self-care
Acute deterioration	Ketoacidosis	Preventable by education
Late symptoms	Blindness	Avoidable by good control
Late complications	Myocardial infarction	Reduced risk with good control

However, with the treatments available for the management of diabetes it is only the rare patient who continues to be troubled by acute symptoms or related acute complications. Unfortunately, as discussed in detail in Chapter 2, diabetes is also characterized by the insidious development of damage to many of the organs of the body; damage that does not occur in non-diabetic people and is clearly related to the metabolic disturbance. The degree of metabolic disturbance required for the development of these late complications is highly variable, but it is clear from those non-insulin-dependent patients who present with complications that such damage can occur in the absence of symptoms. This has now been confirmed in studies in which progression of tissue damage has been monitored over years in conventionally treated, asymptomatic patients. The consequence of this situation is that delivery of diabetes care must be directed towards prevention of tissue damage, and that this care has to be delivered in and by an asymptomatic patient. Organization of care is then found to be largely preventative rather than classical remedial medicine (Table 3.1).

Primary Prevention of Diabetes

Where the aetiology of types of diabetes is not clearly understood, as in forms of 'tropical' diabetes, primary prevention is clearly not possible. Much secondary diabetes in the industrialized world is related to alcohol-related pancreatitis, and its prevention will not be discussed further here.

Prevention of Type 1 diabetes

As discussed in Chapter 1 the mechanism of the pathogenesis of Type 1 diabetes appears at present to be auto-immune, and we have no useful understanding of triggering events. Intervention to interrupt the auto-immune process has been attempted with classical immunosuppressive agents, but without significant effect (Table 3.2). There is now some evidence from appropriately controlled trials that cyclosporin can arrest the development of diabetes in some of those presenting with the condition (secondary prevention). It does appear, however, that the process is only checked by the drug and not reversed, so that treatment would have to be indefinite. Cyclosporin is a fairly toxic drug, difficult to administer safely, and at present the overwhelming consensus is that insulin therapy and acceptance of some risk of long-term tissue damage from diabetes are a preferable course of action.

Type 1 diabetes can now be identified in advance of clinical diagnosis by serum complement-fixing islet cell antibody determination. However, the test is not easy to perform in large numbers, and its organization is not a practical proposition except possibly where family members are already affected. The test would need to be repeated at minimum intervals of two years.

Prevention of Type 2 diabetes

Although genetic factors are important in the aetiology of Type 2 diabetes (see Chapter 1), it is also clear that the quality of the environment has an enormous impact on the degree to which genetic predisposition is expressed as diabetes. However, genetic determination of individuals at risk is not possible at present, except on the simple basis of family history, an approach which could only identify a proportion of such individuals. Even in at risk family members, however, the precise feature of the environment that would need to be modified remains unclear. It remains a fine judgment whether the advice of low sugar, low fat, high fibre diets, recommended worldwide by nutrition advisory committees, may in some circumstances represent too high a social burden for some people relative to the health risk involved. It is furthermore uncertain that dietary factors (rather than say activity level) are important in determining the development of diabetes in a genetically susceptible individual, although dietary changes will certainly ameliorate the metabolic disturbance once clinical diabetes has developed. Family members are, however, well advised

Table 3.2 Status of secondary prevention of Type 1 diabetes with immunosuppression

Management	Comment
Prednisolone, azathioprine, cyclophosphamide	Not effective Unacceptable degree of side effects
Plasmapheresis	Not shown to be effective
Cyclosporin	Effective in a proportion of patients (? depending on how early it is started) Must be maintained continually Toxicity too great for routine use
Nicotinamide, altered diets	Effective in animal models No clear benefit in humans

to reduce risk factors (for example, smoking, obesity, high serum lipid concentrations) for conditions associated with diabetes.

Screening for diabetes

Primary prevention must be distinguished from screening for diabetes which has the aim of detecting asymptomatic individuals who already have the condition, in order that they can be offered advice on the prevention of long-term tissue damage. Screening is justified where the prevalence of a condition is high enough to justify the expenditure of resources on testing a largely fit population, where identified patients can be offered suitable management, and where resources exist to offer such management to all identified individuals. In diabetes there are many populations in industrialized societies where prevalence is high enough to justify screening, but in some societies philosophical problems of changing dietary habits in asymptomatic patients are a real barrier to effective management. Furthermore, in many nations the resources are not available to advise and manage a vastly increased population of people with identified diabetes.

Screening can, however, be useful where the screening physician is also the provider of diabetes care at the primary care level. Screening in these circumstances can be selective, not only for age group, but also for individuals with circumstances associated with diabetes, such as family history, obesity and arterial disease.

Screening cannot be reliably performed using urine tests. A 2-h postprandial blood glucose test is probably satisfactory for this purpose, but a single value so obtained is never diagnostic and must be confirmed.

Targets for Therapy

Overall Aims of Treatment

The aims of the management of the diabetic patient have evolved at an increasing rate during the 20th century (Table 3.3). Up to 1921 efforts were directed, at least in what we would now recognize as the insulin-dependent patient, to prolongation of life in the face of a severe catabolic state, with the

Table 3.3 The historical development of targets for the management of diabetes

---
1. Prolongation of life (up to 1921)
2. Treatment of acute symptoms (1921 onwards)
3. Prevention of acute complications (1921 onwards)
4. Control of blood glucose levels (1960s onwards)
5. Prevention of microvascular complications (1970s onwards)
6. Prevention of macrovascular complications (1970s onwards)
7. Normal duration and quality of life (1976 onwards)

ever-present risk of deterioration into ketoacidosis. With the advent of insulin therapy the risk of acute metabolic death was enormously reduced, and attention seems to have swung initially to giving insulin with the minimum of inconvenience to the patient (meaning once daily injections), and then to the prospects for therapy with oral agents in the non-insulin-dependent patient. Throughout this period attention was directed to maintaining the patient free of symptoms, this including avoidance of hypoglycaemic problems induced by therapy.

In the fourth stage, gathering pace in the 1960s and 1970s, increasing attention came to be paid to the hypothesis that metabolic control, or rather blood glucose level control, was related to long-term tissue damage in diabetes, and hence towards the end of this period emphasis swung back to achieving good control, helped by the advent of satisfactory tools (glycosylated haemoglobin and self-blood glucose monitoring) for its measurement. With attention turning to the nature of the metabolic disturbance actually resulting in tissue damage, the philosophy of therapy turned towards the need to normalize all aspects of metabolism and not just blood glucose control, and with this came the realization that the true aim of treatment must be to restore physiological plasma insulin profiles.

The impetus of self-blood glucose monitoring, together with the overall change of emphasis to self-management by the patient rather than treatment of disease by the doctor, have led to further changes in aims towards treatment satisfaction and more recently achievement of normal quality of life. At present, however, there remains a payoff between current quality of life as disturbed by the consequences of therapy and its side-effects, and future quality of life as determined by the morbidity of long-term tissue damage.

Metabolic targets for Treatment (Table 3.4)

The setting of metabolic targets for treatment is complicated by:

1. The uncertainty over what level of metabolic control gives protection against long-term tissue damage.
2. The lack of measures of metabolic control with the exception of those related to glucose itself, and to lipids.
3. The impracticability of achieving normal metabolism in the average insulin-treated patient, and in many non-insulin-treated patients.

Although the evidence is as yet weak and fragmentary it does suggest that maintenance of glycosyslated haemoglobin concentrations below mean +4 standard deviations of the normal range (the quoted normal reference range is usually mean ±2 standard deviations) will protect the vast majority of insulin-dependent patients from the so-called microvascular complications of diabetes. It is, however, unclear what percentage of patients would remain at risk. Furthermore, glycosylated haemoglobin is an average measure of blood glucose concentration, and a level of say 8.0% implies prolonged periods of

Table 3.4 Metabolic targets in the management of diabetes

	Good	Acceptable	Poor	High risk
HbA_1* (above normal mean)	<2 S.D.	2 S.D.–<4 S.D.	4 S.D.–<6 S.D.	>6 S.D.
Glucose (venous plasma, mmol/l)				
Fasting	<5.5	5.5–<6.7	6.7–<9.0	>9.0
Post-prandial	<6.7	6.7–<9.0	9.0–<11.0	>11.0
Mean	<6.0	6.0–<7.5	7.5–<10.0	>10.0
Cholesterol (serum, mmol/l)				
Fasting or fed	<5.2	5.2–<6.5	6.5–<7.8	>7.8
Triglycerides (serum, mmol/l)				
Fasting	<1.7	1.7–<2.2	2.2–<3.5	>3.5
Body mass index (kg/m^2)				
Male	<25.0	25.0–<27.0	27.0–<30.0	>30.0
Female	<24.0	24.0–<26.0	26.0–<29.0	>29.0

S.D. Standard deviation.
*Glycosylated haemoglobin assays are not always comparable, and hence classification is given in terms of the local normal reference range (but this is also dependent on a good assay). For HbA_1 (normal <7.5%) the cut-off between acceptable and poor will be around 8.75%, and for HbA_{1c} (normal <6.0%) it will be 7.0%.

marked hyper- and hypoglycaemia in some patients, but more constant blood glucose levels in others. While this level may, therefore, be regarded as acceptable in some patients, it remains important to strive for lower levels where these might be achievable.

There is a further problem with reliance on glycosylated haemoglobin as the sole target for good metabolic control. While studies in insulin-dependent patients suggest normalization of serum lipid concentrations at the degree of control suggested above, many non-insulin-dependent patients retain significant degrees of hypertriglyceridaemia and to a lesser extent hypercholesterolaemia. Furthermore, it is known that even people with impaired glucose tolerance (who have glycosylated haemoglobin concentrations overlapping the normal range) carry an increased risk of ischaemic heart disease. Nevertheless, as insulin itself may be a risk factor here, it may only make sense to achieve absolutely normal blood glucose concentrations in those patients who are not insulin-resistant through dietary indiscretion and obesity.

Many national and international groups have published targets for serum lipid concentrations in non-diabetic subjects. These have now been adopted for people with diabetes (Table 3.4).

Targets for Detection of Late Problems Due to Diabetes

Even if all diabetic patients could have their metabolism normalized from now on, problems of late tissue damage, with serious consequences, would, on our present understanding, continue to appear for years to come. Even the most perfect diabetes service must therefore aim to detect problems related to diabetes at a stage where management can be effective. This implies not just the ability to screen for retinopathy, impairment of renal function and neuropathy, but also the organization to ensure that review is actually effected at regular intervals for each and every patient.

Educational Targets

If self-management is to be effective then clearly diabetic patients must be both knowledgeable and motivated to look after themselves. Treatment satisfaction, quality of life, metabolic control and appropriate action when complications are present (in foot care, for example) will all be dependent on patient education. Detailed targets for education are discussed below.

Self-care, Education and Monitoring

The need for self-care

A number of features in the management of diabetes conspire to ensure that this management is largely delivered by the patients themselves with the medical service only acting as advisor.

1. Dietary management is a cornerstone of the treatment of all non-insulin-dependent patients, and is a key feature of the management of the insulin-treated patient. Dietary management can only be successfully achieved by the person actually consuming the food, and on an hour-to-hour basis. Except therefore where patients are institutionalized, they will usually be responsible for most of their own management, although relatives may have a major role to play. The diabetes service can only advise and educate.
2. Monitoring of diabetes, as day-to-day assessment of blood glucose control, can only give effective information about changes occurring between days and within days when performed regularly by the patient (or a relative). For all the usefulness of measures of glycosylation, they can only give average control over a period of weeks.
3. Insulin therapy is unusual amongst medical treatments in:

   (a) Requiring precise measurement of dosage by the patient;
   (b) Requiring self-infliction of pain at fixed times of day;
   (c) Interacting in complex and often erratic ways with everyday events such as eating and exercise.

   Use of insulin therefore requires both understanding and self-discipline.
4. Unpredictable events requiring changes in treatment routine (for example, intercurrent illness) may occur when help is not easily available (for example, on holiday), and may demand both initiative and understanding if acute deterioration is not to occur.

Education for People with Diabetes

Diabetes is an unusual condition in that it combines two major difficulties in securing patient motivation to deal with the disease. Firstly, diabetes is a chronic, asymptomatic condition, which continues to do its damage unannounced, while providing no immediate reward to the patient for trying to ameliorate the processes leading to long-term complications. Secondly, and unlike hypertension, for example, management of the insidious biochemical disturbance affects many important aspects of the way people live, and is not merely limited to complying with tablet dose schedules. In the non-insulin-treated patient the major management is dietary (see Chapter 4), and almost by definition this means maintaining a major change in the eating and drinking habits ingrained over a lifetime. Patterns of calorie consumption are a major part of human social behaviour in industrialized societies, and changing them often has significant consequences for lifestyle and perceived quality of life. Furthermore, for the insulin-treated patient additional adjustments in timing of eating habits are often necessary, levels of activity cannot be ignored in the quest for good control, and a good standard of injection technique needs to be maintained. Additionally, hypoglycaemia may provide a strong negative influence on the desire to keep blood glucose levels down.

Accordingly it is unreasonable to expect people with diabetes to achieve and then maintain the behavioural changes needed to cope with the condition unless significant knowledge can be gained and applied by the patient. Many patients will also require considerable and continuing support if they are to be able to apply their new learning to the way they live their lives.

In addition to supporting behavioural change considerable amounts of information are required in order to deal with the complexities of modern life. Examples are appropriate foot care to cope with changing fashions and while on holiday in the sun, insulin injection regimens for shift work or transcontinental journeys, and assessing food composition in restaurants and supermarkets.

Knowledge Needed by the Diabetic Patient (Table 3.5)

The knowledge needed by the diabetic patient may be divided into six categories:

1. Knowing about the condition It is unreasonable to expect a patient to take active steps to manage their condition without knowing what it is, and what are its consequences. This requires some explanation of the nature of diabetes, an explanation which can be usefully tailored to the type of diabetes and the planned treatment. As many patients will read further about the condition it is important for them to be aware that other types of diabetes exist, or serious misinformation may be gained. It is morally and probably legally necessary for adult patients (or parents) to be aware of the likely risk of long-term tissue

Table 3.5 Educational targets for people with diabetes

The patient should be aware of:
1. The meaning of 'diabetes'
2. The chronic nature of the condition
3. The possibility of long-term complications
4. The relationship of complications to control
5. Interactions with other risk factors (e.g. smoking)
6. Their own level of control (HbA_1)
7. The need for special care before and during pregnancy
8. Risks of diabetes appearing in any children

The patient should know how to:
1. Obtain help in emergencies
2. Cope with intercurrent illness
3. Monitor own glucose levels
4. Choose foods appropriately when shopping and eating out
5. Cope with changes in activity level
6. Maintain good foot care and choose appropriate shoes
7. Recognize acute foot problems
8. Adjust and use therapy appropriately
9. Cope with foreign travel and changes in time zones

The patient should know of:
1. Driving health laws and regulations
2. Insurance implications and how to obtain advice
3. Consequences of diabetes for employment
4. Consequences for high risk sports
5. National diabetes associations
6. Local support groups and meetings
7. Health care concessions for people with diabetes

damage from diabetes, and the forms of damage to health that result. The quest for good control otherwise becomes meaningless.

2. Food and drink   All people with diabetes will need to be able to recognize those foods which contain a high proportion of free sugar, those which are high in cholesterol or saturated fatty acids, and those which provide fibre, while the insulin-dependent patient will also need to be able to estimate carbohydrate equivalents. Again knowledge about food in isolation from knowledge about the reasons for advising healthy eating is likely to be largely wasted. Particular problems which must be addressed include the use of artificial sweeteners, interpreting labelling of prepacked foods, providing variety within a healthy diet, ethnic foods, 'diabetic' foods and alcohol.

3. Foot care   Foot care deserves special educational attention because of its high morbidity, and high resource implications. Topics to be covered include daily inspection, suitable footwear, dangers of going barefoot, use of creams, care of nails and the role of chiropody. Every patient needs also to be clear as to the action to be taken should inspection reveal a suspected ulcer or other medical problem.

4. Self-monitoring Understanding of the need for self-monitoring of blood glucose levels will to some extent overlap with knowledge of the need for tight control of diabetes, but techniques for self-monitoring, how they are to be used and the importance of proper interpretation of results obtained requires dedicated training sessions. Patients must be made to understand that it is sometimes necessary for them to insist that their doctors and nurses take the trouble to review and interpret such results.

5. Injection technique, and problems of insulin therapy Insulin treated patients can only be expected to give injections with care if they understand the significance of changes in dose, depth of injection, and timing of injections. Furthermore, considerable explanation is required of the nature of hypoglycaemia, and how to avoid it without compromising good control. It is also probably wise for patients taking tablets to have some knowledge of hypoglycaemia and its management, but this will need to be tailored to their particular requirements. Insulin dose adjustment also needs to be carefully taught to be both safe and useful.

6. General knowledge This should include an appreciation that people with diabetes can have normally varied and full lives. Additionally, however, knowledge of diabetes support groups locally and nationally is needed, how to obtain special advice from the diabetes services for new situations or emergencies, and the significance and regulations governing diabetes and driving motor vehicles.

Changing Behaviour and Lifestyle

While it is well recognized that better informed patients can achieve better control and lead a fuller life than ill-informed patients, it is also clear that where education programmes are organized the worst controlled patients are often among the best informed. A likely explanation is that considerable educational reinforcement is given to these patients, although an alternative explanation is that a personality which aids learning may in some individuals also inhibit the application of that knowledge. Either way the point is made that knowledge by itself does not guarantee the desired behavioural change. Indeed in some people the change in lifestyle demanded by knowledge of diabetes may be so great as to create insuperable psychological or psychosocial barriers, a circumstance in which 'non-compliance' may be seen as a useful protective mechanism.

A number of influences other than knowledge will therefore affect whether a patient suitably alters their lifestyle. Positive influences can include praise and approval from professionals, relatives and peers, and it is important that opportunities are grasped by these groups to reinforce desirable behavioural change. Self-praise, commonly called self-esteem, is very effective in many

Table 3.6 Features which suggest that appropriate behavioural adaptations are occurring in people with diabetes

At clinic visits	At home
Improvement in metabolic control	Resumption of normal recreational activities
Appropriate weight control	
Volunteering of self-test records to professionals	Ability to travel and eat out
	Appropriate management of acute health crises
Enquiry after HbA$_1$ and cholesterol results	
	Appropriate foot care
Interest in results of annual review	Membership of diabetes associations

people, and can also be strengthened by careful manipulation of minor successes.

Negative reinforcement of failure to achieve desirable changes is often less effective, and stands the risk of alienating the patient from their advisor. It is probably therefore only effective where the relationship between the professional and the patient is already strong through past contact, but even then displeasure will have to be limited by social norms. A commonly used variant of negative reinforcement is to threaten patients with future ill health if they do not change their habits. Fear can certainly be effective in this role in some people, but in others it may carry significant psychological morbidity. More often, however, the tendency of people to live mainly in the present, and with scant regard for the future, means that the concept of future ill health is simply too remote to influence current behaviour. This is a particular problem with the adolescent patient.

Some pointers to success in motivating the individual patient are given in Table 3.6.

Psychological Influences on Living with Diabetes

A significant literature now exists on psychological influences within diabetes, ranging from possible effects on the aetiology of Type 1 diabetes, through to effects on absorption of insulin. While it is clear that a patient's psychological state will have a significant influence on what they gain from a consultation or teaching session, or whether they are subsequently capable of altering their behaviour in a physiologically desirable way, there are as yet no instruments (such as questionnaires) which allow individual patients to be usefully classified at diagnosis or thereafter.

A good deal of information is also available on types of personality, and their interaction with diabetes. In clinical practice an occasionally useful distinction is between those patients who see their disease as part of themselves, and in need of management by themselves, and those patients who see the condition as something external to themselves, and to be managed by doctors, drugs and devices. The latter patients often grasp at new ideas, but fail to use them properly through inability to make a consistent personal effort to effect them.

72 Delivering Optimal Care to the Patient with Diabetes

The former patients are often reluctant to try new ideas, and sometimes suffer considerable guilt if they are unsuccessful in reaching the targets demanded of them.

The Educational Process

The consultation

The hospital consultation is a poor situation for teaching and learning. Many doctors find it difficult to avoid conducting a consultation along traditional lines, concentrating on medical matters and issuing instructions to patients. The patient often adopts a matching mentality, while the stress of the occasion reduces their ability to learn. The time allotted to hospital consultations is often relatively short, and even that time is often taken up by the perceived need to make medical assessments and deal with medical problems related to diabetes. To have any success education within the consultation must allow sufficient time to relax the patient, discover relevant elements of their home and work circumstances, and talk over an area of knowledge. It is rare for diabetes education to be delivered in any systematic fashion over a series of consultations.

A particular problem arises in the initial consultation when a stunned and stressed patient is often asked to take on board a concept of diabetes, the importance of control, a host of dietary information, details of monitoring techniques, plus miscellaneous other comments. In these circumstances retention of knowledge is very poor.

Teaching sessions

A better method of imparting information is to arrange for patients to attend a series of teaching sessions, conducted by someone with training in both education and diabetes. At present this is usually a specialist nurse. While it is possible to arrange these sessions to form part of a residential course over 3–5 days, this needs considerable resources, and a better approach is to arrange for patients to come to the diabetes teaching unit for a series of meetings. The topics to be covered are given above, but for the non-insulin-treated patient the emphasis will need to be on control of food intake, and for the insulin-treated patient, living with insulin injections. Clearly these sessions will involve personnel other than the specialist nurse, and can include practical events such as a visit to the hospital canteen. An outline of objectives to be met by such teaching is given for non-insulin-treated patients in Table 3.5.

Group teaching in this way has the additional advantage of being efficient with medical time, and of allowing patients to meet others with similar problems and going through the same learning process. It is not suitable for all patients, however, occasionally for educational reasons, and sometimes because of inability to conform to group norms. Patients referred to the diabetes service will not usually be expecting such sessions, and unless formally instructed to come (given an appointment) they may regard them as peripheral to their condition.

It should be noted that teaching sessions do not obviate the need for individual instruction where the circumstances demand it. This will apply particularly to starting insulin therapy in the home, initial instruction in monitoring techniques, aspects of foot care individual to the patient, and interpretation of self-monitored blood or urine tests.

An education course must be made available to every newly diagnosed diabetic patient. Knowledge does atrophy, however, and patient circumstances change, thus altering areas of relevance within the teaching course. It is suggested that some educational reinforcement is provided on a yearly basis, or biennially if formal arrangements can be supported.

Diabetes groups

In addition to group teaching sessions more informal meetings of diabetic patients in a supervised group has been suggested as a way of dealing with some of the stresses of living with diabetes. On these occasions it is hoped that discussion with peers will lead to new insights into a patient's own knowledge and behaviour in dealing with the condition, thus leading to improvements in control and quality of life. Such sessions generally take the form of guided discussion within a particular area, and may need careful handling if the objectives are to be fulfilled, and if destructive influences are to be avoided. Such sessions are of most use in patients who have had the condition for some time, and it can be helpful to try to loosely match the people taking part for broad age group, type of diabetes and social attainment. It remains unclear to what extent such sessions are an efficient use of medical time, or indeed achieve their objectives.

Informal group meetings (support groups) may be particularly useful in the younger diabetic patient, who may feel particularly isolated and alienated because of diabetes. The prevalence of diabetes at this age is such that any young person is unlikely to know another with the condition.

Aids to teaching

Diabetes teaching needs to make use of all modern aids to achieve maximum success. Within limits a teaching session is likely to be more successful if it switches between a video, a talk (overhead projector or flip chart), a demonstration (examples), and a discussion, than if only one medium is used. This implies the need for purpose built accommodation.

Learning may also be more successful in an informal environment (youth club, for example) under some circumstances, and in practical situations such as the supermarket and canteen.

Assessing Knowledge and Behaviour

Administration of teaching sessions for patients is probably of little value unless some attempt is made to assess its outcome in terms of a gain in knowledge or change of behaviour.

Assessment of education about diabetes implies design and implementation of knowledge questionnaires, a task that cannot be undertaken lightly. Questionnaires are only useful if:

1. The questions distinguish adequately those people with knowledge from those who do not have it. A question that was too easy or too difficult would always be answered 100% correctly or incorrectly, and therefore would not discriminate the level of knowledge.
2. The questions are relevant to and understood by the patient to whom it is administered. Dietary questions about doughnuts or kiwi fruit may be unanswerable by sectors of the population, and medical terminology is not comprehensible by many people.
3. The questions address a field of knowledge relevant to what has been taught.
4. The construction of questions is such that they are interpreted by the patient in the way intended by the person designing the questionnaire, and that the questions do in fact test the area of knowledge intended.
5. Administration of the questionnaire avoids the possibility of assistance in its completion, distractions when completing it, or bias occurring through the behaviour of an observer.

Although these observations may seem straightforward, design of questionnaires rapidly becomes fraught with difficulties, and it is often easier to adopt a previously validated questionnaire. Unfortunately population differences between clinics may mean that validity cannot be generalized. The problems of administration of questionnaires are best solved by the patient completing them alone in a side room, either on paper or directly into a microcomputer.

Behavioural assessment is even more difficult, although hopefully some influence on the level of metabolic control should be discernible. Some information can be gained by scoring weight change, type of shoes, carriage of glucose, membership of diabetes organizations, attendance at clinic appointments, and rates of consumption of tablets. However, these may not be adequately related to the more important variables of dietary behaviour and administration of insulin. Non-recording of self-tests may be a useful pointer, but completion of records has been shown to be too unreliable to be a positive finding.

Self-monitoring of Blood Glucose Control (Table 3.7)

Self-monitoring of blood glucose control fulfils a number of functions. The choice of technique to be used by a patient, and the intensity to which it is used,

Self-care, Education and Monitoring

Table 3.7 Aids available for self-monitoring of blood glucose control

Semi-quantitative blood glucose reagent strips
Finger pricking devices
Semi-quantitative urine glucose reagent strips
Record diaries
Urine ketone reagent strips
Reagent strip blood glucose meters
Electrochemical blood glucose meters
Blood glucose meters with memory and clock/date facility
Microcomputer programs for data transfer and analysis

will depend on which functions the physician (and patient) feel are important for that individual.

1. Self-monitoring provides feedback to the patient on how well blood glucose control is being maintained, and therefore supplements information given by the physician on glycosylated haemoglobin level, blood lipids and weight. Self-monitoring has the advantage, however, of being performed on a much more frequent basis, and can therefore provide feedback on behaviour on a much more immediate basis. This can be particularly useful in providing positive support in the early phase after instituting new treatment. However, in the patient with stable and well-controlled diabetes such monitoring need not be very frequent, occasional post-prandial urinalysis often being sufficient in non-insulin-treated patients.
2. Self-monitoring of blood glucose provides the only means by which changes in blood glucose concentrations throughout the day can be assessed in the patient's normal environment. Because blood glucose concentrations are highly variable from day-to-day in insulin-treated patients, a high frequency of observations are necessary to discern patterns on which insulin doses can be adjusted.
3. Self-monitoring also provides a means by which patients can investigate the effects of changes in lifestyle on blood glucose control. Thus, even urinalysis will detect dietary indiscretion of significant quantity in otherwise aglycosuric patients, while insulin-dependent patients can experiment for themselves in matching changes in insulin dosage to meals.
4. Blood glucose monitoring provides a method for distinguishing true hypoglycaemia from possible symptoms of a similar nature.
5. Self-testing should be used to monitor control during intercurrent illness, and to maintain a check of integrity of insulin delivery in those patients using insulin infusion systems. Hyperglycaemia in either event should be accompanied by self-monitoring for urinary ketones.

Self-urinalysis for glucose

The use of semi-quantitative reagent strips has considerably improved the usefulness and convenience of home urinalysis, which can often be performed simply by holding the strip in the urinary stream for a couple of seconds, and timing development of colour. The important distinction for clinical purposes is between aglycosuria and glycosuria above 1.0 g/l, as only the former indicates absence of hyperglycaemia. The test is therefore used post-prandially to confirm aglycosuria and therefore maintenance of satisfactory blood glucose levels. The validity of the results should be confirmed by glycosylated haemoglobin estimations, to detect renal threshold problems or mis-recording of results. Where such problems are encountered, or where persistent glycosuria is recorded due to inadequate control, then a move to self-blood glucose monitoring may be indicated as part of the management of resolving the problem.

Self-blood glucose monitoring

Self-blood glucose monitoring may be performed with glucose oxidase reagent strips, read visually or with a meter, or glucose oxidase sensor based meters (Table 3.7). Reagent strips have the major advantage of high portability, although a percentage of patients have problems with colour matching. Meter reading gives confidence to some patients, and most meters can now incorporate some kind of memory system which can be used to analyse validity of results, and present the results in a more useful fashion than the familiar record diaries. The newer sensor-based systems may be convenient and portable enough to replace both systems, if reliability, accuracy, precision and cost prove acceptable.

None of these systems will function properly without adequate training of patients, and technique should be reviewed regularly. All results should be recorded (together with any related information) in a record diary, and patients told to insist that such results are examined at every visit to their medical adviser.

For stable non-insulin-treated patients the frequency of testing can be quite low (once per week after the largest meal) if the glycosylated haemoglobin estimation is also good. However, where insulin doses are to be adjusted against the records, tests must be recorded at all times of the day, on representative days, in each week, although a higher rate of testing is desirable. Increased rates of testing will be needed to cope with periods of exercise or illness, and tests may be performed every day, four times a day, by those patients desirous of adjusting each insulin dose individually.

Some test strips develop colour to an endpoint, which is then relatively stable. Such strips can be brought up to a clinic within 24 h, and used to audit some aspects of technique. Diary records are unfortunately notoriously unreliable. This has been confirmed by patients issued with meters covertly containing memory chips. Clues to such problems include the completion of record diaries in neat writing with a single pen, and discrepancies from glycosylated haemoglobin values. Where patients are issued with memory meters they should be informed of this, as it obliges them to learn to present to medical staff and themselves the real extent of their monitoring and hyperglycaemia.

The Diabetic Service

Core Services

A diabetes service as described here is assumed to be capable of providing all diabetes services for the population under its care. It needs to be recognized that efficient diabetes care cannot be given by individual physicians, unless they have unusually good access to specialist diabetes support services.

The core of any effective diabetes service consists of two elements, namely, medical staff with support facilities, and an educational service with appropriate teaching aids. Experience appears to show that it is difficult for medically qualified staff to suppress their training in concentrating on medical aspects of disease, and that diabetes education is therefore better undertaken by trained paramedical staff outside the regular diabetic clinic (see above). Nevertheless, nearly all Type 2 diabetic patients have medical conditions in addition to diabetes, and are often undergoing therapy which has consequences for the diabetes. In the Type 1 patient regular adjustment of insulin dosage can often be undertaken by patients themselves, and certainly with skilled nursing advice, but the complexities are sufficient for regular medical review to be advisable. Provision of education through specialist nursing staff has the additional advantage of allowing the possibility of assessing the patient's self-management at home, and arranging for initial teaching, for example, of injection technique, to be given in that more appropriate environment.

Centralized diabetes services may be based on the local hospital, or in a purposely adapted centre in the community. Hospital-based services may have the advantage of easier access to both support services such as chiropody and dietetics, as well as to diagnostic facilities and other medical specialties. Diabetes care centres in the community may, however, encourage the development of a different type of service, with the emphasis on education and adaptation of lifestyle, and away from the concept of a disease to be managed

Table 3.8 Modern role of the specialist diabetologist

Developing service policy
Implementing appropriate advances in care
Obtaining adequate recources
Liason with other specialties
Provision of specialist advice
   1.   To other professionals
   2.   To patients
Teaching and training

by doctors. Whatever provision is made it is important that medical, educational, dietetic and chiropody services are made available on one site, if effective communication is to take place between the staff concerned, and patient inconvenience is to be avoided.

Other Medical Services

Special provision needs to be made for the medical care of diabetic patients in a number of common situations. These fall into two categories: (a) care for people who develop problems through their diabetes, and (b) care for people with diabetes and other medical problems (Table 3.9).

The latter category includes the review and diabetic management of any patient undergoing surgery or a related procedure. Experience has shown that proper diabetes management is only effected if specialist care is available both before and after the procedure, and during the convalescent period. Pregnancy in the woman with diabetes becomes a medical rather than a physiological condition, and it is vitally important to the health of both mother and fetus for appropriate diabetic care to be reviewed every 1–2 weeks. Details of the management in both these circumstances are given in Chapter 5.

Because of the consequences of late tissue damage, people with diabetes also need easy access to ophthalmological services with facilities for photocoagulation, to nephrological services providing dialysis and transplantation, and to vascular surgeons. Cardiological services experienced in the investigation and if necessary surgical management of ischaemic heart disease should also be available.

Combined clinics with other specialities have been established in a number of circumstances (Table 3.9), but apart from joint obstetric/diabetic clinics and to a lesser extent foot clinics (involving vascular surgeons and chiropodists) and adolescent clinics, they are not a common feature of diabetes care.

Table 3.9 People with diabetes in need of special care and services

Patients with special needs
Children
Adolescents
The elderly sick
Pregnant women
Those with complications
The house bound

Type of joint clinics
Paediatric clinics with psychologists
Pre-pregnancy and pregnancy clinics
Vascular and foot clinics
Adolescent (joint paediatric/adult) clinics
Annual review/eye screening clinics

Table 3.10 Appropriate organization of care

> Regular review clinic
> Annual review clinic
> New patient clinic
> Specialist clinics
>   Adolescent/pregnancy/vascular/eye
> Walk-in and emergency services
> Educational services

Organization of Clinical Practice

Three major forms of organization of the clinical practice of diabetes may be recognized, any of which may be medically satisfactory if properly effected. These are traditional clinic-based practice, diabetes centre-based practice, often highly dependent on specialist nurses, and community care by general practitioners.

Organization of traditional clinic practice (Table 3.10)

The operation of a successful traditional clinic-based practice can be broken down into three major roles. Regular review of the patient every two to four months involves the doctor in coming to understand the home and work circumstances in which the patient manages their diabetes, reviewing the home and clinic evidence of the quality of blood glucose control, judging the appropriateness of current therapy and advising adjustments where necessary, dealing with associated and other medical conditions, and giving or arranging appropriate management for previously identified complications (see below).

The second role of a traditional service is that of identification of problems arising from diabetes at any early stage. This is perhaps best organized as an Annual Review function, as experience shows that without some form of discipline (including appropriate forms) these vital checks are omitted, particularly if it is intended that they are performed at the same visits as regular reviews of care. Details of an annual review clinic service are given below.

Thirdly, even a clinic-based service will need to provide facilities and staff for education and training of patients. Provision of a diabetes specialist nurse allows not only more careful training of monitoring and injection techniques, but also formal education to help integrate diabetes self-management with lifestyle, and initiation of insulin therapy in the most appropriate environment, the home.

The diabetes centre and specialist nurse-based service

These types of service may be regarded as still being at an early stage of evolution. Provision of a diabetes centre is believed to provide a number of advantages over a hospital- or office-based service:

1. Facilities appropriate to diabetes education can be made available throughout the week.
2. A diabetes centre enhances the idea of diabetes as a condition to be managed by the patient, rather than treated by the hospital or doctor.
3. Members of the diabetes management team can be brought together on one site.
4. The centre can be permanently staffed to provide free and emergency access for patients to diabetes personnel on an informal basis.
5. Equipment needed for diabetes care, and the records needed for its organization can be held where they are actually required.
6. The centre can act as a resource centre for non-specialist referral (dietary or educational) of patients being managed by community practitioners.
7. Diabetes specialist nurses can use the centre as an office and organizational base.

Where services are so organized, and where staffing is appropriate, it may be suitable for patients to be seen by diabetes specialist nurses at some visits, rather than doctors. This again will transfer the ambiance of the consultation towards appropriate self-management of diabetes in the context of the education offered by such personnel.

The major disadvantage of a diabetes centre can be that it removes the patients from hospital facilities (such as ECG services and radiological departments) that are often needed because of the high prevalence of other medical problems in these people. There can be similar problems for medical staff with responsibilities within the hospital.

Community care

Patients with any form of diabetes can be looked after by enthusiastic general practitioners, but few as yet are familiar with the radical changes that have taken place in the concepts of management of diabetes, and fewer still are familiar enough with the intricacies of insulin pharmacokinetics to adjust doses expertly. Nevertheless, the care to be offered to people with non-insulin-treated diabetes is fairly easily standardized (see below) in a way that is well within the experience of most general practitioners. Adequate care in general medical practice will depend as much on proper organization of records, and systems for identifying defaulters, as does clinic-based care. Many studies have shown that people with diabetes discharged to practitioners with no organized system of care are generally neglected.

A major problem of community- or office-based care can be the lack of access to adequate educational, dietary and chiropody services. Unless these are made available it is inevitable that care will be less than first rate.

The Diabetes Consultation

The diabetes consultation can be fairly complex, but fortunately it is also fairly easily organized to avoid neglect of important items. As discussed above consultations are best divided into regular and annual review functions (Table 3.10), and although less satisfactory these can be combined at one visit if suitable record forms are used. The approach to the newly diagnosed patient is dealt with in Chapter 1.

The Regular Review Clinic

Regular review of diabetic patients will need to be at intervals of between one and six months, depending on whether treatment and control are stable or changing, and how much support the patient has been found to require.

After welcoming the patient initial enquiry should be into possible disturbing factors at home or at work and including holidays. Without this information any changes in control may be misinterpreted. For the same reason it is then important to know whether any changes in other aspects of health might have occurred since the last visit. After these preliminaries attention should move directly to the records of self-monitoring to emphasize their importance, and to use these together with other information on metabolic control for further patient education. Usually it will then be necessary to record details of current therapy and hypoglycaemia, so that the patient can be led into suggesting appropriate changes in dietary, insulin/drug and exercise management. Specific enquiry into diet should also be made at every consultation, and at this point consideration given to whether referral to the dietician or diabetes specialist nurse is desirable.

Attention should then turn to diabetes-related problems uncovered at the annual review (see below), and in particular to whether repeat fundoscopy is required, further foot care advice needed, or treatment for hypertension or ischaemic heart disease adjusted. In-depth discussion may be needed for problems of impotence, or where renal albumin excretion has been found to be increased.

Finally attention should be paid to other active medical problems, and a suitable time interval to the next appointment agreed with the patient.

Figure 3.1 illustrates a typical record form.

Annual Review

The annual review should begin with an assessment of corrected or pinhole visual acuity, so that mydriatic drops can be instilled for later fundoscopy. It is useful to make this visit the occasion to review in detail all drug therapy, including the appropriateness of timing of sulphonylurea tablets. Attention should then turn to symptom review for impotence/amenorrhoea (in appropriate age groups), neuropathy, peripheral vascular disease and ischaemic

NEWCASTLE HEALTH AUTHORITY DIABETES CLINIC

Normal/absent = 0; abnormal/present = 1; not done/asked = 9; or number

Hospital (F = 1, R = 2) ⬜	Urine	glucose	⬜ + = 1
Surname ⬜⬜⬜⬜⬜⬜⬜⬜⬜⬜⬜		ketones	⬜ ++ = 2
Firstname ⬜⬜⬜⬜⬜⬜⬜⬜⬜		protein	⬜ etc
Number ⬜⬜⬜⬜⬜⬜		blood	⬜
Date ⬜⬜⬜⬜⬜⬜⬜	Weight (kg)		⬜⬜⬜⬜

Comment AGE ⬜⬜   Year of diagnosis ⬜⬜

Including other conditions Last AR ⬜⬜⬜⬜⬜⬜
and drugs

TESTS (O, U = 1, Bl = 2, both = 3) ⬜ Number/ ⬜⬜
                                              mo

	Fast	PostB	PreL	PostL	PreD	PostD	PreBd	Night
Lo	⬜⬜	⬜⬜	⬜⬜	⬜⬜	⬜⬜	⬜⬜	⬜⬜	⬜⬜
Hi	⬜⬜	⬜⬜	⬜⬜	⬜⬜	⬜⬜	⬜⬜	⬜⬜	⬜⬜

DIET (= 1; not = 0) SFD ⬜ MFD ⬜ HFD ⬜
CHO ⬜⬜⬜⬜⬜⬜⬜⬜

INSULIN/DM DRUGS: Code ⬜
(none = 0, diet = 1, sulph = 2, met = 3, both = 4,
insulin = 5, oth = 6)
Insulin/drugs 1: _____ 2: _____

Doses	AM	⬜⬜.⬜	⬜⬜.⬜
U or mg	MD	⬜⬜.⬜	⬜⬜.⬜
	PM	⬜⬜.⬜	⬜⬜.⬜
	Bed	⬜⬜.⬜	⬜⬜.⬜
	Bsl	⬜⬜	

HYPOGLYCAEMIA last month   AM PM EVE NT
nil = 0 ⬜   self-treated ⬜⬜ ⬜⬜ ⬜⬜ ⬜⬜
                other-treated ⬜⬜ ⬜⬜ ⬜⬜ ⬜⬜

Action from last AR BP: lie = 1, sit = 2, sta = 3 ⬜   ⬜⬜/⬜⬜
FEET:
FUNDI:

Changes INVESTIGATIONS
HbA1 ⬜⬜.⬜   Chol ⬜⬜.⬜
Fructosmine ⬜⬜.⬜   TG ⬜⬜.⬜
Write in other tests done   Creat ⬜⬜⬜

AR needed/requested ⬜   To dietician ⬜   Observer initials ⬜⬜⬜
To diabetes sister ⬜   To chiropodist ⬜   Next visit (weeks) ⬜⬜

Fig. 3.1 A typical form used in a regular diabetes clinic. The form assumes that annual review (AR) information is collected in a separate clinic (see Fig. 3.2).

heart disease. Enquiry should also be made for chiropody attendance, and smoking and alcohol habits.

Examination should concentrate firstly on the feet, to include skin condition, deformities and shoes, and taking the opportunity to impart some education about care and risks. More specifically peripheral pulses should be checked, together with peripheral sensation. Unfortunately pain and temperature sensation can still only be qualitatively tested, but large fibre function, although less relevant to ulceration risk, should be quantified with vibrometers.

All injection sites should be inspected in insulin-treated patients, fundoscopy performed, and blood pressure checked in a standardized position. At present tests for autonomic neuropathy do not have enough predictive value or clinical significance for them to be worth performing on a routine basis.

Finally serum lipid concentrations are checked (non-fasting), together with serum creatinine, and a screening pre-breakfast urine sample sent for albumin estimation by a sensitive assay, expressed as a ratio of urinary creatinine.

Annual review is only useful if the results are adequately recorded on well-designed forms, if appropriate action is subsequently taken on identified problems, and if appropriate recall procedures are in place to ensure the annual appointments are issued and attended. Figure 3.2 illustrates a typical record form.

Audit of Diabetes Care

Introduction

The structure of care suggested above demands a degree of facilities and organization that are not easily maintained. It is suggested that if an optimum service is to be provided on a continuing basis then continuing audit of activities is necessary. This is also likely to reveal the successes and failures of the service, and hence help in resource planning.

Audit is classically thought of as being of facilities (to include staff and staff training), of process and of outcomes. Diabetes audit will be particularly concerned with process and outcomes audit. While audit is useful internally, to be rigorous it should be reviewed by others, most usefully by physicians with an interest in diabetes. Audit by other groups, including patients, can also be revealing.

Process Audit

Classical medical audit is often process audit—were the right decisions, investigations and interventions pursued? In diabetes, process audit takes on a more distinct form because of the protocols of care and structured annual review suggested above. A suggested collection of data fields is given in Table 3.11. Audit asks the question (for example) what percentage of patients are

NEWCASTLE HEALTH AUTHORITY
DIABETES ANNUAL REVIEW CLINIC 1

Absent/Normal = 0, Present/Abnormal = 1; Not asked/known = 9; Or instruction

Hospital (FH, RVI) Number	☐☐☐☐☐	Year diagnosed ☐☐
	☐☐☐☐☐☐☐☐	Post code ☐☐☐☐ ☐☐☐☐
Surname	☐☐☐☐☐☐☐☐☐☐☐☐	
Used name	☐☐☐☐☐☐☐☐☐☐☐☐	

Date	☐☐☐☐☐☐	Weight (kg)	☐☐☐.☐
Age	☐☐☐	Height (cm)	☐☐☐
		BMI	☐☐.☐

Visual acuity	R	☐.☐☐	Albustix protein	☐
(>6/60 = 7/00)	L	☐.☐☐	24 h albumin	☐☐☐☐.☐
with glasses		☐	Microalbumin	☐☐☐
known glaucoma		☐	MSU (abnormal = 1)	☐

Diet
- Calories ☐☐☐☐
- Carbohydrate (g) ☐☐☐
- SFD (=1, none = 0) ☐
- Modified fat (=1, none = 0) ☐
- High fibre (=1, none = 0) ☐

Insulin (syr = 1, pen = 2, pump = 3) ☐ Dose (U/day) ☐☐☐

Oral agents Sulphonylurea: tolb = 1, glib = 2, glip = 3, glic = 4, other = 5
☐ Dose (mg/day) ☐☐☐☐.☐
Metformin (= 1) ☐ Dose (mg/day) ☐☐☐☐

Drugs (taken = 1, none = 0; please write in names and doses)
- Non DM drugs ☐
- Anti-lipid ☐
- Anti-anginal ☐
- Anti-BP ☐
- Oral contraceptive ☐

Habits
- Smoking (cigs/d; pipe/cigars = 98) ☐☐
- Alcohol (units/wk; >90 = 91) ☐☐

Symptoms
- Neuropathic pain/parathesiae ☐
- Impotence/amenorrhoea >6mo age <40 ☐
- Claudication ☐
- Angina ☐

DM Clinic Number of forms last 12 mo (GP clin = 98) ☐☐

Attended
Chiropody	☐	Dietician	☐
Opthalmology	☐	Vascular	☐
Cardiology	☐	Nephrology	☐

Admissions
	Date (mo/yr)	Hospital	Diagnosis
1.	☐☐☐☐☐		
2.	☐☐☐☐☐		
3.	☐☐☐☐☐		

Fig. 3.2 A typical form used in an annual review clinical. Collection of data on treatment type, age, year of diagnosis and admissions, allows the data to be used for audit purposes as well as review of the patients complication and health status.

DIABETES ANNUAL REVIEW CLINIC 2

Normal = 0; Abnormal = 1; not done = 9; or instruction

		R	L
Feet	Deformity/poor skin	☐	☐
	Ulcer/gangrene	☐	☐
	Ischaemia	☐	☐
Circulation	Absent DP and PT (= 1)	☐	☐
	Amputation (toes = 1; foreft = 2; bk/ak = 3)	☐	☐
	Doppler	☐☐☐☐	☐☐☐☐
Nerves	Impaired pinprick	☐	☐
	Biothesiometer (>50 = 51)	☐☐	☐☐
Skin	Injection sites (lipoH = 1; lipoA = 2; oth = 3)		☐
Eyes	Cataract	☐	☐
	Fundi (abnormal = 1; not visualized = 8)	☐	☐
	Microaneurysms (<5 = 1, >4 = 2)	☐	☐
	Other background	☐	☐
	Venous abnorm/soft exudates/IRMA	☐	☐
	Macular/perimacular lesions	☐	☐
	New vessels	☐	☐
	Advanced diabetic retinopathy	☐	☐
BP	Lying (1st/5th)	☐☐☐☐☐☐☐	
Blood	HBA$_1$, Fructosamine	☐☐.☐	☐.☐☐
	Creatinine	☐☐☐☐	
	Cholesterol HDL Chol	☐☐.☐	☐☐.☐
	TG	☐☐.☐	
Action	Smoking		☐
(= 1, none = 0)	Dietary advice		☐
	Diabetes education		☐
	Foot education/attention/chiropody		☐
	Review non-DM drug		
	Write in details and other action needed below		
	Observer initials		☐☐☐

86 Delivering Optimal Care to the Patient with Diabetes

Table 3.11 Examples of measures of diabetes process and outcome audit

Process performed
Education course
Annual review
  Eye screening
  Foot condition
    Pulses
    Neuropathy
  Injection sites inspected
  Blood pressure
  Biochemical tests

Outcomes and outputs
Health status
  Glycosylated haemoglobin
  Cholesterol
  Microalbumin
  Blood pressure
  Retinopathy
  Diabetes education level
Health outcome
  Visual acuity impaired
  Foot ulceration
  Amputation
  Coronary or cerebrovascular disease
  Renal failure
  Erectile impotence
  Quality of life status

receiving an education course after diagnosis, or what percentage of eyes are examined after mydriasis in each year? Indeed since many processes of diabetes care are repeated on an annual basis, it makes sense to analyse audit data yearly, and compare trends from year to year.

Outcome Audit

Process audit makes the assumption that protocols of care, if followed, will achieve the desired result. Outcome audit is intended to look at what end result for the patients' health is actually achieved.

Outcome audit in diabetes is complicated by the chronic nature of the disease, and the very late manifestations of complications. Health outcome in the current year, for example, may reflect health care two decades previously. Thus, as well as true health outcomes (for example, amputation), diabetes outcome audit looks at health status in terms of metabolic indicators (for example, glycosylated haemoglobin) and asymptomatic complications (for example, background retinopathy). A suggested list of data fields is given in Table 3.11. While questionnaires are available for assessment of diabetes knowledge, the instruments as yet validated for measuring quality of life or treatment satisfaction are few, and generally limited in scope.

Data analysis is again best performed on the whole clinic population and on a yearly basis. As well as the current health status of the population with diabetes (Fig. 3.3) the trend between years can be analysed, and trends from year of diagnosis.

Facilities for Diabetes Audit

Retrospective collection of data from unstructured diabetes notes is labour intensive and unreliable. Since, however, diabetes care lends itself to structured note and record taking (Figs 3.1 and 3.2), data can easily be collected prospectively onto forms, and the contents of these entered onto a computer database. Data analysis for audit is then relatively easy. Collection, marking and analysis of questionnaire material for knowledge or quality of life assessment is much more labour intensive, and may not be feasible on a regular basis.

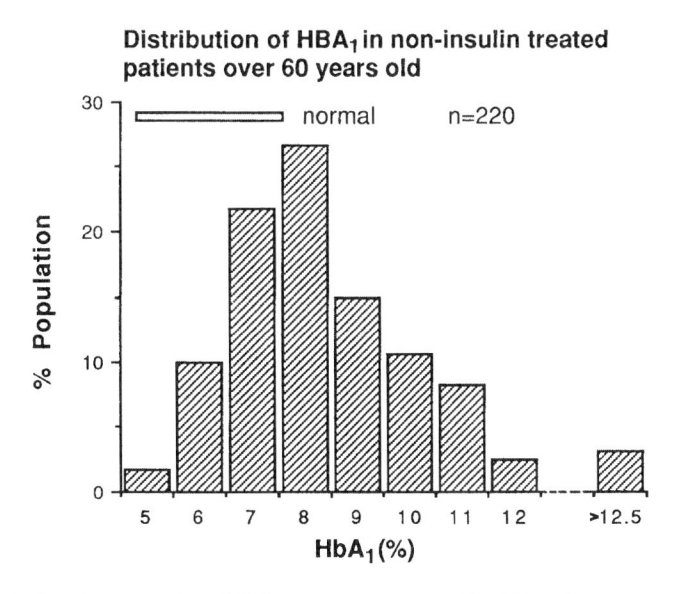

Fig. 3.3 A simple example of diabetes outcome audit. All patients over the age of 60 years were selected for the clinic data base, and their most recent annual review HbA_1 analysed. In this clinic 41% of patients had an HbA_1 above 8.75% ('poor').

Clinic Monitoring of Diabetic Control

Blood Glucose Concentrations

Self-monitoring of blood glucose control is discussed above. When verified by glycosylated haemoglobin estimation it can be a suitable means of testing the overall level of control. Tests are, however, difficult to record quantitatively for analysis of trends in control, unless stored in memory meters and transferred for computer analysis.

Clinic blood glucose estimation is hopelessly unreliable as a means of estimating blood glucose control on a regular basis in the insulin-treated patient. Thus the mean within patient confidence interval for blood glucose at a particular time of day is around ± 7 mmol/l, giving a range of 14 mmol/l around the measured value. Additionally there is only a poor relationship in these patients between blood glucose levels at different times of day, so repeated morning or afternoon estimations may be very misleading. Special indications do arise (the ill patient, or where rows of normal self-test results appear fabricated), but the test is then best performed within the consultation with a reagent strip, when it has maximum education value.

A better case can be made in the non-insulin-dependent patient, particularly as the test is cheap and easy to perform. A normal value (<5.5 mol/l) in a patient on dietary treatment will suggest that good control has been maintained for at least the previous three days, and it can be shown that for in-patients fasting blood glucose concentrations are a good predictor of control over the rest of the day. Unfortunately it is the case that change of dietary behaviour for a week before the clinic visit, plus the stress of the clinic visit, and any change in behaviour necessitated by travel to the clinic itself, can all affect the result obtained in misleading ways (Table 3.12). Furthermore it will be realized that it is impossible to be sure that fasting values are truely fasting, and certainly non-fasting tests are often done on patients who have avoided breakfast to improve their results.

Table 3.12 Problems of within clinic blood glucose estimations

1. Patient stress
2. Unusual day
    (a) Meal times changed
    (b) Activity unusual
3. Single time of day unrepresentative
4. Changes in patient behaviour (eating habits)
    (a) Intentional
    (b) Subconscious
5. High between day variations in insulin-treated patients

Glycosylated Haemoglobin

When exposed to glucose within the erythrocyte the amine groups of the amino acids of haemoglobin slowly react to form a reversible aldimine, which is converted to a stable ketoamine more quickly. The reaction is non-enzymatic and hence only proportional to the concentrations of haemoglobin and glucose. Expressed as a percentage of the haemoglobin present in the blood the amount of glycosylated haemoglobin will therefore be proportional to average blood glucose concentration, always assuming that the time of exposure of the average haemoglobin molecule to glucose (half the lifespan of the erythrocyte) is unchanging.

Percentage of haemoglobin glycosylated is then a useful measure of blood glucose control averaged over 6–8 weeks. Glycosylation affects the charge carried by the haemoglobin molecule, which can therefore be separated from native haemoglobin A by various forms of ion-exchange chromatography, electrophoresis, or high performance liquid chromatography (HPLC). If this is done carefully then three derivatives of haemoglobin A can be detected (A_{1a}, A_{1b}, A_{1c}), of which HbA_{1c} is the glycosylated component. Routine laboratory assays may separate this component alone, or total HbA_1 which is higher by around 1.5% of haemoglobin.

These assays are dependent on the major haemoglobin component being haemoglobin A. If this is not the case then overall charge may vary and the assays will be invalid. Examples are in the neonate (due to haemoglobin F), and some rare haemoglobinopathies. In these circumstances assays for total glycosylation by chemical means of affinity chromatography are more appropriate. Not even these assays will be of use if erythrocyte turnover is abnormal, for example, in most anaemias, clinical haemoglobinopathies, renal and liver failure, and with some types of artificial heart valve.

To be useful glycosylated haemoglobin needs to be assayed very precisely as the range from good to very poor control (say from 7.5 to 10.0% for total HbA_1, or a difference of 2.5%) is only around 30% of its total concentration (Fig. 3.4). This kind of difference is easily disguised by short-term changes in the unstable (aldimine) intermediate, which must therefore be removed before assay.

In clinical use the test has proved indispensible in all types of people with diabetes, and should be performed at every clinic consultation unless the immediately previous results show consistent stability of control.

Glycosylated Serum Proteins and Fructosamine

Albumin is glycosylated in the same way as haemoglobin. Because of its short serum half-life glycosylated albumin has been proposed as a means of looking at short-term changes in control. In practice, however, measures of control over longer periods are more useful, and the assay is no easier to perform.

More recently it has been proposed that glycosylated proteins can be

HbA₁ (%)

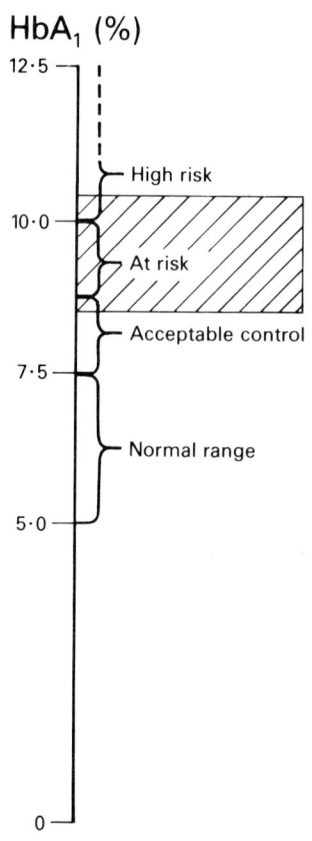

Fig. 3.4 Diagram to demonstrate the need for very precise HbA$_1$ measurements. The shaded area runs from acceptable through to high-risk. It covers only a small range of values (8.5–10.5%), and yet will contain the majority of patients.

measured as serum reducing activity under defined conditions; the test is referred to as fructosamine, and is cheap and easy to perform. Fructosamine certainly bears some relationship to average blood glucose concentration, but at the time of writing it is not fully validated.

Further Reading

Alberti, K.G.M.M. and Gries, F.A. (1988). Management of non-insulin-dependent diabetes mellitus in Europe: a consensus view. *Diabetic Medicine* **5**, 275.

Day, J.L. and Spathis, M. (1988). District diabetes centres in the United Kingdom. *Diabetic Medicine* **5**, 372.

Dunn, S.M. and Turtle, J.R. (1988). Education. In *Diabetes Annual 4*,

pp. 144–161. Edited by Alberti, K.G.M.M. and Krall, L.P. Elsevier, Amsterdam.
Scott, A. and Tattersall, R. (1986). Self-monitoring of diabetes. In *Diabetes Annual 2*, pp. 120–136. Edited by Alberti, K.G.M.M. and Krall, L.P. Elsevier, Amsterdam.
Scott, R.S. and Beaven, D.W. (1988) Organisation of diabetes care. In *Diabetes Annual 4*, pp. 621–632. Edited by Alberti, K.G.M.M. and Krall, L.P. Elsevier, Amsterdam.
Williams, C.D., Harvey, F.E. and Sonksen, P.H. (1988). A role for computers in diabetes care? *Diabetic Medicine* 5, 177.

4
TREATMENT OF DIABETES MELLITUS

Introduction

The management of diabetes (the medical condition) is a much broader subject than the treatment of diabetes (the biochemical disturbance). Organization of diabetes care to ensure effective patient education, screening for and treatment of long-term complications, and management of associated conditions, are dealt with in the preceding chapter, and are a necessary part of the delivery of treatment for the metabolic disturbance, as described here. Management of special situations (for example, pregnancy, childhood diabetes) and acute complications (for example, ketoacidosis, hypoglycaemic coma) in the diabetic patient are covered in Chapter 5.

It is important to reiterate, however, that in practice modes of treatment such as insulin injections, or dietary prescription, cannot be optimally implemented in the absence of considerable understanding by the patient, not only of the nature of the therapy being offered, but also of the necessity and methods of integrating those treatments into their daily lifestyle. This universal need arises because all aspects of treatment of the metabolic disturbance require modification of the dietary habits of all but the rarest of patients, and because dietary habits are often determined by very strong and sometimes immutable behavioural and social pressures. Insulin injections themselves also impose behavioural changes and discipline alien to many patients, and again will be relatively unsuccessful in controlling diabetes without suitable patient education.

It is unreasonable in this context to expect patients simply to follow a set of rules about food intake, or insulin injections, however careful the instruction, although in rare individuals with old-fashioned respect of perceived authority this may be successful. The educational need becomes more important with the recognition of the asymptomatic nature of treated but poorly controlled diabetes, a situation exacerbated by the negative impact of weight gain when glycosuria is better controlled, and the almost inevitable risk of hypoglycaemia with good blood glucose control on insulin therapy. In general then the therapies discussed below must be delivered in the context not only of adequate training, but also of conversion to the practice and philosophy of better health. Discussion of the long-term consequences of poor control is probably morally obligatory in adults, but whether of positive or negative educational impact will depend on the patient's personality.

Dietary Management

Aims of Dietary Instruction

The underlying aims of dietary management in the diabetic patient is to prevent, or reduce, the risk of health problems both acutely and in the long-term.

Since the specific late tissue damage of diabetes is assumed to be associated with the metabolic disturbance associated with hyperglycaemia (Chapter 2), a primary aim is reduction of high blood glucose concentrations. As obesity

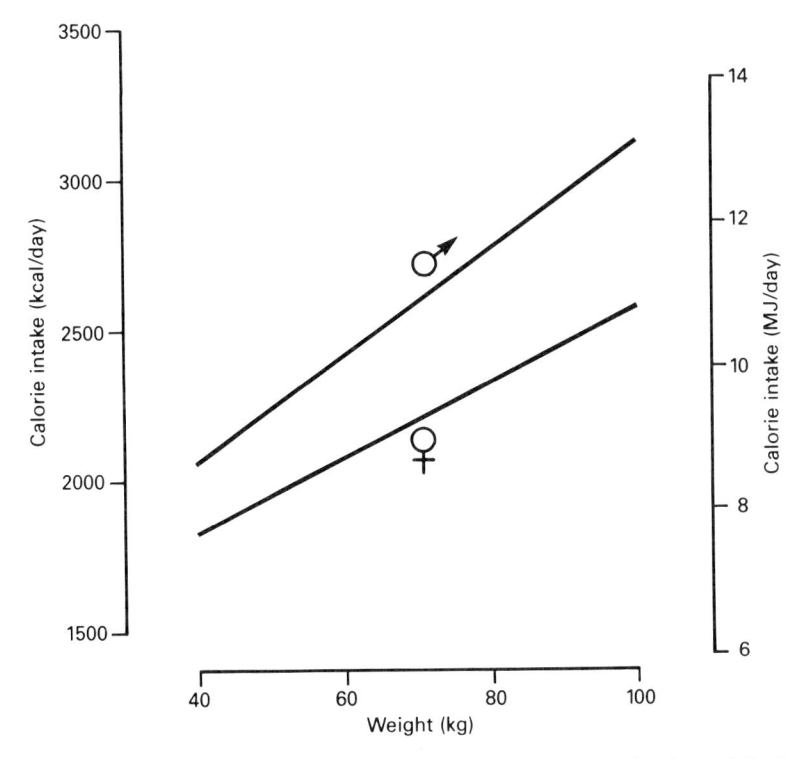

Fig. 4.1 The relationship between energy requirement and body weight in men and women in middle age. This assumes light activity typical of people in industrialized nations; continuous activity through the day increases requirement by about 15%. In people over retirement age calorie requirements tend to fall by around 300 kcal/day.

increases the requirement for insulin delivery from the pancreas, control of calorie intake as well as some forms of carbohydrate intake is desirable (Fig. 4.1). Given that the incidence of major arterial events is considerably higher in the diabetic population than the already high levels in the general population of industrialized nations, it is also sensible to attempt to control the amount and pattern of fat intake. As part of this overall change in the balance of food intake towards the type of healthy diet recommended for the whole population, it then also makes sense to encourage a high fibre intake, and to reduce reliance on artificial sweeteners.

More specific aims will relate to particular patient circumstances. Modification of high alcohol intake will reduce calorie intake considerably, reduce free sugar load if beer is the favoured drink, reduce risks from post-alcohol hypoglycaemia, lessen the progression of pancreatic and liver damage, and control hyperlipidaemia induced by alcoholic hepatitis and poor diabetic control. Adequate carbohydrate intake should be maintained during illness and may help to inhibit the development of ketogenesis, and through hyperglycaemia will result in earlier detection of out-of-control diabetes. In childhood and pregnancy adequate calorie intake must be ensured to support increased physiological requirement. Attention to protein intake may be desirable in patients developing diabetic nephropathy, and certainly in those with established renal failure.

Delivery of Dietary Advice

The role of the dietician

The hospital or community dietician classically has provided most of the dietary instruction delivered to newly diagnosed diabetic patients, and much of the follow-up deemed to be necessary for continuing obesity. Dieticians are unrivalled as sources of detailed dietary information but this is not what is required by the majority of patients.

To be effective the dietician must:

1. Have received instruction in, and be appreciative of, the difficulties and methods of altering dietary behaviour, as well as of imparting dietary knowledge.
2. Be part of the diabetes care team, rather than a separate hospital service to whom 'recalcitrant' patients are referred.
3. Be provided with appropriate information as to the status of the patients with regard to biochemical measures of metabolic control (glycosylated haemoglobin, lipids), changes in drug therapy or insulin treatment, and doctors' and specialist nurses' assessments of patient performance.
4. Be well informed on changing views of the role of dietary management in diabetes.

Patients will then benefit from talking with a dietician in the following circumstances:

1. Newly diagnosed patients should be seen with full referral details, and require assessment (with a report to other members of the team), as well as a course of individually tailored dietary advice.
2. Patients with problems in coming to terms with dietary modification may benefit from counselling at frequent intervals.
3. Annual or biennial review of dietary knowledge is helpful in dealing with changing eating patterns, answering queries arising from information in the lay press, and avoiding atrophy of dietary knowledge.
4. Patients following ethnic diets may not receive adequate follow-up assessment from doctors and specialist nurses, or benefit from group teaching structured for majority populations.
5. Referral is required when the type of ancillary treatment is changed, such as a change in insulin regimen.
6. Where a patient has specific dietary questions or concerns, and in particular requires advice for visiting foreign countries.

Role of the specialist nurse

The diabetes specialist nurse will generally not have had any specific training in giving dietary advice to patients, but should have been instructed in the principles of dietary management of diabetes, and will have the advantage of knowledge of techniques of patient education. Together with a wider knowledge of the individual patient, acquaintance with local dietary habits, and a perception by patients of being on their own level, the diabetes specialist nurse is often in a position to put over ideas that will help with dietary modification in a way that can be more successful than dieticians and doctors. The diabetes specialist nurse will also be able to provide dietary advice in the context of other educational advice given to the patient, such as the response to self-monitoring of diabetes as recorded in patient diaries.

It is possible that, after the initial consultation, dietary advice could be provided more effectively and economically by group teaching and discussion, as organized for other aspects of diabetes education. While it would be the specialist nurse's role to organize and co-ordinate these, the dietician should provide the major dietary educational and material input as a member of the diabetes team.

The doctor

The time available to the diabetes doctor for specific discussion of diet with the patient is often short. Nevertheless it is still usually the doctor who determines the major direction of diabetes management, and as such it is important that doctors should be able to make their own assessments of dietary behaviour, as an important element in making decisions on therapy. Because of a more detailed knowledge of patterns of blood glucose control, it may also be the doctor who can identify specific dietary problems.

Simple Sugars and Sweeteners

Sucrose and glucose

The average consumption of these di- and monosaccharides in developed countries is generally in excess of 1 kg a week. By comparison, primitive societies still following the kind of diet which influenced human biochemical evolution have a negligible intake of these free sugars. Disaccharides are rapidly digested to monosaccharides and these are very rapidly absorbed from the gut. Thus in addition to a major calorie problem, ingestion of simple sugars results in rapid delivery into the circulation of large amounts of glucose. Table 4.1 lists some foods containing clinically significant amounts of free sugars. This is particularly true when sugars are taken in liquid form without food, as in the many higher sugar soft drinks. In people with undiagnosed diabetes it is often the case that the uncontrolled thirst is assuaged with such drinks, leading to marked degrees of hyperglycaemia.

Control of non-insulin-dependent diabetes is therefore often achievable merely by appropriate advice to cease or severely restrict intake of free sugars. It is, however, not self-evident to most people what foods are high in sucrose or glucose. Thus many patients on being told they have diabetes only reduce intake of added sugar and of confectionary, until specific advice is given. Common errors even in educated patients are to assume that natural fruit juices or even the more bitter soft drinks are not high in sucrose.

There is considerable evidence that relatively small amounts of free sugars, when taken with other foods (a moderate portion of preserves on bread, for example), do not cause a large deterioration in blood glucose level, by comparison with the same amounts of the more readily digestible starches.

Table 4.1 Foods containing clinically significant amounts of free sugar

Soft drinks (unless marked 'low calorie')
   Including colas and squashes
Fruit juice
Some alcoholic drinks
   Including beer, liqueurs, some wines
Confectionery
   Including chocolate
Biscuits
Cakes
Sweet tarts and tartlets
Jam and other preserves
Honey
Syrup
   Including fruits canned in syrup

However, the behavioural difficulty of controlling such moderation is not easily solved by many patients.

Free sugars should also be restricted in patients reliant on exogenous insulin. Aside from the excess calorie load, which can often be a problem in people needing snacks between meals, the rate of absorption of these sugars is faster than the rate of absorption of subcutaneously injected unmodified insulin, again resulting in unnecessary post-prandial hyperglycaemia. Glucose-containing tablets, drinks, or other liquids do, however, form the basis of portable means for management of hypoglycaemia.

Fructose and sorbitol

Fructose is present naturally in some fruits and vegetables, where it is of little dietary significance to people with diabetes. Where fructose is used as a sweetener it will have little impact on blood glucose levels acutely, being only converted to glucose intracellularly.

Sorbitol is also a naturally sweet sugar, not easily converted to glucose. As such it is present in many proprietary foods sold as being suitable for people with diabetes. Most of these foods are, however, very high in calorie content and thus not suitable for the majority of Type 2 diabetic patients, while the taste of sorbitol is not acceptable to some patients, and others develop diarrhoea. These foods are also expensive, and in general better avoided.

Consumption of large amounts of fructose or sorbitol is probably not desirable biochemically over long periods of time. If sweet foods must be taken then one of the artificial sweeteners should be recommended.

Artificial sweeteners

The artificial sweeteners have no significant calorific value and cause no problems specific to people with diabetes. They are, however, not without problems; some are unsuitable for cooking, while others are of unacceptable taste to some people.

Use of artificial sweeteners will maintain a patient's 'sweet tooth' when taken regularly, and lead to a failure to detect by taste foods containing sugar. They are therefore better avoided where possible.

Complex Carbohydrates

Complex carbohydrates are conveniently divided into two groups, depending on ease of digestion. Indigestible carbohydrate, better known as dietary fibre or roughage, can itself be further divided into mainly cellulose-containing foods (for example, bran, vegetable fibres), and glutinous fibres (for example, gums, pectins). Digestible carbohydrate consists mainly of starch, and is generally found naturally in association with indigestible carbohydrate in seeds and vegetables (for example, beans, rice, potato). Primitive diets are very high in unrefined carbohydrate, up to 85% of calorie intake, with dietary fibre forming a high proportion of this.

Digestible carbohydrate

Starch is consumed in raw or cooked form in many fruits and vegetables. In general cooked foods are more easily consumed and therefore taken in larger amounts. They are more quickly digested and the glucose is absorbed more quickly into the circulation. Wheat flour starch is incorporated into a wide range of prepared foods (for example, bread, biscuits), although unfortunately in preparation the flour is often mixed with large quantities of undesirable food, such as fat (for example, pastry, cakes) and sugar (for example, biscuits, cakes, puddings). In some cases the method of cooking the starch itself renders it undesirable (for example, potato crisps, potato chips).

It is now recognized that a proportionately high consumption of unrefined carbohydrate is not deleterious to blood glucose control in the insulin-treated patient or the reasonably well controlled non-insulin-treated patient. Furthermore, advice to consume as much complexed carbohydrate as can be tolerated (usually 50–60% of calories) avoids substitution of carbohydrate calories with less desirable fat, and tends to lead to earlier satiation with lower overall calorie consumption. An added advantage of a high carbohydrate diet is that it almost inevitably also increases dietary fibre intake to some degree.

It will be recognized on *a priori* grounds that it is unlikely that starch in the different forms of cereals, bread, vegetables, fruits and pasta will be absorbed from the gut at the same rate, especially after modification by cooking. As people with diabetes are relatively unable to remove absorbed carbohydrate from the blood, and incapable of modifying this by appropriate insulin delivery, total excursion of blood glucose concentrations from baseline will be reduced if absorption of the digested starch is spread over time. Furthermore, the metabolic and hormonal response itself will be modified by other nutrients present in the food, particularly amino acids. Accordingly it has been suggested that it is possible to construct a relative index (the 'glycaemic index') of blood glucose excursions for different foods, thus documenting the quite fast absorption of boiled potato and white bread, slower absorption of more complex cereals, and relatively slow absorption of pasta. However, the reason for the beneficial qualities of pasta remain elusive, but illustrate the problem of the glycaemic index, namely, that it deals with individual foods, while normally dietary intake entails considerable mixing of food types.

For insulin-treated patients it is desirable that carbohydrate intake at different meals remains constant on a day-to-day basis, or for the more sophisticated insulin regimes that the amount of carbohydrate intake is determined by the patient and used to adjust insulin dosage. In order for there to be variety in dietary intake it is then necessary to have a system of equivalents or exchanges. In the United Kingdom this is based on 10 g carbohydrate portions, equivalent to a small slice of bread or a medium-sized apple. It should be noted that this system is not universal, some European carbohydrate units being 25% larger. Dietary carbohydrate prescriptions to match different insulin regimes are discussed below.

Dietary fibre

As discussed above raising carbohydrate intake to the moderate levels normally tolerated (but termed 'high carbohydrate diet') will also raise the intake of indigestible structural carbohydrate to a moderate degree. It is unclear whether raising the intake of these forms of fibre further [by the use of wholemeal flour in cooking, eating the skin of vegetables and fruits where possible, taking high bran foods ('high fibre diet')] will result in improvement in blood glucose control *per se*. However, such measures are likely to be accompanied by changes in attitude to eating which will decrease fat intake and probably total calorie intake. Furthermore, these forms of fibre are probably beneficial to large bowel function, and may improve the serum lipoprotein profile.

The viscous fibres have a much more pronounced effect on the function of the gut, and in smaller quantities have significant effects on blood glucose excursions. Unfortunately the gums are much less pleasant to take with food in any quantity, and when sufficient quantities are taken they are much more likely to lead to abdominal discomfort and flatulence. While to some extent these problems can be overcome by the gradual introduction of prepared products such as guar granules or tablets, none is wholly satisfactory and they do tend to detract from attention to conventional dietary measures.

Dietary Fat

Appropriate advice on dietary fat intake is important to diabetic patients for a number of reasons:

1. Fats contain a disportionately large amount of calories per unit weight, and hence contribute easily to obesity.
2. Fats are easily consumed in quite large quantities with low satiation.
3. Advice to restrict calorie intake in the form of free sugars may result in replacement of calories as fat in combination with starch (as in pastry or biscuits).
4. Even moderately raised lipid levels are associated with significant elevations of cardiovascular risk in the general population, with diabetic patients running two to four times the general risk.

Dietary fat prescription for people with diabetes does not differ from the advice given for healthy eating for the general population. Fat intake in primitive diets is very low, many times lower than the 30% of calories that seems to make food unpalatable in industrialized society. Intake should therefore be restricted to the tolerated level. In general this implies:

1. Avoiding food cooked in added fat.

Table 4.2 Foods containing large amounts of fat

High in saturated fat
Dairy products
Milk and cream
Butter and cheese
Biscuits and cakes
Pastry
Many cooking fats and oils
Chocolate
Some nuts including peanuts
Hard margarines
High in polyunsaturates
Soft margarines
Many vegetable oils
Fish and fish oils
Some meat (e.g. venison)
High in monounsaturates
Olive oil

2. Avoiding high fat foods (pastry, chocolate, some nuts).
3. Avoiding dairy fat products (cream, milk, cheese), and substituting low fat equivalents (skimmed milk, cottage cheese).
4. Using low calorie spreads instead of butter on bread.
5. Avoiding meat products such as sausages and paté.

Table 4.2 lists some foods containing large amounts of fat.

In addition to these measures to control overall fat intake it is desirable to control intake of high cholesterol foods, and those containing high proportions of saturated fatty acids. This will again suggest avoidance of dairy products, nuts and chocolate, but additionally means:

1. Using vegetable oils for salad dressings and the like; these will be high in poly- or monounsaturates.
2. Use of polyunsaturated margarines rather than butter.
3. Eating fish and poultry rather than red meat and pork.
4. Restricting the consumption of egg yolk.

It will be noted that even vegetable-based salad dressings are inappropriate for the overweight in any quantity (but may be necessary for palatability). The same is true for polyunsaturated, low cholesterol margarines.

Dietary Protein

Protein intake is not a problem in diabetes, except insofar as many protein products are associated with undesirable amounts or quality of dietary fat. A high carbohydrate, high fibre diet with some fish and poultry will inevitably be of adequate nutritional quality for all patients.

A true low protein diet may reduce the rate of progression of early or established diabetic nephropathy. At the time of writing this has yet to be established in longitudinal studies.

Alcohol

The problems of high alcohol intake by people with diabetes have been discussed above. Where alcohol must be taken then it is desirable that the calories are subtracted from food intake (on another occasion) in the obese, and that the carbohydrate in beer is counted at half rate in the insulin-treated patient, given that the alcohol is itself hypoglycaemic. Ideally drinking should be restricted to 1 unit (250 ml beer, 1 glass wine, 1 measure spirits) per day.

Patients must be warned that alcohol is potentially hypoglycaemic, and that warning signs may not be noticed under its influence. Alcohol, insulin treatment and driving are a high risk combination.

Oral Hypoglycaemic Agents

Types of Oral Hypoglycaemic Agents

By far the largest group of oral hypoglycaemic drugs in clinical use are the sulphonylureas, the development of which stemmed from the observation of Loubatières of the pancreatic effects of sulphonamide derivatives. Although the earliest drugs of this series (so-called first generation agents) have been in use for some decades now, and although the newer more potent agents (second generation) are now nearing or beyond their patent life, the properties and indications for use of all these drugs are essentially the same, and they can be considered as one group. The second major group of drugs are the biguanides. The hypoglycaemic effect of guanidine was again discovered by serendipity early in the 20th century, but it was too toxic for clinical use. The biguanides were developed later to retain these hypoglycaemic effects without the toxic problems.

More recently other approaches have been made to the problem of lowering blood glucose concentrations in diabetic patients, although none is yet formally established in regular clinical practice (Fig. 4.2 shows the possible sites of action of oral hypoglycaemic agents):

1. The use of lipid lowering drugs (fibrates or nicotinic acid derivatives) is being promoted not only to reduce the risks of accelerated macrovascular disease in diabetic patients, but also to reduce plasma triglyceride and fatty acid concentrations, and thus promote glucose disposal.
2. Drugs which inhibit digestion of starch and sucrose in the gut, namely, the alpha-glucosidase inhibitors. These will slow or even reduce absorption of glucose from the gut, and hence reduce post-prandial hyperglycaemia in people who cannot mount an effective insulin response.

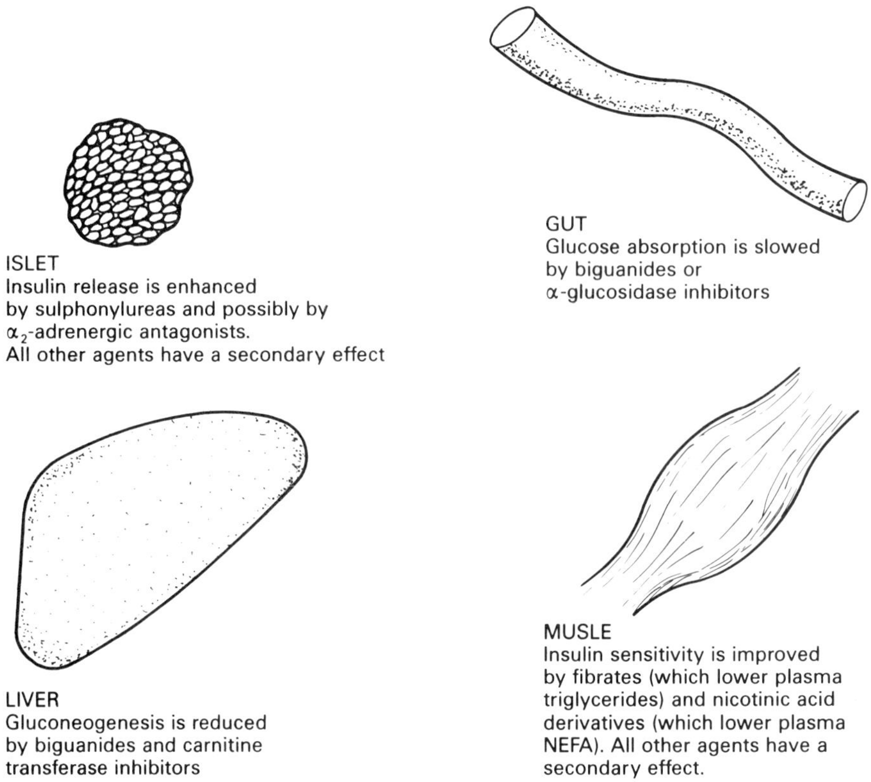

ISLET
Insulin release is enhanced by sulphonylureas and possibly by α_2-adrenergic antagonists. All other agents have a secondary effect

GUT
Glucose absorption is slowed by biguanides or α-glucosidase inhibitors

LIVER
Gluconeogenesis is reduced by biguanides and carnitine transferase inhibitors

MUSLE
Insulin sensitivity is improved by fibrates (which lower plasma triglycerides) and nicotinic acid derivatives (which lower plasma NEFA). All other agents have a secondary effect.

Fig. 4.2 An illustration of the probable sites of action of oral hypoglycaemic agents. Any effective drug that lowers blood glucose levels will improve insulin secretion and insulin action as a secondary effect.

3. It is possible to reduce the rate of hepatic gluconeogenesis with the use of drugs which block fatty acid transfer across the mitochondrial membrane (carnitine palmitoyl transferase inhibitors), thus altering the mitochondrial and cellular metabolite balance. Such agents are as yet experimental, and although sometimes dramatically hypoglycaemic suffer the problem of causing marked increases in plasma non-esterified fatty acid levels. They are not considered further here.
4. Alpha-adrenergic antagonists have been tested for hypoglycaemic effects because of the inhibitory effects of the respective agonists on insulin secretion. It does seem that such agents potentiate insulin secretion, but this can only be demonstrated *in vitro*, and it is therefore unclear what their pharmacological action might be. Again, use of these drugs is as yet experimental, and is not considered further.

Sulphonylureas

Classification of sulphonylureas

A large number of sulphonylurea drugs is now available, and some of the more widely used are listed in Table 4.3. Although the older drugs tend to be less potent, in practice there is a gradation of potency from tolbutamide to glibenclamide (glyburide), with newer and yet more potent agents being tested. Theoretically the less potent agents should carry a greater risk of non-hypoglycaemic-related side-effects (because of the larger drug load), but in practice these only seem to be a problem with the antidiuretic effects of chlorpropamide. There is no evidence for greater efficacy (as opposed to potency) of any one sulphonylurea agent over the others.

A more useful classification of sulphonylureas is by duration of effect (Table 4.3). In this respect, in the commonly used group of agents tolbutamide and glipizide can be regarded as short-acting, with little acute effect beyond 6 h, glibenclamide (glyburide) intermediate-acting with marked effects in the period 3 to 6 h, gliclazide long-acting with effects beyond 12 h, and chlorpropamide very long-acting with effects well into the next day. It should, however, be recognized that these estimates may not be appropriate where routes of metabolism and physiological state of the patient are abnormal, and in particular glibenclamide and chlorpropamide can produce marked hypoglycaemia days after the last administration of the drug in the presence of renal impairment.

Sulphonylureas are used as chronic therapy, and their cost varies considerably. Cheapest, where available off patent, are tolbutamide, chlorpropamide and glibenclamide (glyburide). Non-proprietary preparations of glibenclamide need careful assessment for bioavailability, as the drug is not well absorbed, and formulation can make a difference to rate and extent of absorption.

Table 4.3 A classification of sulphonylurea drugs

	Starting dose mg		Maximum dose mg	
	Doses/day	Amount/dose	Doses/day	Amount/dose
Short-acting				
Tolbutamide	2	500	3	1000
Glipizide	1	5	3	10
Glibenclamide*	1	2.5	2	10
Gliquidone	1	30	3	180
Intermediate-acting				
Gliclazide	1	80	2	160
Long-acting				
Chlorpropamide	1	100	1	350

* The pharmacodynamics of glibenclamide are changed in the presence of renal impairment; it may then behave as a very long-acting agent.

Action of sulphonylureas

Tolbutamide is an effective and fast insulin secretogogue when injected intravenously, or added to cultured islets, and indeed it is the basis of some tests of islet B-cell function. All the sulphonylureas subsequently developed also promote the insulin secretory effect of glucose at the islet B-cell. However, a combination of three factors has cast doubt in some minds on whether potentiation of insulin secretion remains the major clinical effect of these agents in chronic treatment:

1. A good proportion of patients started on sulphonylureas continue to show a decline in islet B-cell function (and deterioration of diabetes) after the first month of therapy. This makes it difficult to demonstrate continuing effects of the drugs on insulin secretion in any study population.
2. Where treatment is successful in the diabetic patient blood glucose levels are of course lower. As blood glucose is itself one of the major determinants of the rate of insulin secretion, it becomes difficult to demonstrate continuing effects of the sulphonylurea without the more sophisticated investigation of raising blood glucose levels acutely with feedback controlled glucose infusion (hyperglycaemic clamp).
3. In any circumstances where diabetes control is improved beyond 2–3 weeks, and whether achieved by dietary management alone, insulin or oral agents, improvement occurs in a number of physiological and biochemical variables. These include, for example, measures of insulin binding to its receptors in target tissues, and measures of the cellular uptake and metabolism of glucose. This has led some researchers to conclude that direct extrapancreatic effects of sulphonylureas are an important part of their clinical action. In all however the evidence is as yet unconvincing.

Problems of sulphonylurea drugs (Table 4.4)

The major problem encountered in effective sulphonylurea therapy is hypoglycaemia. This problem is compounded by low awareness amongst doctors and patients, the similarity of hypoglycaemic symptoms in the elderly to symptoms of other health problems, the lesser frequency of the condition compared to insulin-treated patients, and the duration of action of chlorpropamide [and glibenclamide (glyburide) in the presence of renal impairment].

In the more elderly patient, hypoglycaemia most commonly takes the form

Table 4.4 Problems of sulphonylurea therapy

Hypoglycaemia (common except with tolbutamide)
Fluid retention (chlorpropamide)
Alcohol intolerance (chlorpropamide)
Interactions with protein-bound drugs (including anticoagulants)
Hypersensitivity reactions (rare)
Cholestasis (rare except with tolbutamide)
Blood dyscrasias (rare)

Table 4.5 Risk factors for hypoglycaemia in the elderly patient on sulphonylurea therapy

1. Absence of obesity
2. Incidental diagnosis of diabetes
3. No previous trial of dietary therapy alone
4. Low–normal glycosylated haemoglobin
5. Erratic eating habits
6. Unaccustomed exertion
   (shopping, gardening, moving house)
7. Failure to identify symptoms
   (not educated, mild glycopenic symptoms)
8. Inappropriate timing of therapy
   (not at meal-times)
9. Confusion over multiple therapy
10. Renal impairment

of shaking and disequilibrium occurring late morning or early afternoon after exercise (often only walking to the shops or gardening), and often interpreted as the need to sit down and have something to eat. Direct questioning will often be necessary to elucidate the symptoms, and a glycosylated haemoglobin concentration in the normal range should prompt suspicion. Particularly at risk seem to be the thinner elderly patient in whom diabetes is picked up incidentally, and who is started on drug therapy inappropriately before time has been allowed for dietary instruction to have its complete effect (Table 4.5).

More serious reactions are seen where meals are omitted, perhaps because of illness or surgery, and where the patient is taking a very long-acting preparation, has renal impairment, or where the tablet is incorrectly continued. These patients can suffer severe and prolonged hypoglycaemia, which can be life-threatening if not adequately treated. Management involves frequent blood sampling (hourly), with continuous glucose infusion, and prolonged observation (4 days with chlorpropamide) after stopping the infusion.

Two of the more important problems of sulphonylureas are the fluid-retaining properties of chlorpropamide, and its tendency to cause idiosyncratic reactions after alcohol consumption. Occasional patients, affected by diabetic/ischaemic heart disease, can retain large amounts of water when treated with chlorpropamide, and be diuretic-resistant. A change to a second generation sulphonylurea (glipizide, or glibenclamide which is mildly diuretic) will resolve the problem. A second group of patients find that while taking chlorpropamide they are unable to consume alcohol without marked flushing particularly of the face. Although this is now believed to be related in some way to acetaldehyde production from alcohol, the exact mechanisms are unclear. It is not any longer believed that the phenomenon is related to risk of diabetic complications.

Some concern has been expressed that agents promoting insulin secretion will increase peripheral insulin concentrations, and hence increase any risk from a direct effect of insulin on the arterial wall, as suggested by associations between insulin concentrations and major vessel disease in epidemiological studies. This view received some support from the results of the University Group Diabetes Program (UGDP) study which suggested increased cardiovascular death with tolbutamide therapy. In practice the reduced blood glucose concentrations and improved insulin sensitivity achieved with sulphonylurea therapy generally result in better metabolic control without higher plasma insulin concentrations, while the results of the UGDP study cannot be regarded as experimentally sound enough to influence therapeutic decisions.

Probably all sulphonylurea drugs have a small association with dermatological problems, blood dyscrasias and gastrointestinal side effects, but these are very uncommon.

Choice of sulphonylurea

The choice of sulphonylurea will to some extent be dictated by local circumstances, such as experience with a particular agent, licensing of individual drugs in different countries, and the resources available to pay for them. Although there is a belief by some physicians that chlorpropamide and glibenclamide (glyburide) have a maximum hypoglycaemic effect greater than that of some other agents, in practice changing patients ill-controlled on other tablets to these drugs is without benefit. These two drugs also appear to be the most likely to give symptomatic and serious problems of hypoglycaemia. In the case of glibenclamide (glyburide) this may reflect its very widespread use at unnecessarily high initial dose levels, and the unexplained prolongation of its effects in the presence of renal impairment.

Tolbutamide appears to be relatively safe in these respects, and has the advantage of being cheap. Where its large tablet size and frequent, preprandial dosage are not a problem (the majority of patients), it would appear to be the agent of choice, with glipizide the more potent and easily taken alternative. Glibenclamide (glyburide) has more of a reputation for causing weight gain than either of these agents, although here again this may simply reflect its effectiveness in reducing urinary calorie loss as glucose in conventionally used doses. It has been suggested that gliclazide is superior in minimizing weight gain, but satisfactory comparative data are lacking. Evidence that any of these agents have specific effects on complications or coagulation factors (as distinct from effects as a result of changes in metabolic control) is as yet very weak.

It has been suggested that the longer acting agents have the advantage of promoting basal insulin secretion, rather than post-prandial insulin secretion. This is assumed to be an advantage because of evidence that the defect of insulin secretion in Type 2 diabetes is largely one of basal supply. Careful inspection of this evidence suggests that in reality all insulin responses, prandial as well as basal, are impaired. In practice no clinical advantage has yet been

Oral Hypoglycaemic Agents 107

demonstrated for sulphonylurea regimens either designed to affect mainly prandial glucose responses or mainly basal blood glucose concentrations.

The second generation agent gliquidone is entirely metabolized by the liver, and its degradation products are excreted in the bile. It may therefore be a useful alternative to tolbutamide in patients with marked renal impairment.

Clinical use of sulphonylureas

Sulphonylurea therapy is indicated in the patient with non-insulin-requiring diabetes who is judged to have failed an adequate trial of dietary therapy. In general it is not possible to reach this conclusion in the newly diagnosed patient without a minimum of three months dietary management alone, with at least three clinic visits, and adequate education on diabetes and diet from diabetes specialist nurses and dieticians. It must also be assumed that without adequate self-monitoring (post-prandial urinalysis is often satisfactory in these patients) the patient will not derive appropriate feedback information on their own performance. The commonest error in sulphonylurea therapy is to start treatment unnecessarily early, and convey the impression to the patients that the tablet is the treatment for diabetes, rather than just being ancillary to proper dietary management.

Sulphonylureas are generally not used in pregnancy, to delay insulin therapy in the younger patient, or to achieve rapid improvements in diabetic control for other medical purposes (for example, surgery, infection). Occasionally in the thinner, weight-losing, newly diagnosed patient not consuming large quantities of high sugar drinks, it is justified to move rapidly to maximal doses of sulphonylureas to demonstrate that insulin therapy is really required. This is best achieved if the patients monitor their own blood glucose concentrations.

It is important to stress the continuing role of dietary management when starting these drugs. For longer or medium-acting agents dosage should begin once daily with the lowest clinically effective dose (Table 4.3). The short-acting agents are better started twice daily. Additional tablets are then added in the evening for medium-acting preparations, and before the midday meal for short-acting preparations, before increasing dosage at the original meal-times. Short- and medium-acting agents should be taken 30 min before meals when possible. It is important to remind patients that the evening dose of a twice daily preparation should be taken before the main meal, and not in mid-evening as so often assumed.

Assuming that it is judged that an adequate trial of dietary management has been successfully accomplished, and this may take over a year in some obese patients, then sulphonylureas should be started (in any patient likely to live five years) if glycosylated haemoglobin is judged to be above the risk level for microvascular complications. A sensible recommendation, admittedly based largely on studies in insulin-treated patients, is that HbA_1 should be kept no higher than 4 standard deviations above the normal population mean (the upper limit of the normal 'range' is +2 SD). When glycosylated haemoglobin estimations are not available, keeping the less satisfactory fasting blood glucose concentration below 6.7 mmol/l may suffice. Dosage should therefore be adjusted approximately bimonthly to achieve these aims.

Sulphonylurea therapy will generally have a significant impact on blood glucose control in all but those patients who have absolute insulin deficiency. Thus even patients who continue to abuse calorie intake will respond initially with reduced blood glucose concentrations, and hence reduction in glycosuria. Unfortunately if calorie loss is thus reduced without reduction in calorie intake then weight gain is inevitable until the patient stabilizes at a new level (Fig. 4.1). Contrary to anecdotal opinion improvement in blood glucose control is, however, generally maintained in these patients, and this reduction in risk to future health should far outway any increased problems from a few kilograms of weight gain. Troublesome weight gain may be promoted by some of the more effective short- and medium-acting sulphonylureas, if patients become somewhat hypoglycaemic around lunch-time.

Sulphonylureas can be used successfully in combination with metformin (see below). Their use in combination with insulin therapy in patients retaining endogenous insulin secretion is more controversial, although theoretically attractive, and cannot at present be recommended. Similarly suggestions of their use in off/on therapy alternating with insulin injections over periods of weeks cannot be endorsed as sensible clinical management.

Biguanides

Problems and action of biguanide drugs

A major mechanism of action of phenformin, the first biguanide to be widely used clinically, is the inhibition of hepatic gluconeogenesis. Although the drug was therefore an effective hypoglycaemic agent, a consistent metabolic effect was to raise blood lactate levels, through a failure of the liver to convert endogenous or exogenous lactate into glucose. Although this led to some concern that phenformin worsened other aspects of metabolism while improving blood glucose metabolism, a more serious problem proved to be lactic acidosis in conditions (tissue hypoxia) where lactate production was markedly raised. As lactic acidosis has a very high fatality rate, phenformin has been withdrawn from sale in many countries.

Metformin and buformin are still widely available, reflecting a lesser propensity for causing hyperlactataemia and lactic acidosis. Nevertheless, these remain real clinical problems, and care should be taken not to prescribe these agents in the presence of factors decreasing their plasma clearance, in particular renal impairment, in conditions increasing the risk of tissue hypoxia (for example, ischaemic heart disease, major surgery), or when liver metabolism is already disturbed.

It might be gathered from the decreased risk of lactic acidosis that these latter two agents are less effective as inhibitors of gluconeogenesis. Indeed it is generally believed that their major hypoglycaemic action is not mediated by an effect on the liver. Another possible site of action is to delay and interfere with glucose absorption from the gut. This effect may be the cause of the disorders of intestinal motility reported by a high proportion of patients taking these drugs, and generally manifested as looseness of stool, or frank diarrhoea.

As discussed above all means of treatment which improve blood glucose control can be demonstrated to affect insulin secretion, receptor insulin binding and glucose metabolism after 2–4 weeks of effective treatment. Studies which purport to demonstrate that biguanides act by directly improving these variables in patients should therefore be interpreted with caution. Evidence that biguanides have some specific antilipolytic action at the adipocyte is also very weak.

Clinically, high doses of these agents can make patients feel less well, particularly if there is accompanying gut disturbance, to the extent that some patients become relatively anorexic, and may thus lose weight more easily. Given that such therapy could only possibly be justified in the very short term, and then with patient consent, its clinical role is very limited.

Clinical use of biguanides

Biguanides are effective hypoglycaemic agents when used in adequate dosage, and in patients with only moderately raised glycosylated haemoglobin concentrations they are as effective as sulphonylurea therapy. Since, however, sulphonylureas are widely regarded as being more physiological in their mode of action, and less toxic, biguanides are not generally used as first-line tablet therapy. Biguanides do, however, have a reputation for causing less weight gain than sulphonylureas, and may therefore be the more logical therapy in patients needing psychological support in dealing with obesity. They do, however, appear to be less effective in controlling blood glucose levels and therefore glycosuria in the very poorly controlled patient. Interestingly many of this last group of patients are markedly overweight, with the result that biguanides are generally prescribed for just those patients in whom they are least effective.

A second role for biguanides is as ancillary therapy in patients who have failed to achieve targets of blood glucose control on dietary therapy with sulphonylureas. Again they may be effective when given to patients whose overall control is only 1 to 2% of glycosylated haemoglobin above the upper end of the normal reference range. However, addition of biguanide therapy to sulphonylureas in patients whose control is already very poor will simply impose a further period of unsatisfactory control before the necessary change to insulin therapy is instituted.

It is mandatory to check renal function yearly in patients taking biguanides, and stop their use if plasma creatinine shows signs of rising towards the upper end of its normal reference range. More frequent checks are appropriate in patients at risk of renal impairment. Biguanide therapy should also be stopped a minimum of 3 days, and ideally a whole week, before major surgery.

Other Hypoglycaemic Drugs

Hypolipidaemic agents

Hypertriglyceridaemia is very common in patients with less than adequately controlled diabetes, often in association with hypercholesterolaemia. The management of hyperlipidaemia as such in diabetic patients is discussed in Chapter 5. However, recently attention has turned towards the possibility that reduction in plasma triglyceride or non-esterified fatty acid levels might improve a patient's sensitivity to insulin, and therefore improve blood glucose control. The postulated mechanism would be to reduce availability of non-esterified fatty acids to muscle tissue and the liver, and thereby enhance glycolysis and inhibit gluconeogensis through changes in intracellular metabolites.

The extent to which this treatment is effective in the diabetic population is unclear at present, and although licensed and very widely used in hyperlipidaemia there must remain an element of doubt about the long-term use of fibrate drugs. It also remains unclear whether the nicotinic acid derivatives (for example, acipimox) can reduce non-esterified fatty acid levels for long enough to make a useful contribution to blood glucose control. These approaches to hyperglycaemia should therefore be reserved at present to those patients with hypertriglyceridaemia.

Alpha-glucosidase inhibitors

As discussed above the mechanism of action of these drugs is to inhibit digestion of glucose containing polysaccharides from the gut. Glucose is delivered to the gut in two main forms, namely, the starches and as sucrose, the former undergoing a series of digestive steps before absorption of the free glucose into the blood stream. The term alpha-glucosidases therefore covers a spectrum of enzymes, and to be effective clinically any one inhibitor must block both the starch and sucrose pathways. The most successful candidate in these respects is acarbose, with high activity towards both maltase and sucrase, and relatively low activity against amylases.

Large doses of acarbose very effectively inhibit carbohydrate digestion in the upper gut, and for 2–4 h thereafter while digestion continues in the ileum. Unfortunately undigested carbohydrate passing to the colon is a useful substrate to colonic flora, with resulting abdominal symptoms and possible interference with large bowel function. At present it is unclear that this agent, or any other glucosidase inhibitor, has significant effects on blood glucose control at doses which are tolerated by patients.

Insulin Therapy

Available Insulin Preparations and their Classification (Table 4.6)

The history of insulin therapy since 1923 is echoed by the different ways available insulin preparations can be classified (Table 4.7). The earliest improvements in insulin formulations were the steady decrease in pancreatic

Table 4.6 Classification of available insulin preparations

Short-acting (peak 2–6 h after injection)
1. *Unmodified*
   Synonyms: unmodified, soluble, regular
   Formulation: neutral solution
   Species differences: very little, beef is longer acting than pork or human insulin
   Proprietary names*: Actrapid, Velosulin

Short- and intermediate-acting
1. *Pre-mixes*
   Formulation: neutral solution + suspension, e.g. 30/70 unmodified/NPH
   Species differences: very little
   Proprietary names*: Initard (50/50), Mixtard (30/70), Actraphane (30/70)

Intermediate-acting
1. *Neutral protamine Hagedorn (NPH)*
   Synonym: isophane
   Formulation: neutral suspension
   Species differences: very little
   Proprietary names*: Insulatard, Protaphane
2. *Lente*
   Synonym: insulin–zinc suspension (30/70 amorphous/crystalline)
   Formulation: neutral suspension
   Species differences: marked, human insulin is shortest acting and beef is much longer
   Proprietary names*: Monotard
3. *Ultralente (human species)*
   Synonym: insulin–zinc suspension, crystalline
   Formulation: neutral suspension
   Proprietary names*: Ultratard

Long-acting
1. *Ultralente (bovine)*
   Synonym: insulin–zinc suspension, crystalline
   Formulation: neutral suspension
2. *Protamine–zinc insulin*
   Formulation: neutral suspension
   Species differences: only beef insulin is available

*Proprietary names: Insulin manufacturers sell their products under different names in different areas of the world. It cannot even be assumed that the same proprietary name is not used for an entirely different product in different countries. The names of some products are therefore not given above, while those given are in worldwide use outside N. America.

112 Treatment of Diabetes Mellitus

contaminants in the insulin vial, improvements that had particular momentum in the 1920s and 1970s, but continued throughout the intervening decades. The 1930s and 1940s (to 1951) were periods of development of extended-acting insulin preparations, a field that has subsequently lain fallow until very recently. The 1970s saw greater interest in the species of insulin used clinically in many parts of the world, culminating in the early 1980s with the availability of human sequence insulin. The late 1980s and early 1990s are witnessing the development of analogues of insulin, possibly to become the biggest revolution in therapy since 1921.

Purity of insulin preparations

The major advance in the purification of insulin from extracts of animal pancreas was the discovery in 1922 by Walden in Indianapolis and Shaffer in St Louis of the isoelectric precipitation of insulin at mildly acidic pH. As insulin could be reprecipitated and redissolved more than once, and as contaminant substances not precipitated would be reduced in proportion at each step, this

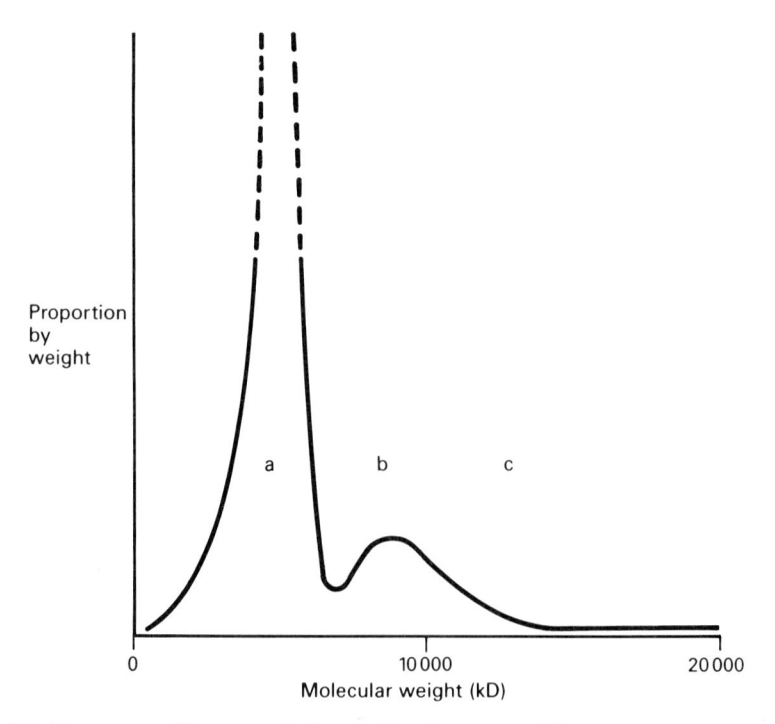

Fig. 4.3 Diagram to illustrate the impurities in recrystallized insulin, according to molecular size. Peak 'a' contains the insulin, but also insulin derivatives such as desamidoinsulin, and other pancreatic peptides (e.g. glucagon). Peak 'b' contains mainly proinsulin, but also proinsulin derivatives (splits), and preproinsulin. Higher molecular weight compounds (peak 'c') are contaminant pancreatic proteins.

Table 4.7 Possible means of classifying insulin formulations

1. Insulin species
   Human, porcine, bovine, analogues
2. Purity
   Recrystallized (conventional), highly purified
3. Duration of effect
   Short-, intermediate-, long-acting
4. Preparation
   Unmodified, neutral protamine Hagedorn (NPH), insulin–zinc suspensions, protamine–zinc

allowed purification of insulin by so-called recrystallization to around 95% purity. This recrystallized insulin was the basis of the bulk of insulin supplies used clinically before the 1970s, and is still sold in the less technologically advanced parts of the world.

After repeated recrystallization most of the higher molecular weight pancreatic proteins are removed, together with a considerable amount of the proinsulin from islet B-cells. Nevertheless, the bulk of the remaining contaminants is proinsulin, accompanied by much smaller amounts of preproinsulin, proinsulin derivatives, insulin derivatives and several other pancreatic peptides. Proinsulin (and preproinsulin), being of higher molecular weight, can be separated from insulin by gel filtration, resulting in the insulin preparations marketed in the 1970s as 'single peak' insulin (Fig. 4.3).

Further purification to remove remaining proinsulin, and other pancreatic hormones, requires the use of ion-exchange chromatography on an industrial scale. By these techniques it is possible to reduce contaminants to effectively undetectable levels, although some insulin derivatives will remain, and indeed may increase in concentration in later parts of the production process and in storage. These insulin preparations were variously known as single component, monocomponent or rarely immunogenic, but they are now more widely known as 'highly purified' preparations.

When insulin production switched to the new technologies (see below), pancreatic contaminants became irrelevant. However, exclusion of contaminants from bacteria or yeast is, if anything, of even greater importance, and all insulin formulations use sophisticated chromatographic techniques to obtain preparations of very high purity.

Extended-acting insulin preparations

After the 1920s extending-acting (intermediate- and long-acting) insulin preparations were developed in response to the perceived desirability of treating diabetic patients with less than the minimum of two to three injections per day needed with unmodified (soluble, regular) insulin.

Protamine zinc insulin, first reported in 1936, achieved considerable popularity as a once daily injection, having a duration of effect well in excess of 24 h. In its conventional form this insulin was highly antigenic, however, with local injection site problems (lipoatrophy) occurring in up to 30% of patients. Even in its more highly purified form its popularity has not continued, perhaps because of rather erratic absorption, and although it is still available it is now used by few patients. In recent years insulin manufacturers have made a number of attempts to improve on the principle of the retarding effect, but consistency of manufacture or erratic subcutaneous absorption have stopped further commercial development.

Isophane or NPH Neutral Protamine Hagedorn insulin is a stable form of the protamine insulin introduced by Hagedorn in 1936. Protamine is a very regular protein with a high content of basic amino acids. When mixed in appropriate conditions in the correct ratio with insulin in the presence of phenol and *m*-cresol stable crystals are formed. The mechanism by which these crystals dissociate after subcutaneous injection is not understood, to the extent that it has been proposed that the process might be enzymatic, or merely physicochemical. Protamine is obtained from fish sperm, and is remarkably non-antigenic because of its smooth sheet-like structure. The duration of effect of isophane (NPH) insulin preparations will depend on dose, but in the doses commonly used in patients a single injection will be enough to prevent blood glucose concentrations rising above normal in the fasted patient for 8 to 12 h. This duration of effect appears to be independent of the species of insulin used in the complex.

Ultralente insulin consists of regular crystals of an insulin–zinc complex. This was part of a series of insulin–zinc suspension preparations introduced by Hallas Møller in 1951, in an attempt to find a commercial alternative to NPH, and produce a preparation without other foreign proteins. Unlike NPH the duration of effect of ultralente is highly dependent on the species of insulin used in the complex, and extends to well over 24 h for the bovine preparation. Human ultralente is again dose dependent for duration of effect, but can only control basal blood glucose levels for up to 10–16 h. Bovine ultralente gave erratic blood glucose control, probably secondary to poor and variable bioavailability from subcutaneous tissue, and has been withdrawn from many markets. Human ultralente, with shorter subcutaneous residence time, is rather better in these respects, although like all other extended-acting preparations its day-to-day absorption does seem to be very erratic.

Lente insulin consists for the most part (70%) of the same insulin–zinc crystals found in ultralente insulin. The other 30% of the insulin–zinc complexes are in the form of an irregular suspension that more easily dissociates on dilution of its zinc supernatant. As, dose-for-dose, lente has less of the slower dissolving complexes, its apparent duration of effect is shorter, and is comparable for the human preparation to isophane preparations. The amorphous component of the complexes should, however, mean that there is a greater hypoglycaemic action than ultralente in the period 2–7 h after injection. As with ultralente, bovine preparations will have a much longer duration of action, and porcine preparations have a slightly, but detectably, longer effect than human preparations.

Semilente insulin consists only of the amorphous insulin–zinc complexes. There is no clinical indication for its use.

Pre-mixed insulin preparations (insulin mixtures) are now almost always combinations of isophane insulin with unmodified insulin. The correct manufacture of isophane insulin involves the precise matching of protamine and insulin ratios to form the isophane crystals, and once this has taken place it is possible to add extra insulin, which then remains in the free state. There is some evidence that loose coupling of the free insulin to the crystals can subsequently occur, but this is believed to be rapidly reversible on dilution. The most popular ratio in clinical use is 30:70, unmodified: isophane, but preparations from 10:90 to 50:50 are also available.

Insulin analogues are presently in clinical trial, but most of these new insulins are short-acting. Insulin analogues are made by substituting base pairs in the DNA of the insulin gene, so that when inserted in yeast an insulin with a novel amino acid sequence is produced. Care has to be taken not to render the molecule inactive, or antigenic, in clinical use. Short-acting analogues are produced by interfering with dimer and hexamer formation, thus enhancing diffusion within subcutaneous tissue, resulting in faster absorption. Long-acting analogues depend on increasing the insolubility of the molecule at tissue pH, thus delaying its residence in subcutaneous tissue. It is not yet possible to discuss the actual benefits or problems associated with the use of these compounds.

Problems of Insulin Therapy (Table 4.8)

Poor metabolic control

The problems of hypoglycaemia and poor metabolic control are discussed in other sections. Insulin absorption and the erratic nature of insulin adsorption are addressed later in this chapter.

Immunological problems

Insulin preparations given subcutaneously are antigenic. At one time it was felt that this was principally a problem of using animal species insulin in humans, despite evidence that when impure human insulin is used experimentally an insulin antibody reaction is elicited. However, most of the antigenicity is probably derived from the proinsulin and derivatives delivered with pancreatic-derived insulin, animal proinsulins being much more chemically divergent than insulin itself, and proinsulin antibodies cross-reactive with insulin. Thus with the improvements in purification technology mentioned above, the antigenicity of insulin preparations decreased considerably. There is no evidence, however, of clinically significant immunological problems where highly purified animal insulin is used from the time of diagnosis.

Interestingly, human insulin is also antigenic when given subcutaneously.

Treatment of Diabetes Mellitus

Table 4.8 Problems of insulin therapy

Poor blood glucose control (including hypoglycaemia)
  Erratic insulin absorption
  Erratic dose measurement or delivery
  Erratic or inappropriate patient lifestyle (diet, exertion)
  Damaged injection sites
  Inappropriate dose distribution

Immunological problems
  Immunological insulin resistance (rare)
  Local (injection site) reactions and lipoatrophy
  Lipodystrophy
  Systemic allergy (rare)

Injection site problems
  Lipohypertrophy, thickening and scarring
  Lipodystrophy
  Local infections

Social problems
  Limitations on flexibility of eating
  Availability of facilities for self-injection
  Concern of parents, colleagues and teachers
  Travelling
  Driving, leisure and jobs
  Insurance

Psychological problems
  Denial of disease
  Injection phobia

Other
  Insulin oedema

Indeed, it requires very large studies to distinguish genetically engineered human insulin from highly purified porcine insulin in this respect. A possible explanation is the antigenicity of the insulin derivatives formed after the synthesis of the insulin, during manufacture and storage. Insulin antibody assays can detect antibodies in around 50% of patients treated with human insulin from diagnosis, but this detection rate is limited by assay sensitivity and the true antibody stimulation rate is probably much higher. Again, however, patients treated with these insulins from diagnosis do not suffer clinically significant immunological problems.

Local (injection site) reactions
Local immunological reactions were common in the early days of insulin therapy when insulin preparations were very impure, but they are now rare. Both immediate and delayed reactions could occur, but they were generally reported to improve with continued treatment. Local reactions to insulin need to be distinguished from irritative phenomena arising from the use of impure spirit to clean injection sites or from substances added to the insulin by

disturbed patients, and chronic injection site infections (see later). Rarely, injection site reactions may be due to the other constituents of the insulin vial (for example, zinc, protamine, *m*-cresol, phenol), and carrier media are available from manufacturers for exclusion testing. Management of milder immunological reactions is by switching to a human insulin preparation, and for more serious reactions by proceeding as for systemic allergy.

Injection site lipoatrophy
This is also very rare with treatment using highly purified porcine or human insulin. With recrystallized bovine insulin it was common, and often of great cosmetic significance. At the active edge of a lipoatrophic area it was possible to demonstrate the presence of insulin–antibody complexes by fluorescent techniques. Management again is by changing to highly purified insulin preparations, but where these are not easily available, it is necessary to inject well away from the atrophic area. Past recommendations to inject into the atrophic area, or into its edge, should be ignored.

Systemic insulin allergy
Allergic reactions are also now rare in developed nations. Classically they were caused by intermittent insulin therapy with recrystallized insulin in the elderly patient with an infection of some kind. Systemic allergy takes the form of acute anaphylactic responses, and can be managed by normal clinical measures. Desensitization can be successful in some cases, and this is one situation where human sequence insulin may have an advantage over porcine insulin. These reactions can occur to highly purified preparations if the patient has previously been exposed to less purified animal preparations, and in parts of the world where supplies of highly purified insulin are limited it makes sense to reserve these for patients treated with insulin for short periods (for example, peri-surgically or due to infected feet or pregnancy).

Immunological insulin resistance
Resistance had become uncommon even before the highly purified insulin preparations were introduced, and it now needs very large numbers of patients to show any relationship between insulin dose and insulin antibody titre. Except when patients have been exposed to recrystallized insulin, other causes of high insulin dosage (for example, adolescence, overtreatment, infection, pregnancy) should demand attention first, but even in those patients without these problems high serum insulin antibody titres are very unlikely. Management is by changing to highly purified insulin preparations.

Injection site lipohypertrophy, disorganization, and scarring

Lipohypertrophy is a local metabolic response to injected insulin. It is found to be common, when actively sought. Even in patients without evident subcutaneous fat hypertrophy, ultrasonography of injection sites will often reveal

118   Treatment of Diabetes Mellitus

increased thickness, with areas of fat interleaved between disorganized fascial planes and scar tissue. The phenomenon is of clinical significance since insulin absorption is significantly disturbed from these sites when compared to a standard subcutaneous injection. At present, however, it remains unclear whether this is just alteration of the rate of absorption and hence duration of action, or whether, as is likely, erratic and unpredictable absorption occurs, possibly with loss of bioavailability.

Lipohypertrophic and thickened injection sites should be actively sought at least yearly in all patients. When present advice should be given to inject over a wide area within any one site, and to avoid the affected area. The cosmetic results of lipohypertrophy can be socially disastrous for those desiring holidays in the sun.

Insulin oedema

Insulin oedema is an ill understood phenomenon. It is usually seen in patients who have newly started on insulin therapy. The patients are often in some form of continuing physiological disturbance in addition, perhaps as a result of a chronic slow onset of their diabetes, or as a result of pregnancy. In high concentrations, above those found physiologically after meals, insulin can be shown to have effects on cellular ion transport, and perhaps on renal glomerular haemodynamics, but the exact relevance of these to the observed generalized tissue oedema is unclear. Management is by reviewing whether other factors which exacerbate fluid retention are present, reducing insulin dosage where possible, and awaiting resolution of the problem.

Injection site infections

Injection site infections are rare, perhaps rarer than might be expected on *a priori* grounds. A probable reason for this is the high content of preservatives needed to ensure sterility of reusable vials containing protein. The most commonly used preservatives in insulin vials are now phenol and *m*-cresol (or both), and it is these that account for the characteristic odour of insulin formulations. Injection of quite large innoculates of bacteria into an insulin vial results in their quite rapid death. Injection site infection therefore suggests very poor hygiene, either of injection sites or syringes/needles, or of tampering with the contents of the insulin vial.

A variety of organisms have been reported as involved in injection site infections, including the common skin pathogens. Other reports are of various *Mycobacteria* species and unusual *Streptococci* species.

Social and psychological problems

Some of the social problems of insulin injection therapy are given in Table 4.8. Many of these relate to hypoglycaemia, but frequent problems are encountered over employment, schooling and travelling (Chapter 3). It can be very helpful for professionals to counsel teachers and factory sick room staff about the needs of people on insulin injections, even if just to find a suitable venue for giving midday injections. Travelling and insurance (as well as driving) can be particular burdens to the diabetic patient if not adequately discussed. Useful advice is available from patient associations.

Insulin therapy poses particular problems for the parents of diabetic children, often to a greater degree than to the child itself. Particular attention needs to be given to ensuring that parent–child relationships develop appropriately during adolescence, by encouraging transfer of responsibility for diabetes to the child, and giving help in arranging periods of independence, for example, at diabetes camps.

True psychological problems (for example, denial of disease, injection phobia) are fortunately rarely severe enough to place health at risk acutely, although they can be worth seeking out where control is unexplainedly erratic. Nevertheless, management of these problems is often disappointing.

Subcutaneous Absorption of Insulin

Insulin was never intended by evolution to be delivered subcutaneously, being secreted physiologically into the portal vein. Subcutaneous delivery has certain consequences which alter the pharmacodynamics of the substance when compared to portal intravenous delivery, and which have important consequences for insulin injection therapy. Possible effects and problems of depot injections might be expected to include:

1. Alteration of the time course of effect of a substance.
2. Effects on bioavailability.
3. Effects on (1) and (2) of changes in local conditions, such as blood flow.
4. The consequences of absorption into the peripheral circulation rather than the portal vein.
5. Local metabolic effects of subcutaneously injected insulin which seem to be limited to the lipohypertrophy discussed above.

Time course of subcutaneous absorption of insulin

After subcutaneous injection of unmodified (soluble, regular) insulin there is a delay of around 10 min before insulin becomes detectable in the circulation. This presumably corresponds to the time required for those insulin molecules adjacent to blood capillaries to diffuse across the endothelial barrier.

Plasma levels then rise to peak concentrations at around 60–120 min from injection, a rise which may be compared to the physiological peak occurring some 30–45 min after beginning a meal (Fig. 4.4). There are two determinants of this rate of rise. Firstly, plasma concentrations partly reflect the time needed to fill the body insulin distribution space to a higher concentration. This process

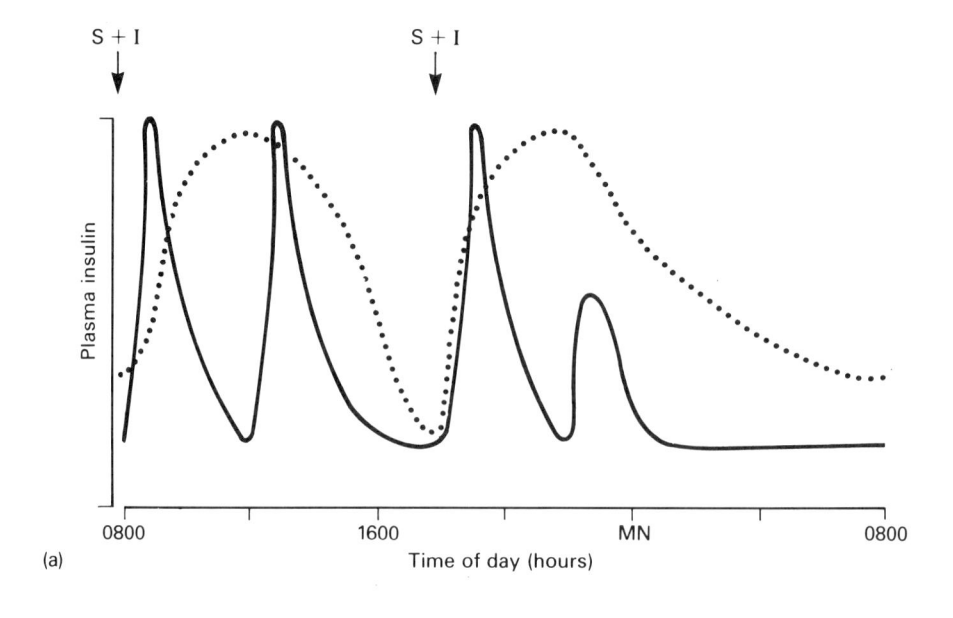

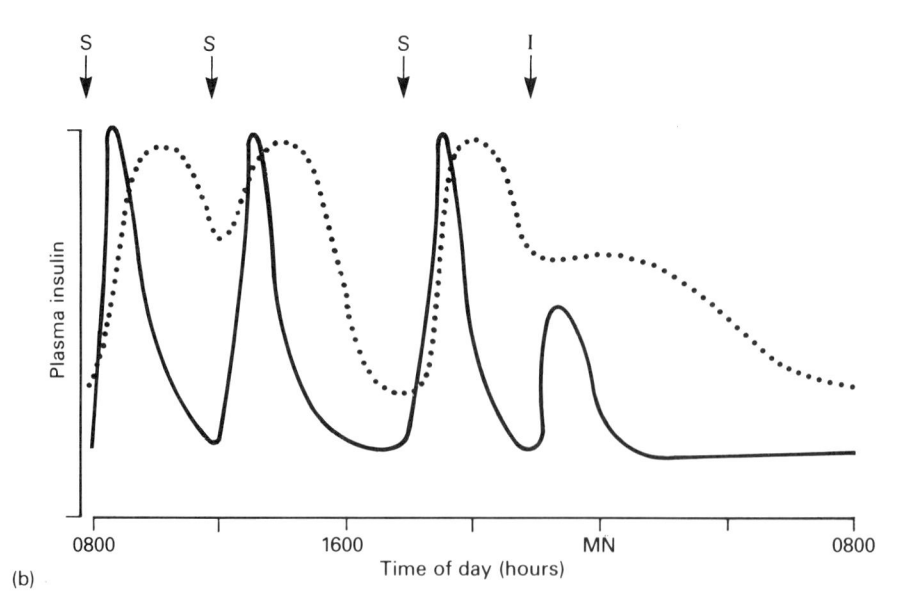

Fig. 4.4 Profile of plasma insulin concentrations in normal subjects (———) given three major meals a day, and in diabetic patients (-----) treated (a) with twice daily injections (↓) of short- (S) + intermediate-acting (I) insulin, or (b) with short-acting insulin before meals and intermediate-acting insulin before going to bed. Note that insulin concentrations are always slow to rise after meals, and remain very high in the post-prandial period and in the early part of the night. Although insulin concentrations appear high at the end of the night, tissue insulin insensitivity results in blood glucose levels that are actually rising rapidly. MN, midnight.

would take about fives times (25 min) the plasma half disappearance time (5 min) if all the insulin in the injection depot were immediately available for absorption across the endothelial barrier. The extra delay beyond 25 min is believed to be caused by the necessity for insulin to diffuse within the tissue before becoming available for capillary absorption, and will be lengthened by the presence of insulin in the higher molecular weight hexameric form in the high concentrations of the subcutaneous depot. A major influence on absorption will therefore be available capillary density, namely, the number and proportion of subcutaneous capillaries carrying blood at the time. A further consequence is that any disruption by scarring of subcutaneous tissue will lead to further delays in the time to peak absorption rate, and evidence suggests that the time to peak concentration (taken from studies of subcutaneous injection in normal subjects) is significantly longer again in insulin-treated patients.

Subsequent to the peak concentration, plasma insulin levels fall with a half time of around 50–60 min, but again this may be slower in insulin-treated patients. The consequence is that insulin concentration remains very high in the period 3–5 h after injection, when compared to the rapid fall in concentration which has occurred by the end of the second hour in the physiological response (Fig. 4.4). As a result, and allowing for the slow switch on and switch off of the peripheral effect of insulin, significant effects of insulin will continue in skeletal muscle for at least 6 h after subcutaneous injection, and will have effects above basal on the liver for perhaps nearly as long, even under ideal conditions.

Absorption of extended-acting insulin preparations will be further delayed by the rate of dissolution of the complex, as discussed above in the section on insulin preparations. Once dissociated from the complex, however, the free insulin pool is subjected to the same influences as a subcutaneous depot of unmodified insulin.

Factors altering the rate of absorption

It will be understood from the above section that any factor reducing the diffusion path of insulin, or speeding that diffusion, will change the absorption rate. Thus, aiding the dispersion of insulin within subcutaneous tissue will shorten the time to peak concentration by making insulin available to a greater capillary surface area, something that can be achieved by injection site massage or by the use of an injection gun. Other experimental approaches have included the use of a sprinkler needle to disperse the insulin further at the time of injection itself. Dispersion will also be faster for the monomeric insulin analogues.

Increasing the rate of blood flow in subcutaneous tissue will increase both the surface area available for absorption, and decrease the diffusion distance from the depot. Thus warming and cooling the injection site can have dramatic effects on the absorption of unmodified insulin. Similarly exercise will enhance absorption through increased subcutaneous blood flow, as well as by massaging the injection site particularly if this is over the thigh.

It has been unclear whether those factors which alter the rate of absorption of unmodified insulin might also influence absorption of the extended acting preparations, except insofar as they will inevitably affect the insulin already released from the insulin complex but not yet absorbed into the circulation. More recently studies in which injection site characteristics have been altered for longer periods of time do confirm that dissolution of the complexes can be altered by skin temperature and exercise, although the role of blood flow is as yet unclear.

It is possible that it is variations in capillary density which account for the differences in insulin absorption rates between injection sites. It is well recognized that use of the subcutaneous tissue of the abdominal wall results in faster (and therefore more physiological) absorption of unmodified insulin than from the thigh, with the arm being an intermediate site. The consequence is that rotation of injection sites at random will result in more erratic blood glucose control. An ideal choice is the abdominal wall in the morning (when fast absorption is needed to overcome fasting hyperglycaemia), and the thigh in the evening (to extend insulin action to the next morning).

Design and Use of Subcutaneous Insulin Regimens

Multiple injection regimens

The ideal insulin regimen would deliver insulin into the circulation at the same rate as would occur physiologically. Since physiological insulin secretion is regulated on a minute-to-minute basis, and since the events which affect insulin requirement (principally food intake and exercise) are difficult to predict accurately in advance both in timing and degree, this will be difficult to approximate until continuous glucose sensing becomes available. The alternative is to give insulin injections frequently during the day when most changes in requirement occur, and to cover basal night-time requirements with a single injection before bed.

Examination of the physiological insulin profile (Fig. 4.4) reveals that insulin delivery rises and falls rapidly with each meal, and is very constant overnight. As discussed in the section on insulin absorption (above) neither of these requirements can be met by injection of available insulin preparations, even if it were the case that requirements could always be predicted up to the time of the next injection. Nevertheless, injection of unmodified insulin before each main meal will come as close as currently possible to imitating physiological insulin delivery, particularly if the injection is given 30 min before the meal, thus partially compensating for the slow rise in plasma insulin concentrations after injection.

Such a multiple injection regimen has other consequences (Fig. 4.4). When the interval between injections does not exceed 6 h the slow absorption of the so-called short-acting preparations will cover basal requirements in the post-absorptive phase when digestion is complete. Indeed insulin concentrations remain relatively high, and hence post-prandial snacks are required in the well-controlled patient to avoid hypoglycaemia. Because each injection is given before a meal it is generally easy for patients to adjust the unit dosage if they feel that food intake will differ from usual. At lunch-time, for example, a 50% reduction in food intake appears to require a 50% reduction in dose, although individuals can experiment for themselves with the aid of self-monitoring of blood glucose. When a normal dose of insulin has been taken at the meal beforehand it is also possible to take the next meal later than normal, but patients taking larger doses of insulin may find they need an extra snack to tide them over if hypoglycaemia is to be avoided. It is similarly relatively easy to deal with predictable periods of severe exercise (see below).

Basal insulin supply during the night is then probably best given as human ultralente insulin before going to bed, although the advantage over isophane (NPH) used at this time is not proven. Both these preparations are erratically absorbed, and if occasional night-time hypoglycaemia is to be avoided it will be necessary to settle for much less than perfect pre-breakfast blood glucose concentrations.

Physiologically about 50% of total insulin secretion is required for control of basal metabolism. In patients, as discussed above, meal-time insulin injections will provide some of this requirement. Nevertheless, experience suggests that the basal night-time injection needs to be around 50% of total daily dose, if reasonable fasting blood glucose control is to be achieved. The meal-time dose distribution will depend on relative carbohydrate and calorie contents, any hang-over of insulin absorption when the interval between meals is under 6 h, and the blood glucose concentration immediately before each meal. In the authors' own practice, with a moderate breakfast, working lunch and main evening meal, the distribution is often then around 2:1:2.

Meal-time insulin injections of unmodified insulin are best given by a pen-injector, combining the roles of cartridge and syringe in a device with excellent portability. Such devices are not suitable for ultralente preparations, which must be given by conventional syringe (see below).

Twice and thrice daily injection regimens

Twice daily injection regimes are still very widely used. Their major advantage is that two injections per day are the minimum needed if the extended-acting insulin preparation is to have any hope of controlling blood glucose concentrations overnight without causing problems during the day (Fig. 4.4). Twice daily regimens are therefore based on giving mixtures of unmodified (soluble, regular) and either isophane (NPH) or lente insulin, both before breakfast and before the main evening meal. Theoretically lente insulin should have a rather longer duration of effect, and therefore give better fasting blood glucose control, but may complex the unmodified insulin when mixed with it in the syringe. However, in large-scale clinical trials regimens based on lente and isophane preparations cannot be distinguished at any time of day. It is also possible to use human ultralente in this role, and although theoretically this should give less adequate insulin delivery at lunch-time, in clinical practice the effect is not detectable.

Unlike multiple injection regimens (see above) the morning extended-acting preparation must make a significant contribution to insulin delivery from lunch-time through the afternoon. This may give less satisfactory blood glucose control in some patients, but is not detectable in the whole population, who therefore have very similar glycosylated haemoglobin concentrations on the two types of regimen. Delivery of both morning and afternoon insulin in one injection does, however, make the regimen much less flexible, particularly in terms of midday meal carbohydrate intake, afternoon exercise, and in the timing of the evening meal. Additionally it is much less easy for patients (and doctors) to understand the relationship between lunch-time or afternoon blood glucose levels and the components of the morning insulin dose, thus reducing the potential for self-adjustment of doses.

Experience would suggest that initially one-third unmodified to two-thirds extended-acting insulin should be a reasonable ratio of doses in the easily regulated patient, with approximately equal split of dosage between morning and evening. However, self-monitoring of blood glucose should lead to modification of these ratios, for a number of reasons.

1. Distribution of carbohydrate intake will vary between patients. A very small breakfast may sometimes require omission of the morning unmodified insulin, for example.
2. Regular exercise at a particular time of day will alter insulin requirements.
3. Diurnal variations in insulin sensitivity can have a dramatic impact on morning/afternoon versus evening/night insulin requirement.
4. Failure to control fasting blood glucose levels (through night hypoglycaemia after increasing evening extended-acting dosage), can necessitate corrective increases in morning unmodified insulin dosage.

This last problem is the major cause of hyperglycaemia in the insulin-dependent population, with over 80% of patients having their highest average blood glucose concentrations of the day before or immediately after breakfast. The problem is emphasized by the observation that asymptomatic night-time hypoglycaemia occurs in a very high percentage of patients on these regimens, and is nearly universal in patients who go to bed with glucose concentrations below 7.0 mmol/l. A sensible approach to the problem is to increase evening doses of the extended-acting insulin slowly, but only in those patients without a history of recent night-time hypoglycaemia, and with monitoring of 0300 h blood glucose levels where possible. Bed-time blood glucose concentrations below 7.0 mmol/l should be an indication for extra carbohydrate. Where these measures fail then consideration should be given to moving the injection of the extended-acting preparation to bed-time (thrice daily injections), which can be done without change in doses.

Absolute dosage requirement will also vary enormously between patients. In general a useful starting dose in the hyperglycaemic but well patient will be 12 U morning and evening, but care must be exercised in the unduly thin patient, those with a history of pancreatic disease, and patients with renal impairment or adrenal insufficiency. Patients recovering from ketoacidosis, toxic from infection, stressed by critical illness or grossly obese, may require much higher doses.

Interprandial snacks are needed on twice daily injection regimens, particularly in the morning if a high corrective dosage of unmodified insulin is combined with the normal dose of an extended-acting preparation. However, blood glucose monitoring may suggest, contrary to established opinion, that afternoon snacks are not necessary, or are even unnecessarily hyperglycaemic, in some less active patients.

Twice daily injection regimens are usually given by syringe injection. Where 100 U/ml insulin is used, and provided the injection is given immediately after drawing up into the syringe, the insulin formulations may be mixed in the syringe, even when using lente preparations. It is recommended, however, that unmodified preparations are drawn up before complexed preparations, to avoid the risk of contaminating the unmodified insulin vial with the contents of the other vials. Insulin should be given from the smallest syringe that will hold the dose to be given, as dose markings are more widely separated on such syringes, thus improving precision in drawing up the doses. Plastic disposable syringes may be reused while the needle stays sharp, provided the needle cap is replaced after excess insulin is expelled. Alcohol swabbing of injection sites is unnecessary, but rules of simple hygiene should be observed.

Adjusting Insulin Doses

Adjustment of insulin dosage is as much an art as a science, if only because a number of important factors relevant to the determination of doses (for example, sensitivity of different organs to insulin, degree of variability of absorption, variations in behaviour) often remain unknown and inaccessible. Certain principles should, however, be borne in mind when adjusting doses:

1. The nature of subcutaneous insulin absorption precludes achievement of physiological insulin delivery. Perfect control of immediate post-prandial hyperglycaemia will, for example, inevitably cause hypoglycaemia later.
2. Adjustment of dietary content and timing may be more appropriate than adjustment of insulin dosage.
3. Hypoglycaemia is tolerated to varying degrees by different patients. The aim of insulin therapy may be said to be to obtain the best possible blood glucose control, but this aim will usually be compromised by hypoglycaemic events. The frequency and severity of such hypoglycaemia, and the degree to which it is tolerated by individual patients are therefore major determinants of the levels of blood glucose control which can be achieved.
4. As insulin absorption is seldom consistent on a day-to-day basis, and as patient behaviour is also erratic, it is only by averaging several days results

126 Treatment of Diabetes Mellitus

that changes in blood glucose control may become apparent. Insulin dosage changes should be around 10% or more of current dosage, if psychologically acceptable to the patient.

5. Duration of effect of an insulin preparation is proportional to dose. Thus a high morning dose of isophane (NPH) (say 18 U) can be contributing as much insulin throughout the next night as a lower evening dose (8 U). Similarly a high morning dose of unmodified (soluble, regular) insulin will act through much of the afternoon.

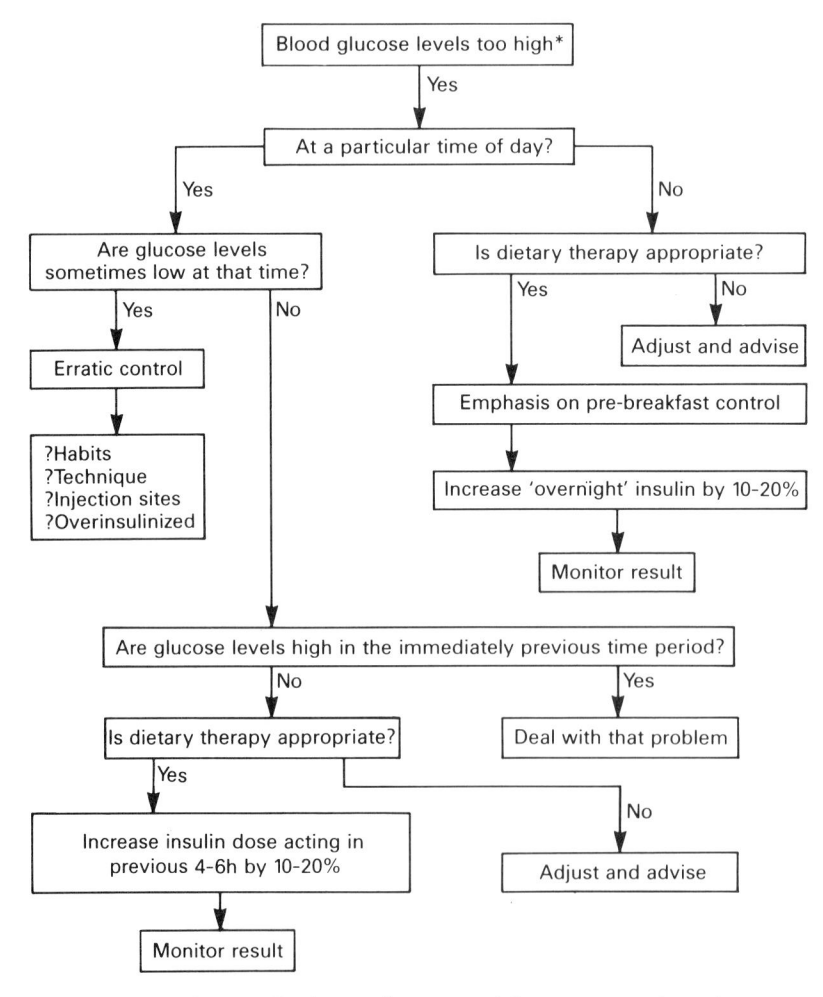

Fig. 4.5 Algorithm for insulin dose adjustment. It is an assumption of the application of such an algorithm that blood glucose control is in a steady-state, that blood glucose concentration data is available from a series of different days, and that the blood glucose self-test results are known to be reliable. Although set out for dealing with high blood glucose levels, the algorithm can be applied with suitable substitutions to low blood levels.

6. However, when the insulin dose distribution is balanced, it is generally possible to attribute blood glucose control at the end of any 4–8 h period as resulting from the effects of a particular component of the insulin regimen. In this way it can be determined which insulin dose needs adjusting.
7. An exception to point 6 is when blood glucose on entry to any period of time is grossly abnormal. High blood glucose concentrations at lunch-time may simply reflect high blood glucose concentrations before breakfast (rather than an inadequate morning unmodified insulin dose), and thus demand adjustment of the evening extended-acting insulin preparation.
8. Regular changes in life-style (resting or active weekends, weekly sport, shift work) demand a separate insulin dose distribution.

From these principles follows the adjustment algorithm given in Fig. 4.5. It should be emphasized that no amount of adjustment of insulin dose will help if the blood glucose monitoring results are unreliable, insulin doses are not given precisely, or variations in food intake and timing are erratic.

Hypoglycaemia

This section deals with hypoglycaemia induced by insulin injections. Hypoglycaemia from other causes is dealt with in Chapter 6.

Hypoglycaemia is a frequent problem in insulin-treated diabetes, particularly in those patients without endogenous insulin secretion in whom it is almost inevitable if tight blood glucose control is attempted. The frequency of patient-detected hypoglycaemia is around three episodes per patient month, but in any one month half the patients may not have a reaction, while others may sense and deal with as many as 30 episodes. For many patients, but by no means all, hypoglycaemia is an unpleasant experience and to be avoided if at all possible, while night-time hypoglycaemia is often a subject of fear. It is important for medical personnel to recognize the importance of the significance and timing of hypoglycaemic events to any individual patient, rather than just recording the frequency.

Hypoglycaemia is usually recognized by the classical symptoms and signs of sympathoadrenal activity and/or neuroglycopenia. Either may predominate in individuals. In elderly patients the symptoms may be rather different, perhaps just of unsteadiness or hunger, and may require differentiation from other cardiovascular or neurological disturbance. Timing of the events, relationship to exertion, and response to food may be useful indicators. Where patients are doubtful about whether they are hypoglycaemic then a self-blood glucose test is very helpful, but it may be wise to do this only after taking extra carbohydrate. Blood tests at the time may also be useful in relation to night-time symptoms such as sweats, or when waking with recurrent headache. Hypoglycaemia does occasionally present as epilepsy, and where the EEG is abnormal the fits will often respond to anti-epileptic therapy if they persist despite adjustments to insulin therapy.

Insulin-induced hypoglycaemia occurs when plasma insulin concentrations remain abnormally elevated for long enough to reduce the prevailing blood glucose concentrations to below normal. Given the nature of insulin absorption this is particularly likely to be the case 3–5 h after injection of unmodified (soluble, regular) insulin, and in the early hours of the night (see above). Blood glucose concentrations will fall when hepatic glucose production remains suppressed by insulin at a time when glucose delivery from the gut has ceased. The additional peripheral action of insulin on glucose disposal in muscle is of much less significance. Many factors will enhance hypoglycaemia:

1. Stimulation of non-insulin-dependent glucose disposal by exercise. Vigorous exercise may promote this for many hours afterwards.
2. Delaying or missing meals or snacks.
3. Alcohol, through inhibition of hepatic gluconeogenesis.
4. Excessive insulin dosage.
5. The failure of the counter-regulatory hormone response to hypoglycaemia, which occurs commonly after 5–10 years of diabetes, and leads to failure of the normal warning symptoms.
6. Autonomic neuropathy, pancreatic disease, adrenocortical insufficiency, liver failure.

Frequent hypoglycaemia will call for review of insulin dosage, food and exercise habits, and lifestyle. It will then be managed simply as an important contribution to blood glucose records.

Hypoglycaemia needing physician/hospital intervention is clearly of more importance, and occurs at a rate of 0.1–0.2 events per patient year in the insulin-treated population. When spasmodic it can nearly always be related to one of the exacerbating factors listed above, and to failure to detect warning symptoms. A single event may therefore require appropriate counselling, rather than insulin dose adjustment.

Asymptomatic (biochemical) hypoglycaemia is more common in well-controlled patients than symptomatic hypoglycaemia. The definition of hypoglycaemia in these circumstances is not generally agreed, but cerebral performance can be shown to deteriorate below a blood glucose concentration of 3.0 mmol/l. Curiously many insulin-treated patients appear to function normally well below these levels, although in part this observation may reflect a failure to test them formally. It is normal practice to ignore isolated blood glucose records down to 2.0 mmol/l where symptomatic hypoglycaemia is not a problem, but consistent results of this order are associated with a high likelihood of hypoglycaemic coma. More worrying are unrecognized periods of prolonged and recurrent asymptomatic hypoglycaemia at night, very common in patients with normal bed-time blood glucose concentrations, or pre-breakfast levels below 7.0 mmol/l. At present, however, there is no evidence of long-term damage from these problems, most clinicians relying on anecdotes about intellectually active patients who have remained mentally sharp throughout a lifetime of recurrent hypoglycaemia.

Death from hypoglycaemia does occur, and is well recognized in association with alcohol abuse and suicide. Whether death from hypoglycaemia occurs in other circumstances has proved very difficult to ascertain, there being no reliable measurement of plasma post-mortem glucose concentrations. Vitreous glucose concentrations are now known to be unreliable. Sudden death in insulin-treated patients does occur, but its relative frequency in relation to non-diabetic deaths is not known, and there is no evidence of a connection with any known factor related to diabetes or insulin treatment.

Exercise

Exercise is probably beneficial to people with diabetes, in improving insulin sensitivity, and is regarded as an important part of life by many people, particularly the young. Unfortunately exercise does give rise to problems of blood glucose control in any patient taking insulin who is adequately controlled. Physiologically the response to exercise includes a massive increase in non-insulin-dependent glucose disposal to muscle, with a marked drop in insulin secretion, and thus an increase in hepatic glucose production to maintain blood glucose concentrations. The diabetic patient suffers a double disadvantage in that subcutaneous insulin has already been given, and delivery into the circulation cannot therefore be reduced, while exercise itself will often increase subcutaneous blood flow and massage the injection site, thus actually increasing plasma insulin concentrations. At a time therefore when glucose requirements are markedly increased, hepatic glucose production falls, and blood glucose concentrations plummet.

When injections are given twice daily, modification of insulin dosage in anticipation of exercise will often result in hyperglycaemia at other times. In practice therefore exercise of short duration is better managed by quickly absorbed carbohydrate given beforehand, the amount (15–50 g) being determined by duration and intensity of exercise, and adjusted by response as monitored by blood glucose concentrations. For longer periods of exercise, or very vigorous exercise, it may be appropriate to adjust insulin dosage in anticipation. This adjustment may be as little as 10% off for light gardening, to 50% down for a day's fell walking. Sports where some risk is involved may demand further reductions for the sake of safety.

Exercise may be associated with late hypoglycaemia (even next day), apparently due to changes in insulin sensitivity.

Adjustment of Insulin Dose during Illness

Insulin dose requirements are very variable during illness, changing very little in some patients, while doubling with minor illness in others. Insulin requirements never fall during illness, and mistaken reduction in dosage is a common cause of ketoacidosis. Carbohydrate intake must be maintained at all times as this helps control ketonaemia, and as a rising blood glucose concentration is a useful signal that diabetes is no longer adequately controlled. Patients unable to maintain carbohydrate intake need medical assistance.

Increased insulin requirement during illness is caused by the increased output of the stress hormones, all of which have adverse effects on glucose metabolism. Patients may need to increase insulin dosage in steps as great as 20% per injection, until blood glucose concentrations begin to come under control, insulin doses have doubled without effect (when medical assistance is required), or vomiting or ketonuria intervene. Clearly these measures require adequate patient education, and competent and frequent blood glucose monitoring. Unfortunately it is during illness that many patients find it most difficult to bring themselves to do frequent self-testing, with the result that insulin dosage is often not increased fast enough.

Many patients fear hypoglycaemia when their insulin doses have been increased, even if blood glucose estimation shows this not to be of concern. Usually then doses are dropped rapidly at the first sign of requirements decreasing again, but prior advice should be given that reductions in steps of up to 20% per injection may be needed, once the original stress has been removed.

Socio-legal Consequences of Insulin Therapy

The risk of hypoglycaemia, however remote in any individual, should impose certain restrictions on any patients taking insulin. Some of these, including legal restrictions on holding various forms of transport licences, cannot be challenged. Additionally it makes sense for insulin-treated patients to avoid some hazardous occupations dependent on continuous self-reliance, such as scaffold work, deep sea diving, or the armed forces. While many patients do continue in potentially hazardous jobs, it is necessary to assess and advise such patients continually on their suitability for their posts. There is evidence that people with insulin-treated diabetes do not have worse work attendance records than the general population, but when they are off work it tends to be for longer periods.

Appropriate advice must also be given to patients who wish to engage in dangerous sports, such a scuba-diving, hang-gliding and rock climbing. In many cases national and local clubs will have rules excluding insulin-treated patients from active membership.

In many countries patients taking insulin will be required to obtain medical reports if they are to continue to hold licences to drive light motor vehicles. This should not be a problem unless hypoglycaemia is unpredictable or very frequent. Insurance companies will often charge extra premiums for insulin-treated patients (based on risk experience) who wish to drive.

Other Ways of Giving Insulin

Insulin infusion pumps

Insulin may be delivered subcutaneously from portable insulin infusion pumps, worn 24 h a day (Fig. 4.6). These pumps use only unmodified (soluble, regular)

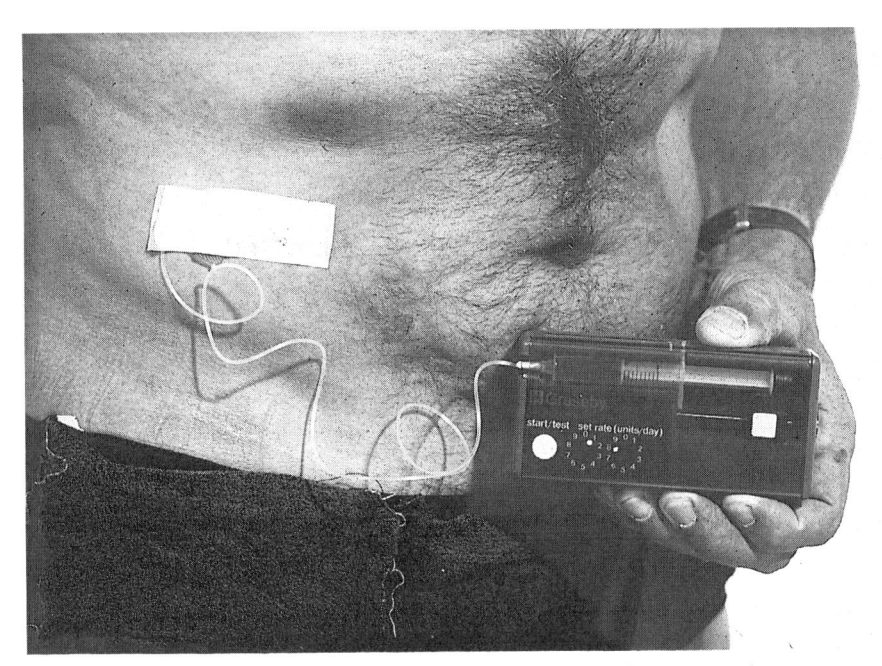

Fig. 4.6 Continuous subcutaneous insulin infusion. The pump is worn permanently, normally on a belt or in a shoulder pouch, and delivers insulin throughout the day and night via the plastic cannula to a needle placed subcutaneously. The buttons and dials on the pump allow adjustment of basal delivery rate, and delivery of meal-time boluses.

insulin, with delivery divided into a basal rate and a facility for supplementary bolus delivery before the main meals. In this sense pump therapy approximates to multiple injection therapy, with the major difference being that overnight insulin delivery is provided by infusion. Theoretically this should give more physiological night-time plasma insulin concentrations and hence better blood glucose control.

In regular clinical practice overall glycosylated haemoglobin concentrations are, however, little different, perhaps because night-time hypoglycaemia is also less marked with pump therapy. As a result it is difficult to recommend these devices for regular clinical use, given their cost and the inconvenience of carrying them around. There is no clear single clinical indication for their use, though some authorities still believe that they can be useful if recurrent serious hypoglycaemia occurs on injection therapy.

The principles of dose adjustment and dose distribution are very similar to those of multiple injection regimens. The major concern with these pumps is that ketoacidosis can be more common without repeated and continuing patient education. This must include more frequent blood glucose estimation when unwell, and self checks for urinary ketones. There is also the danger that pump breakdown or catheter failure may go unnoticed without careful monitoring, which therefore needs to be more consistent than in the injection-treated patient. Pumps should not be used on people with brittle diabetes, or those seeking an external solution to the problems of their diabetes.

Unusual Routes of Insulin Administration

Intramuscular insulin administration is discussed in the section on ketoacidosis (Chapter 5). Intravenous and intraperitoneal insulin administration have a very limited role at present in the rare patient who appears unmanageable for whatever reason on subcutaneous injection therapy. Both routes are associated with reactions to long-term cannulae, resulting in major vein thrombosis or local encapsulation, often with obstruction of insulin delivery. When used for any length of time these routes should only be employed where implantable insulin infusion pumps are available to units experienced in their problems.

Nearly every natural orifice of the human body has been explored as a potential site of insulin delivery. In all cases bioavailability of insulin delivered to these sites remains poor, and absorption highly erratic. Even intranasal insulin, where a considerable part of the dose (10–20%) is absorbed if adjuvants are used, cannot hope to give adequate control, and would of course be severely disturbed by upper respiratory tract infections.

Insulin is a peptide, and hence digested in the gut. Attempts to wrap it up in lipid particles to protect the molecule from digestion have as yet met with no success.

Pancreas and Islet Transplantation

Pancreas transplantation has made great strides in recent years, with graft function rates in the few centres doing many procedures a year reaching or exceeding 60% at 12 months, and 40% at 4 years. The major technical problems have been coping with the exocrine secretions, and preventing splenic vein thrombosis. Continuing graft function has also been helped by reduction of cold ischaemia time, the use of cyclosporin to spare steroid treatment, and the use of heparin to reduce early thrombosis. Identification of rejection episodes is difficult, however, and considerable reliance has been placed on the function of kidneys transplanted in parallel. Pancreatic transplantation does not seem to put the success of the renal graft at risk.

Since immunosuppression carries risks as high or higher than diabetes, pancreatic transplantation alone cannot be considered a treatment option for the average Type 1 diabetic patient. When immunosuppression has not been used (for example, identical twin part-organ transplants) the graft has ceased to function after about 6 weeks, suggesting recurrence of islet B-cell damage. In any case graft availability rate will never be high enough to meet the demands of all insulin-treated patients. There may, however, be a role for joint kidney–pancreas transplantation in patients with diabetic nephropathy.

Islet transplantation, or islet B-cell transplantation, has not yet been successfully carried out in many humans. Harvesting human islets still has a yield of below 30%, and availability of the preferred fetal material is very limited. Islets offer the potential advantage over pancreatic transplantation of culture *in vitro* to increase B-cell mass many times, and of manipulation *in vitro* to reduce antigenicity. Attempts are also being made to transplant animal islets within membranes that prevent recognition of foreign antigen.

Further Reading

Arky, R.A. (1986). Diet and diabetes. In *Diabetes Annual 2*, pp. 49–68. Edited by Alberti, K.G.M.M. and Krall, L.P. Elsevier, Amsterdam.

Frier, B.M. (1986). Hypoglycaemia and diabetes. *Diabetic Medicine* **3**, 513.

Home, P.D., Thow, J.C. and Tunbridge, F.K.E. (1989). Insulin treatment: a decade of change. *British Medical Bulletin* **45**, 92.

James, W.P.T. (1984). Treatment of obesity: the constraints on success. *Clinics in Endocrinology and Metabolism* **13**, 635.

Lebowitz, H.E. (1987). Oral hypoglycaemic agents. In *Diabetes Annual 3*, pp. 72–93. Edited by Alberti, K.G.M.M. and Krall L.P. Elsevier, Amsterdam.

5
SPECIAL SITUATIONS IN DIABETES MANAGEMENT

Pregnancy in the Diabetic Woman

Natural History of Diabetes during Pregnancy

Diabetes and pregnancy occur together in three separate circumstances. The most obvious of these is a pregnancy occurring in a woman with pre-existing diabetes, which given the age of most pregnant women will generally be insulin-treated. However, diabetes may also be diagnosed during pregnancy (and persist after it) partly by chance association and partly because already developing diabetes may be precipitated by the metabolic stress, and come to notice through increased medical attention. Finally, diabetes may appear during pregnancy, only to disappear post-partum, although these women are highly likely to develop diabetes again in later years. This last type of diabetes is classified as gestational diabetes.

Diabetes during pregnancy is an important condition, carrying risks to both the mother and the developing fetus (Table 5.1). Prior to the availability of insulin it was unlikely that a woman with pre-existing diabetes would conceive, but should she do so then maternal death through decompensation into ketoacidosis was likely. Even with the availability of insulin, risks to the

Table 5.1 Problems associated with diabetes during pregnancy

Maternal	Fetal	Neonatal
Pre-eclampsia/eclampsia	Congenital malformations	Hypoglycaemia
Hypertension	Macrosomia	Respiratory distress syndrome
Ketoacidosis	Intrauterine death	Polycythaemia
Progression of retinopathy/nephropathy	Risks from polyhydramnios	Jaundice
Urinary tract infection/chronic pyelonephritis		Hypocalcaemia
Necrotizing fasciitis (rare)		

mother's health through pre-eclampsia and hypertension are more common in diabetes, as is polyhydramnios. The presence of nephropathy will add to the risks of pregnancy, while changes in control during pregnancy may accelerate or precipitate proliferative retinopathy.

The fetus of a diabetic mother is probably at risk from the time of conception, but at the very earliest stages any damage is likely to curtail further development. In the stage of organ formation, however, especially between weeks 4 to 10, metabolic disturbance can lead to abnormal development, either serious enough to result in fetal death, or to form the basis of a congenital malformation. These include lesions almost specific to diabetes, such as caudal dysgenesis, but more typically there is a higher rate of common malformations, with cardiac disorders accounting for the highest mortality and morbidity after birth. Poor diabetic control in early pregnancy can result in growth retardation at that stage, and also in placental abnormalities which can continue to affect growth, and possibly result in intra-uterine death later in the pregnancy. In the third trimester disturbed maternal (and hence fetal) metabolism leads to the development of a large but immature infant, with the consequent problems of respiratory distress syndrome if the fetus is delivered prematurely, or obstetric problems if delivered at term. The large diabetic baby is believed to result at least partly from overstimulation of the fetal pancreas (which functions from about week 24), and this hyperinsulinaemic responsiveness may result in hypoglycaemia up to 48 h after birth. High titres of insulin antibodies (which cross the placenta) may also increase the risk of neonatal hypogylcaemia.

Aims of Management of Diabetic Pregnancy

The problems of diabetic pregnancy can all be related to the metabolic disturbance. The aim of management is therefore to maintain metabolism as close to normal from before conception until after delivery. Intensive management is particularly worthwhile because:

1. The medical and economic costs of pregnancy are high to both mother and community.
2. Intensive management can largely eliminate both the early and late risks of diabetic pregnancy.

As blood glucose is the most easily measured index of metabolic control, and as no other biochemical substrate is known to be more closely related to fetal outcome, the management aim reduces to normalization of blood glucose concentrations.

Ketoacidosis during pregnancy carries a very high risk of fetal death. A secondary aim is therefore to avoid (or detect early) any acute metabolic decompensation.

Management of Pregnancy with Pre-existing Diabetes

Family planning

Diabetes is a condition requiring considerable self-management, a burden which is significantly increased by the co-existing responsibility of having young children around. It is therefore appropriate to suggest that patients take this into account when planning family size. Appropriate advice should also be given to patients with evidence of development of diabetic nephropathy, in view of the likelihood of the need for dialysis or renal transplantation within a few years, and the quite high possibility that the patient will not be around to care for the child through to adulthood.

Contraceptive advice will in general be the same for people with diabetes as for those without, now that low-dose oestrogen oral contraceptives are in general use, and given their very small effect on glucose tolerance. Contraindications to oral contraceptives, and monitoring of those patients using them are therefore unchanged. Barrier methods of contraception are also entirely suitable for people with diabetes.

Pre-pregnancy counselling

All diabetic women of childbearing age should be reminded yearly of the importance of seeking advice with regard to diabetes before becoming pregnant. In practice human nature dictates that many women will not be in a position to follow this recommendation, so support advice to contact the diabetes service immediately pregnancy is suspected is also indicated.

Pre-pregnancy counselling inevitably makes a woman (or couple) aware of the risks of a diabetic pregnancy, but advice can be given very positively because of the minimal risk of increased problems if good control can be maintained throughout. Even non-diabetic pregnancy carries quite a high rate of problems, however (the congenital malformation rate is around 3%), and it is important not to be overreassuring, or to lay possible seeds of guilt should a malformation occur.

Pre-pregnancy management should strive to attain as good control of blood glucose concentrations as possible. There is almost certainly no added risk of malformation where glycosylated haemoglobin is below mean +4 SD of the normal population mean, and indeed there may be little added risk up to 6 SD above the normal mean. It must be recognized that blood glucose control is the art of the possible, and some women will inevitably become pregnant with less than desirable control.

The degree of metabolic control of a diabetic father at the time of conception appears to have no influence on fetal outcome.

Management of early pregnancy

Pregnant women with diabetes should be seen throughout pregnancy by a joint team of diabetologist and obstetrician. After booking it is important to establish gestational age as closely as possible, and ultrasound examination can additionally be used to detect gross malformations. Careful monitoring of fetal growth should continue throughout pregnancy, with repeat ultrasonography, and initially weekly or fortnightly visits to the clinic. Particular attention should be paid to those risk factors (for example, smoking, alcohol, hypertension) which, like diabetes, can interfere with fetal development. Ophthalmoscopy should be performed throughout pregnancy to detect precipitation or progression of retinopathy.

Management of insulin therapy uses the same techniques as in the non-pregnant patient, but with re-education as to self-blood glucose monitoring and insulin dose adjustment if this has not been done at pre-pregnancy counselling. Intensification of management is mandatory from as early a stage as possible, but however motivated the patient it may not prove possible to achieve really tight control in the first trimester. The level of control as judged by self-blood glucose test results should be confirmed by frequent glycosylated haemoglobin estimation, and admission for optimization of control used urgently where blood glucose concentrations are not ideal.

Tight blood glucose control in the first and second trimesters is associated with a high incidence of hypoglycaemia, and hypoglycaemic coma, particularly if morning sickness is a problem. Maternal hypoglycaemia although undesirable does not present a significant hazard to the fetus.

The occasional patient, not already on insulin therapy, will usually require insulin during pregnancy, and those using sulphonylureas should be converted to insulin at the earliest opportunity.

Management of late diabetic pregnancy and delivery

As pregnancy progresses blood glucose monitoring should continue on a four times a day basis, and clinical assessment should be weekly in the third trimester. Insulin doses rise rapidly as the pregnancy progresses, particularly in those doses used to control day-time blood glucose excursions, and the total dose may rise to 2–3 times the pre-pregnancy dose. Many women become highly motivated to maintain self-care as their pregnancy becomes more evident, while metabolically they become easier to control, possibly through more consistent insulin absorption and a resistance to hypoglycaemia. As in early pregnancy problems of control should lead to admission for in-patient control.

Obstetric monitoring should also be more intensive in the diabetic than non-diabetic patients, particularly in regard to markers of continuing fetal development and well being. Pre-eclampsia and hypertension can be managed conventionally, but administration of beta-adrenergic agonists to inhibit premature contractions, or steroids to promote fetal lung maturity, requires very strict monitoring of blood glucose control and often massive increases in insulin dosage by intravenous infusion.

Delivery should be vaginally unless otherwise indicated and as near term as possible. Where control has been good in the first and second trimester, and near-normal blood glucose concentrations confirmed by glycosylated haemoglobin estimation throughout the third trimester, and where indications of fetal size and development are also normal, the pregnancy should be allowed to proceed to term. In other circumstances delivery is probably better induced at 38 weeks because of the occasional occurrence of unexplained intra-uterine death. Obstetric monitoring in labour will follow local practice for non-diabetic women if control has been good and development normal, but again should otherwise be more intensive and with recourse to Caesarean section at any sign of fetal distress.

Where delivery is planned then insulin and glucose should be given intravenously from induction. Various regimens are possible, and the insulin infusion rate should be modified according to frequent (hourly) blood glucose monitoring to maintain concentrations at 4–6 mmol/l. A useful starting regimen is glucose 10 g/h with insulin 2 U/h. Where spontaneous labour occurs a woman may have had her usual dose of insulin and be at risk of hypoglycaemia on stopping eating. In these circumstances infusion of glucose should be modulated to maintain normal blood glucose concentrations, and insulin infusion commenced when blood glucose concentrations rise above 6 mmol/l at a glucose infusion rate of 5 g/h.

Separation of the placenta is associated with a rapid drop in insulin requirement, which can be halved prospectively. The insulin/glucose infusion is continued up to the time of the first meal, when subcutaneous insulin is restarted according to pre-pregnancy insulin dosage.

The use of insulin/glucose infusion is particularly convenient where the mother comes to Caesarean section, when management can proceed as for other surgery (see below). Again, however, insulin requirements change rapidly after delivery.

Management after pregnancy

Breast feeding should be encouraged in diabetic women, as in non-diabetic women. Lactating mothers will generally increase their calorie intake automatically to cope with the demands of the baby.

Self-management of diabetes often suffers severely when a mother is managing a young baby, and commonly blood glucose control is even worse than before the pregnancy. Careful counselling and advice are often disappointing at this stage, but control will often improve as the baby's habits become more conducive to a regular life-style.

Diabetes Diagnosed during Pregnancy

Diagnosis of diabetes during pregnancy poses particular problems, mainly because a much higher proportion of possible cases have a relatively mild degree of disturbance of glucose intolerance than do newly diagnosed non-pregnant patients. Most cases are still picked up by positive routine urinalysis, which should result in blood glucose estimation (2 h after the last meal), and a glucose tolerance test if this is equivocal (between 6.0 and 8.0 mmol/l), or if the glycosuria is heavy or detected fasting. Risk factors for diabetes in pregnancy include previous glucose intolerance, a family history of diabetes, previous large baby (>4000 g), and previous intra-uterine death. In these women timed blood glucose samples should be monitored throughout pregnancy, and especially from 28 weeks. Equivocal results suggest the need for formal testing with a glucose load. It should not, however, be assumed that normal glucose tolerance at say 28 weeks excludes the possibility of diabetes when the pregnancy has advanced to 36 weeks.

The oral glucose tolerance test is best performed in the standard way, with a 75 g load. The criteria for definite diabetes are the same as for the non-pregnant patient. It is generally suggested that women who would fulfill the criteria for impaired glucose tolerance if not pregnant be managed as having diabetes during pregnancy. In practice, given appropriate dietary advice, many of these women will run normal post-prandial blood glucose and glycosylated haemoglobin concentrations, and can then be regarded as not being at increased risk.

Younger, thinner patients diagnosed during pregnancy will often be cases of true Type 1 Diabetes in the prodrome of the disease (see Chapter 1). These patients will generally require insulin therapy during pregnancy, but often come off it for a period of months afterwards. More elderly, overweight patients, possibly with a family history of diabetes, may well be manageable on dietary control alone, but severe calorie restriction is of course contraindicated. Many of these women may be classed as having had gestational diabetes when found to have normal glucose tolerance 6 weeks after pregnancy, but a very high proportion go on to develop Type 2 diabetes sometimes many decades later. Appropriate dietary and risk factor advice, and annual follow-up by a general practitioner, are therefore indicated.

Diabetes in Childhood

Natural History of Childhood Diabetes

Diabetes of onset in childhood is overwhelmingly of the insulin-dependent type (Type 1 diabetes), characterized by islet cell antibodies, an HLA DR 3 and 4 association, and immune destruction of islet B-cells (see Chapter 1). While the peak age of onset is the early teenage years, and the yearly pattern shows a spring peak, diagnosis can occur at any age, and the condition is very rarely congenital. Although childhood diabetes often seems to have an abrupt onset, and often to be associated with an infectious illness, this is now understood only to be because the metabolic stress of intercurrent illness precipitates the condition in an individual with very little functional B-cell capacity after many months or even years of the destructive process. After diagnosis progression of islet B-cell destruction continues rapidly in children, the youngest becoming C-peptide negative within a year.

Diabetes or glucose intolerance is also found in association with a wide variety of genetic syndromes including some glycogen storage diseases, Praeder–Willi syndrome, DIDMOAD syndrome and generalized lipoatrophy (Table 5.2). Insulin treatment will be required where life expectancy is good, and glycosylated haemoglobin concentrations abnormal. However, diabetes (Type 1) in children with Down's syndrome accounts for the majority of cases seen in clinical practice in association with genetic syndromes.

Non-insulin-dependent diabetes similar to the adult Type 2 diabetes is seen occasionally in childhood. It is generally of teenage onset and usually with obviously dominant inheritance. The condition is known variously as Mason-type diabetes, maturity onset diabetes of the young (MODY), or even more horribly as NIDDY (non-insulin-dependent diabetes of the young). This type of diabetes has a reputation for sparing those afflicted from microangiopathy, but several reports indicate that these patients are at risk, and the impression may have been gained simply by comparison to the very poor control previously achieved in Type 1 diabetic children on insulin. Children with Type 2 diabetes should be treated conventionally by dietary measures, adding sulphonylureas and changing to insulin where glycosylated haemoglobin exceeds 4 SD above the normal population mean.

The late tissue damage (complications) of diabetes take many years to develop, and as the majority of children are diagnosed in their second decade of life such complications make a very small impact on paediatric care. Nevertheless, considerable tissue damage does occur in childhood, and any sizeable clinic population will include examples of background retinopathy, microalbuminuria and limited joint mobility in post-pubertal adolescents. Screening for complications has a useful educational impact, and should be performed yearly. Family dietary education, to reduce saturated fat intake and hence later arterial disease, should also begin in the first year after diagnosis.

Table 5.2 Types of diabetes presenting in childhood

1. Type 1 (insulin-dependent) diabetes
2. Secondary diabetes
    Malnutrition related
    Pancreatitis related
3. Non-insulin-dependent diabetes of the young
4. Diabetes in special syndromes (see Table 1.2)

Nutrition and Growth

Children with diabetes will grow normally, provided their metabolic control is not very poor. Indeed it has been the impression that they grow faster than other children, perhaps because in the past quality of diet was better supervised in this group. Again, puberty can be expected to occur at the normal time unless control is poor. If insulin therapy is inadequate then serum growth hormone levels will be raised (although only detectably in the diabetic population as a whole), but as somatomedin C production by the liver is defective normal growth will not occur. Restoration of adequate insulin delivery before puberty will result in a growth spurt, and if puberty is delayed by poor control this can occur even in the late teenage years. Much beyond puberty growth stunting is irreversible.

Nutritional recommendations for young people with diabetes do not differ in balance from those for adults (see Chapter 4). A number of problems do however arise. Calorie intake during childhood rises continuously, and particularly rapidly in early puberty. Even a diabetic child will quite naturally and subconsciously increase their calorie intake accordingly, but if the dietary carbohydrate prescription is not reviewed then conflicts can arise. These tend to be resolved by a combination of increased intake of dietary fat (undesirably) and by gradual changes in the perception of what constitutes an exchange of carbohydrate. Where the parents are strict (or anxious) disciplinarians the potential for family conflict over food is large, often with psychological repercussions for diabetic control. Planned dietary review throughout childhood is therefore important.

Changes in a child's eating pattern towards a modified fat diet are easier if the whole family moves the same way. Care needs to be taken, however, to avoid the possible danger that the diabetic child becomes seen as inflicting a punishment on other family members.

Junk food, often high fat or high sugar, is a nearly universal passion amongst youngsters in industrialized societies. Absolute bans on taking these foods will rarely be effective, and lead to a lack of empathy (and even dishonesty) between the care team and patient. As with adults it is better to find the excuse of special occasions to fulfill these needs as they arise. The wide availability of soft drinks with negligible calorie intake has largely solved the pop and cola problem, while the need for confectionary can be usefully combined with the promotion of strenuous exercise and the avoidance of hypoglycaemia during it.

Management of Diabetes in Childhood

The basic tools and principles of the management of diabetes in young people are the same as in adults (Chapter 4). Basic dietary aspects are discussed above. Children do, however, live a philosophically different style of life from many adults, generally with much more emphasis on the present day, and with a very limited time horizon. In younger children there is often more emphasis on

Table 5.3 Special problems of childhood diabetes

Organic (with poor metabolic control)	Psychosocial	Parental problems
Poor growth	Hypoglycaemia	Overprotection
Delayed puberty	Psychosomatic symptoms	Genetic counselling
Recurrent infections	Brittle diabetes	
	Sibling relationships	
	Peer pressures	
	Injection phobia	

exertion and exercise than in adults, but this often fades in adolescence, when however a variety of other activities lead to an increasingly unpredictable and erratic lifestyle. Young diabetic patients will often more readily adopt (and discard) new ideas and new gadgets suggested for management of their diabetes, and are generally much more honest than adults about the degree to which they are able to comply with dietary or other restrictions, or perform self-monitoring.

Persuading a child of the need for good diabetic control to the extent where it influences behaviour is therefore not easy, and needs to be couched in the positive terms of maintaining good health to be able to take part in whatever activities are currently most popular with the individual. Minor childhood illnesses are common enough to make this appear realistic. Children (like adults) do like to please and be praised, and their inherent honesty makes it more difficult for them to achieve this without appropriate performance. To understand what motivates a particular child it is necessary for members of the care team to have a good appreciation of the current fashions of childhood culture, and to be able to talk sensibly about them. Personal experience of family life and its conflicts are helpful in these respects.

It is inappropriate to threaten children with the bogeyman of late complications. It is however morally indefensible to deny parents the knowledge of these problems, particularly as they will gain partly digested information by reading pamphlets and books. As children grow up they will need to have questions answered about these problems, and an annual screening for complications can be a useful time to introduce information on these aspects.

The potential for psychological problems occurring in both parents and children, and for family conflicts, as a result of diabetes is immense. Such problems are after all not uncommon in the absence of diabetes. Some common examples include:

1. Parental guilt or anger. What have we done to deserve this, or what have we done to inflict this on our child? The importance of environmental factors/genetics will have to be handled differently according to the parents' problem.
2. Will it happen again? A worry in relation to living and planned siblings.

3. Conflicts over food. Eating is a major part of human behaviour, and problems over amounts, timing and nature of food can have major family repercussions if unresolved.
4. Discipline over insulin injections. This can be a particular problem if the child is not self-administering before adolescence begins. Late lie-ins on weekend mornings can be a problem if suitable solutions are not found.
5. Infliction of insulin injections. In younger children this can lead to problems for both parent and child.
6. Fear of hypoglycaemia. Hypoglycaemia is unpleasant, and night-time hypoglycaemia is often associated with a fear that it might cause death. This needs recognition and heavy reassurance.
7. Overprotective behaviour. This can lead to inappropriate restrictions on a child's lifestyle, sometimes manifested in the form of psychosomatic complaints.
8. Manipulative behaviour. Consciously or unconsciously a child may use diabetes to avoid certain activities or obligations.
9. Sibling rivalry. This can become a problem when a child's diabetes becomes a major focus of family life, and the siblings' needs become relatively ignored.
10. Failed loosening of child–parent bonds. It is not unusual for parental care of a diabetic child to continue inappropriately well into adulthood.

Because of these, and other, family and psychological difficulties it is generally recommended that the paediatric diabetes health care team includes a clinical psychologist.

Young people take well to self-blood glucose monitoring, and generally dislike urine testing. They often seem happy to use devices such as memory blood glucose meters and dosage computers for short periods of time. Pen-injectors and multiple injection therapy are if anything even more popular than in the adult population, and such regimens are indicated from the time of diagnosis.

Diabetes in the elderly

Natural History of Diabetes in Old Age

The natural history of glucose tolerance with age is disputed, possibly because it is dependent on social habits. Thus there is little evidence, in those who have not developed frank diabetes, that glucose tolerance changes with age provided weight remains below a body mass index of 25.0 kg/m^2 and activity does not diminish. In many industrialized nations, however, the population gains weight and becomes less active with time, and the proportion of people with abnormal glucose tolerance on screening increases. In these circumstances the life-time incidence of diabetes may reach 10%, although the overall prevalence

144 Special Situations in Diabetes Management

is only 2%, emphasizing that the highest incidence is in the last two decades of life.

Most of this incidence is of Type 2 diabetes, and since the elderly are prone to other medical conditions much is diagnosed incidentally. Nevertheless, Type 1 diabetes with progression to absolute insulin deficiency can occur at any age, although its evolution tends to be much slower in the elderly. Other forms of diabetes (secondary, hormone-induced, tropical) tend to have become manifest at an earlier age.

At the time of diagnosis diabetes will often have been present for many years in the older patient, and as many as 25% will already have evidence of diabetes-related complications. This prevalence of complications often increases considerably in the first five years after diagnosis, for reasons that are not entirely clear.

The types of late tissue damage found in elderly diabetic patients are the same as those in younger age groups, but the pattern is different. Thus the risk of developing end-stage renal failure due to diabetic nephropathy is much less than for young Type 1 diabetic patients, although the absolute numbers of patients (due to the higher prevalence) are similar. Foot problems tend to be much more commonly related to peripheral vascular disease in later life, and accordingly are much more intractable. Similarly the prevalence of ischaemic heart disease, hypertension and cerebrovascular disease is very high in elderly diabetic patients, and they are the commonest cause of death. As with nephropathy, proliferative retinopathy is relatively uncommon in the elderly diabetic patient, but this is more than balanced by a large increase in the incidence of diabetic maculopathy, the major cause of blindness in this group.

Management of Diabetes in the Elderly

The principles of management of diabetes in old age are not different from those described for the majority of diabetic patients (Chapter 4). Differences arise because in many elderly patients life expectancy is such that the weight placed on the risk of late complications is reduced, and it may therefore be judged appropriate to reduce the inconvenience and risks of therapy. Some particular problems of the elderly with diabetes are given in Table 5.4 (see also Table 4.5). It is not appropriate to lay down rules in these respects according to age group, as life expectancy can be highly variable even in the eighth decade. Although late complications may be less common it should be recalled that thrombotic problems and infections are more common in the elderly, and that poorly controlled diabetes predisposes to both. Thus although tight blood glucose control may be judged unnecessary, good control remains desirable, with HbA_1 levels kept below 6 SD above the normal mean in all patients.

Dietary therapy is often well tolerated and accepted by elderly patients, but calorie restriction may be very difficult after a life-time of overeating. It does not make sense to apply the full rigours of a modified fat diet to people who

Table 5.4 Difficulties of the elderly patient with diabetes

All patients
Learning/reading problems
Foot care problems
   Through poor eyesight
   Through poor mobility

Non-insulin-treated
Hypoglycaemia on tablet therapy (see Table 4.5)
Rigidity in dietary habits
Confusion over multiple tablet therapy

Insulin-treated
Hypoglycaemia (especially if living alone)
Measuring insulin doses imprecisely
   Through poor eyesight
   Through hand arthritis
Difficulty in learning injection skills
Erratic eating habits

have survived 70 years despite a serum cholesterol level typical of industrialized society.

Sulphonylureas are in general also well tolerated by these patients, though the thinner patient with a milder metabolic disturbance can be very sensitive to these drugs (Table 4.5). Furthermore, renal impairment is common, and hence drug levels can be higher for the same dose. The starting dose should therefore be as small as possible, and only begun after a proper trial of dietary therapy has failed. The first generation agent tolbutamide is an effective and safe choice, except in those who have difficulty in swallowing large tablets, or remembering more than the simplest dosage regimen. It is common to find that elderly patients are not taking their sulphonylureas appropriately, namely, just before their main meals.

Advice should be given about hypoglycaemia to patients taking sulphonylureas as well as to those on insulin. Unfortunately the symptoms of hypoglycaemia in this age group are often non-specific and easily confused with other symptoms common in the elderly. A careful history indicating a relationship of hypoglycaemia to a particular time of day, to increased activity (often just shopping), and alleviated by food, can be of great help. It is important that elderly people well controlled on sulphonylureas do not miss meals.

Metformin is not specifically contraindicated in the elderly, but the high incidence of renal impairment, and the commoner progression to renal impairment, mean that monitoring of renal function must be at least yearly.

Insulin therapy is well tolerated by the elderly. It is a mistake to delay beginning insulin for too long, thereby depriving the patient of precious months of good health. Very many older patients comment on how much better they are after insulin injections have been started. Because many patients have significant endogenous insulin secretion (either having slowly progressive Type

1 diabetes, or sulphonylurea-resistant Type 2 diabetes), a pre-mixed insulin preparation (unmodified + isophane (NPH)) given twice a day often results in very adequate blood glucose control.

Many elderly patients prove able to give their own injections adequately, after appropriate instruction. However, eyesight problems, arthropathy of the hands and poor co-ordination are common in these patients, and injections may have to be given by a visiting nurse. Self-blood glucose monitoring seems less acceptable to elderly patients, perhaps because they often have less personal use for the results. Choice of monitoring will need to be dictated by individual preference.

Annual screening for problems related to diabetes should be performed as for younger patients (Chapter 3). Measurement of visual acuity becomes more important however, as a decrease of one line is often the first indication of maculopathy, which may be difficult to confirm by ophthalmoscopy. Proteinuria (after exclusion of infection) is often more difficult to interpret in the elderly patient with hypertension. Similarly biothesiometry may be of little use when many non-diabetic, non-neuropathic patients have decreased vibration sensation.

Acute Hyperglycaemic Emergencies

Acute metabolic decompensation of diabetes to a life-threatening degree is usually manifested as hyperglycaemia plus dehydration accompanied by acidosis due to high plasma ketone body levels, ketoacidosis. An alternative manifestation is that of hyperglycaemia, hyperosmolarity and dehydration without acidosis. In their extreme forms these states progress to lowered consciousness, and are therefore often given the epithet 'coma', but this is now inappropriate to the majority of cases.

Hyperglycaemic emergencies are probably less common than previously, possibly due to a higher awareness of diabetes amongst family physicians, more appropriate professional and patient education on the handling of intercurrent illness, and more ready access to specialist care. Unfortunately the conditions still carry a significant mortality rate, most of which is probably avoidable with careful and experienced management. Non-ketotic hyperglycaemic emergencies carry a higher mortality than ketoacidosis, possibly because they tend to occur in elderly and already ill patients.

Pathogenesis of Hyperglycaemic Emergencies

Insulin withdrawal in the well and fasting diabetic patient (with no endogenous insulin secretion) will lead to a rise in hepatic glucose delivery into the blood, and hence a rise in blood glucose concentration until glucose disposal again equals input. This occurs at 12 to 18 mmol/l. Blood glucose concentrations will rise further if exogenous glucose is consumed, or if stress hormone production stimulates gluconeogenesis and blocks glucose disposal. Glucocorticoids are probably of most relevance in these respects in infective illness, but in more acute conditions such as myocardial infarction the catecholamines and glucagon may be of more importance. Furthermore, glucagon concentrations will rise in insulin deficiency even in the face of hyperglycaemia. Where stress hormone output is high metabolic decompensation can occur with only relative insulin deficiency.

Marked hyperglycaemia leads to dehydration through osmotic diuresis. The diuresis leads to electrolyte losses, the loss of body potassium being exacerbated by the mineralocorticoid response to dehydration. Nevertheless, in the acute stages plasma potassium concentrations can be high, as early intracellular dehydration and the loss of the effects of insulin on cell membrane pumps lead to a leak of the high levels of intracellular potassium into the extracellular fluid. Deficits equivalent to five or more litres of isotonic saline, and 200 to 600 mmol of potassium are usual. The dehydration leads to poor tissue perfusion, which may impair absorption of any remaining subcutaneous insulin.

Insulin deficiency also leads to the mobilization of non-esterified fatty acids from adipose tissue, and indeed prolonged starvation decreases fat reserves and protects against ketoacidosis. The fatty acid load to the liver, in the presence of insulin deficiency, leads to excessive ketone body production (3-hydroxybutyrate and acetoacetate). High glucagon concentrations will switch fatty acid metabolism in the liver from re-esterification into triglyceride towards oxidation to ketone bodies. Peripheral metabolism of these acids also becomes impaired, and as buffering capacity is consumed plasma and intracellular pH will fall. Stress hormones may have some role in promoting fatty acid mobilization and hepatic ketogenesis, but as these processes can be inhibited even in the ill patient by high physiological concentrations of insulin given therapeutically, it is insulin deficiency that is more important.

The hyperosmolar rather than ketotic state usually occurs in patients with less severe pre-existing insulin deficiency, but it is difficult to demonstrate a difference in insulin concentrations at the time of the emergency. Hyperosmolar states are also more common in populations which tend to assuage their thirst with large volumes of high sugar drinks.

Presentation of Hyperglycaemic Emergencies

Classically these patients are dehydrated and unwell on presentation, but with the realization by patients and doctors of the circumstances in which metabolic decompensation can occur, and with the wide availability of reagent strips for glucose and ketones, referrals are now often of severely hyperglycaemic or mildly acidotic patients who are not markedly dehydrated and not desperately unwell. Dehydration in the ketoacidotic patient will generally be accompanied and exacerbated by nausea and vomiting. Decreased conscious level is a late but important sign indicative of disturbance of brain water and electrolyte metabolism.

Special Situations in Diabetes Management

Acidosis is accompanied by hyperventilation in an attempt to blow off CO_2 to compensate, the breathing being characteristically deeper as well as more rapid than normal. Acetone may be detectable on the patient's breath. Urinary ketones will be detectable in ketoacidosis, and plasma ketones can also be detected with a reagent strip. Plasma bicarbonate should be below 18 mmol/l for the diagnosis of ketoacidois, and is often <5 mmol/l, with blood pH 6.9 to 7.2.

Management of Hyperglycaemic Emergencies (Table 5.5)

Standard management

A high proportion of deaths, particularly in patients with ketoacidosis, are probably avoidable. Management of hyperglycaemic emergencies therefore needs to be both disciplined and thoughtful.

Dehydration should be corrected with isotonic (150 mmol/l) saline, begun at the time that blood is taken for urgent estimation of glucose, electrolytes, HCO_3^-, creatinine and pH. One litre is generally given in the first half-hour, then 1 l/h, and more slowly thereafter until four to five litres have been given according to the state of dehydration. Use of lower concentrations of NaCl (75 mmol/l) is usually contraindicated even when the plasma sodium concentration

Table 5.5 Key features in the management of hyperglycaemic emergencies

Diagnosis
Examination
  Dehydration, Kussmaul breathing, conscious state
  Presence of infection, acute cardiac/arterial event
Investigation
  Blood glucose, ketonuria, ketonaemia, plasma HCO_3^-, blood pH
  Plasma potassium, plasma creatinine
  Chest X-ray, urine microscopy/culture, blood cultures
  Electrocardiogram

Management
Treatment (initial)
  Saline (150 mmol/l)
  Insulin (6 U/h)
  Potassium (20 mmol/l saline)
  Antibiotics
  Gastric and urinary catheters (if indicated)
  Subcutaneous heparin
Monitoring
  Blood glucose (hourly)
  Plasma potassium (2-hourly)
  Plasma sodium, plasma creatinine, blood pH
  Cardiac ECG T-wave
  Central venous pressure (older patients)

is high, as this can lead to a greater risk of cerebral oedema, a major cause of death. In the elderly patient, or those with impaired cardiac or renal function, monitoring of central venous pressure is a useful guide to fluid replacement.

Potassium replacement should be started at the same time as insulin therapy, as 20 mmol/l of saline. Plasma potassium concentration at presentation is not a guide to potassium deficiency, but if it is known to be above 6.0 mmol/l before saline is begun then it may be omitted from the first litre only. A check on potassium concentrations should be made 2 h after starting fluid/insulin therapy, when rapidly falling or low levels will often suggest a need to increase the rate of replacement. Hypokalaemia is a second major cause of death. ECG monitoring of T-wave amplitude provides a useful continuous indication of plasma potassium concentrations. Oral potassium replacement (16 mmol, four times a day) should be continued for two to three days after the emergency, and plasma concentrations measured daily.

Insulin therapy may be given as hourly intramuscular injections (10 U, followed by 6 U/h), or by intravenous infusion from a syringe pump (1 U/ml, 6 U/h). Laboratory measured blood glucose concentration should have fallen at 2 h. If it has not, then injection therapy should be changed to an infusion, and infusion therapy checked for pump malfunction and infusion line integrity, while changing the insulin syringe. An early fall in blood glucose concentration may, however, occur with rehydration alone. Blood glucose is monitored hourly by reagent strip estimation, and the insulin delivery changed to a glucose/insulin/potassium combined infusion (10 g + 5 U + 4 mmol per hour) when blood glucose drops to 13 mmol/l. Blood glucose concentrations should then be maintained at 8 to 12 mmol/l by adjusting the insulin delivery rate if necessary, and subcutaneous injection therapy started when the patient is eating. The initial insulin dosage will need to be 50–100% higher than normally estimated.

Bicarbonate therapy has not been demonstrated to be beneficial, but may be given if blood pH is below 7.0 as two infusions of 75 mmol given over 45 min, each with 20 mmol of potassium. A pH check is advisable between infusions, and a check of plasma potassium 30 min after the infusions. The sodium load is equivalent to 1 litre of isotonic saline; this is one circumstance where the use of 75 mmol/l NaCl may temporarily be justified.

Phosphate depletion is present in ketoacidosis, but specific phosphate replacement is not known to be of any benefit.

Infection may be difficult to detect, especially in acidotic patients, as body temperature is depressed by ketosis, while leucocyte counts are usually elevated. Urine should, however, be screened by microscopy, blood cultures taken and chest X-ray performed (after initiation of fluid/insulin therapy). Broad spectrum antibiotic therapy, such as amoxycillin, should be started intravenously at double normal doses (leucocyte function being severely impaired in ketoacidosis) on any suspicion of infection. Antibiotic therapy should also be started if bladder catheterization is judged desirable. Invasive mycoses, and in particular mucormycosis, are rarely associated with ketoacidosis, but probably require several days of severe insulin deficiency to become established.

An ECG should be performed as silent myocardial infarction may precipitate acute hyperglycaemia. Interpretation can be difficult, however, with very bizarre changes sometimes occurring with electrolyte disturbance.

A decreased level of consciousness at any stage suggests the need for a nasogastric tube and aspiration of stomach contents, as ketoacidosis causes gastroparesis and inhalation pneumonia is then a real risk.

Anticoagulants should be used in any patients in whom mobility is likely to be markedly impaired for more than the 4–6 h of acute management. This is particularly important in patients with the hyperosmolar state, but all diabetic patients in poor control show hypercoaguable features. Subcutaneous heparin is suitable prophylactic therapy.

Other problems in management

Decreasing consciousness level, particularly that occurring after 2 to 4 h of treatment or later, can be assumed to be due to cerebral oedema in the absence of localizing neurological signs at presentation. This is a dangerous condition, not uncommonly progressing to brain death. Delivery of free water (75 mmol/l NaCl, or glucose solutions) must cease, and delivery of isotonic saline slowed particularly if mannitol is used to draw water into the extracellular space.

Adult respiratory distress syndrome also appears to be a feature of patients in whom osmolarity is lowered too quickly through the excessive use of hypotonic fluids.

Persistent acidosis is uncommon, and must not be confused with persistent ketonuria which is acceptable. If acidosis persists then the first presumption should be that insulin delivery is not occurring, and this should be investigated. A persistent anion gap suggests either ketoacidosis or more rarely lactic acidosis. This differential diagnosis is important as lactic acidosis (lactate over 8 mmol/l) requires much more aggressive bicarbonate therapy, until the pH is above 7.20. Measurement of plasma ketones or blood lactate can therefore be useful. Lactic acidosis suggests a major precipitating event, such as a large myocardial infarct. Acidosis without a large anion gap will be hyperchloraemic, is usually relatively mild (pH >7.15) and will correct itself with continuing conventional management.

Abdominal pain can pose a diagnostic problem in patients with ketoacidosis, but it must be emphasized that abdominal pain in the absence of ketoacidosis cannot be due to diabetes. Acute abdominal emergencies can precipitate metabolic decompensation, but it is in any case safer to correct the metabolic state before undertaking laparotomy. An additional diagnostic problem arises through elevation of plasma amylase levels in ketoacidosis. Abdominal pain secondary to ketoacidosis alone resolves rapidly with its treatment.

Preventative Management

Except in the undiagnosed patient (and sometimes even then), every episode of ketoacidosis should suggest an educational or behavioural error on the part of the patient and/or their medical advisors. The commonest errors are not seeking medical help when the patient is unable to eat, not measuring blood glucose and failing to increase insulin doses when unwell, and omitting insulin therapy (or reducing the dose) because carbohydrate cannot be taken. These aspects should therefore be reviewed, and steps taken to avoid similar episodes occurring in other patients. In patients who have recurrent episodes of ketoacidosis an explanation should be sought in the area of psychological disturbance.

Diabetes in Patients Undergoing Surgery and Other Procedures

Consequences of Surgery and Anaesthesia in Diabetes

A surgical procedure carries potentially significant problems for the diabetic patient, with high morbidity and mortality rates recorded in some series. At its simplest a patient dependent on insulin therapy, who needs to be starved for a simple procedure, will need to be given insulin in a manner which minimizes the risk of hypo- and hyperglycaemia. Many patients with diabetes have significant vascular disease, and are therefore at high risk of an acute vascular event, while the presence of undetected autonomic neuropathy can predispose to sudden cardiorespiratory arrest. Vitreous haemorrhage is at least a theoretical risk in any patient with proliferative retinopathy subjected to swings in blood pressure, and a very real risk to the many diabetic patients anticoagulated for cardiac or vascular surgery. Renal impairment is common in people with diabetes, with consequent difficulties over the management of fluid and electrolytes. The nerves of people with diabetes are particularly susceptible to pressure damage and while function usually recovers after short procedures, special care should be taken during anaesthesia to avoid the problem.

In the more markedly insulin-deficient patient failure to increase insulin delivery appropriately can lead to ketoacidosis in the face of the stress hormone response (see below). Lesser degrees of insulin deficiency will be associated with severe muscle catabolism, and poor wound healing. Hyperglycaemia above 13 mmol/l leads to significant urinary glucose loss, and rapidly to osmotic diuresis with consequent disturbance of water and electrolyte balance. In addition, impaired phagocyte function is detectable at blood glucose concentrations over 11 mmol/l, and hence resistance to infection is soon impaired. Ketosis will also impair leucocyte cell function.

The Metabolic Disturbance of Surgery and Anaesthesia

In all people both surgery and anaesthesia can induce very significant metabolic stress, although modern anaesthetic techniques cause much less disturbance than previously, and for the most part can be ignored. The metabolic response to surgery is however greater than can be explained simply by the stress hormone response, and probably, as with infection, also reflects the effects of cytokines released by macrophages.

In the non-diabetic patient the combined effects of glucagon, catecholamines and cortisol lead to stimulation of gluconeogensis and glycolysis, impaired insulin-mediated glucose disposal and marked muscle catabolism, but these effects are partly countered by a rise in insulin secretion, and indeed this overcomes the effects of the other hormones on lipolysis and hence on the fatty acid drive to ketogenesis. In people with diabetes this insulin response will be deficient to a varying degree, the consequences then being hyperglycaemia, protein breakdown, mobilization of fat and excess ketone production.

Pre-operative Management

Many authorities recommend that diabetic patients are admitted two to three days before operation for stabilization and investigation. With modern management however (Chapter 4) perhaps 60% of insulin-treated patients and the majority of non-insulin-treated patients will have glycosylated haemoglobin concentrations within 6 SD of the normal mean, while most of the investigative procedures can be undertaken as an out-patient. Pre-operative assessment will include examination for neuropathy and cardiovascular disease, an ECG and serum creatinine estimation. When patients are in poor control, management in hospital on an intense insulin and dietary regimen for two to three days is still recommended.

The long-acting sulphonylurea chlorpropamide should be stopped two to three days before operation, with substitution of a short-acting agent if necessary. Because of the theoretically increased risk of lactic acidosis, biguanide therapy should also be stopped a few days in advance of operation.

Per-operative Management (Table 5.6)

Pre- and post-operative management of the diabetic patient are easier if the operation is performed early on the morning list. Minor procedures (under 1 h) in patients controlled on diet alone and with normal fasting blood glucose (<5.5 mmol/l) or glycosylated haemoglobin concentrations can be managed by simply avoiding glucose infusions and monitoring blood glucose before and after the procedure. Patients well or only moderately controlled on sulphonylurea therapy can be similarly managed for very short procedures (for example cystoscopy), omitting the drug on the morning of operation and giving a short-acting agent with the first full meal.

Other patients require per-operative insulin therapy, and a wide range of subcutaneous and intravenous regimens have been proposed for this purpose. Intravenous regimens are, however, much more flexible than subcutaneous delivery, and more dependable in the event of poor skin perfusion. Published

Table 5.6 Management of the diabetic patient needing peri-operative insulin therapy

Pre-operative assessment
Current metabolic control
Retinopathy, cardiac disease, renal disease
Neuropathy
Change from biguanides or long-acting sulphonylureas

Day of operation
First on list
Omit morning insulin injection
At 0800 h (latest)
   Begin IV infusion at 100 ml/h of:
     500 ml 100 g/l glucose + 10 mmol K^+ + 15 U unmodified insulin
   Monitor blood glucose at least 2-hourly
     Target blood glucose 5.0–10.0 mmol/l
     Adjust insulin delivery rate as necessary
Post-operatively
   Continue glucose/potassium/insulin infusion if not eating
   Monitor glucose as above
   Monitor electrolytes as necessary
   Beware of fluid overload with renal impairment or prolonged infusion
   Restart insulin therapy with first full meal
   Stop IV insulin 1 h after first meal

These are guidelines only. Individual patients with special problems may require special management. Obese patients may require more insulin IV (e.g. starting with 20 U/500 ml), and thin, elderly patients less (e.g. 12 U/500 ml).

reports of control are comparable for the peri-operative period, but much better for intravenous regimens over the post-operative day.

The infusion should be started at the beginning of the morning, after estimation of blood glucose concentration. A typical regimen uses 3 U insulin + 10 g glucose + 10 mmol K^+ per hour, made up by adding the insulin and potassium to 10% glucose solution. At these concentrations some insulin will be lost to the plastic of the giving set, and the first 50 ml should therefore be run out to waste. Overweight patients poorly controlled on high insulin doses will require a higher insulin infusion rate (4 U/h), while thin patients in good control on small doses of insulin or sulphonylureas are more safely started on a lower rate (2 U/h). In any case blood glucose concentrations should be monitored at a minimum of every 2 h (more frequently if changing), and the insulin dose adjusted according to the projected glucose concentration. Blood reagent strips are adequate for this purpose if appropriate training and quality control procedures are in operation.

Surgery in Special Situations

Emergency surgery can be managed similarly, but if blood glucose concentrations are >13 mmol/l it is to be desirable to use an insulin infusion alone (with potassium in isotonic saline) until this level is regained. Ideally surgery should be delayed until metabolic control can be restored. Surgery in the ketoacidotic patient carries a very high fatality rate, and should be deferred unless there is a balancing risk.

Surgery requiring cardiopulmonary by-pass causes a major degree of metabolic stress and disturbance, exacerbated by periods of hypothermia and rewarming, and sometimes the use of catecholamine infusions. Glucose- or lactate-containing solutions should not be used for the by-pass prime. Insulin requirements often rise dramatically in the post-by-pass and immediate post-operative periods. This is best managed by adjustment of insulin delivery from a syringe pump by means of very frequent blood glucose readings performed by the anaesthetist using a blood glucose meter.

Post-operative Management

Glucose/insulin/potassium infusions can be continued while the patient is not eating, with appropriate monitoring of blood glucose concentrations (2-hourly initially, hourly if unstable, 4-hourly once stable) and adjustment of insulin dosage. Careful monitoring of electrolyte and fluid status is necessary after 24 h or if renal impairment is present, with a reduction in the free water delivery rate if necessary.

Subcutaneous insulin (or sulphonylureas for minor surgery in non-insulin-treated patients) can be given with the first post-operative meal, and the infusion stopped an hour later, when subcutaneous absorption will have begun, and by which time the patient's ability to eat without vomiting will have been confirmed. Increased insulin dosage may be required for several days by patients having major surgery, or those developing complications such as wound infections. The aim should be to maintain blood glucose concentrations in the range 5–10 mmol/l, while avoiding hypoglycaemia.

Dyslipidaemia in People with Diabetes

Introduction

Abnormal plasma lipid and lipoprotein concentrations are very common in people with diabetes, and indeed in the Type 2 diabetic patient they may be found in a majority. These abnormalities may not simply be a reflection of abnormal metabolic control, although the abnormalities found in Type 1 diabetes may largely reflect the adequacy of insulin replacement therapy and the peripheral route of insulin delivery. As discussed in Chapter 1, the Type 2 diabetic patient has, in addition to relative insulin deficiency, a more general metabolic disturbance associated with insulin insensitivity, hypertension and truncal obesity. These abnormalities are associated with combined hyperlipidaemia and a high risk of major vessel disease even in people without diabetes, and hence the high prevalence of raised plasma cholesterol and triglyceride levels in Type 2 diabetes is to be expected.

Although this pattern may be recognized as combined hypercholesterolaemia and hypertriglyceridaemia (phenotype IIb), more subtle distinctions can also be recognized. Thus the total cholesterol concentration may not be particularly high (5.5–6.5 mmol/l) in the patient with well-controlled Type 2 diabetes, but the HDL cholesterol is uniformly low (0.7–1.0 mmol/l), and triglycerides moderately raised (2.5–5.0 mmol/l). Individually these measurements may not be striking, but the risk of arterial disease is high. This may explain the much clearer association of raised triglyceride levels with atherosclerosis in diabetic than non-diabetic people.

Although diabetes is classically associated with a phenotype class IV hyperlipidaemia (isolated hypertriglyceridaemia), this is not common in patients with good or moderate blood glucose control. Diabetes can, however, severely exaggerate the abnormalities found in other types of hyperlipidaemia, in particular phenotypes III (remnant particle disease) and V (chylomicronaemia syndrome).

The mechanisms by which dyslipidaemia occurs in diabetes are unclear and almost certainly complex (Table 5.7). The hypertriglyceridaemia is associated with both increased very low density lipoprotein (VLDL) production and decreased clearance, the latter perhaps reflecting abnormalities of lipoprotein lipase activity. Particles of VLDL may then be only partially metabolized, resulting in high concentrations of atherogenic intermediate density lipoprotein (IDL) particles, and low rates of formation of high density lipoproteins (HDL). Furthermore, the rate of clearance of low density lipoprotein (LDL) cholesterol is reduced, thus increasing its plasma concentration. The role of glycosylation of the apolipoproteins in causing these abnormalities remains to be elucidated.

These abnormalities are, however, those of relative insulin deficiency. In the well-controlled Type 1 diabetic patient conversion of VLDL to HDL may actually be increased, with consequently low–normal levels of plasma triglycerides, and relatively high HDL cholesterol concentrations. The prognostic

Table 5.7 Abnormalities of lipoprotein metabolism in people with diabetes

Lipoprotein	Poorly controlled (all patients)	Tightly controlled (insulin-treated)
VLDL	Production increased Clearance decreased Triglyceride enriched	Production increased
LDL	Clearance decreased Triglyceride enriched	Normal
HDL	Formation decreased Clearance increased	Formation increased

VLDL : very low density lipoprotein.
LDL : low density lipoprotein
HDL : high density lipoprotein.

significance of these changes is unclear. Lipoprotein levels will however deteriorate with the development of early diabetic nephropathy.

Management of Dyslipidaemia in Diabetes

The principles of dietary management of diabetes, their relationship to arterial disease risk, and targets for plasma lipid levels, are discussed in Chapter 4. Education of patients with respect to low saturated fat, low total fat and high fibre diets should receive due emphasis. Hypertriglyceridaemia often responds very well to the reduction in free sugar intake advised for general management of the diabetes.

Because of the increased risks of major vessel disease in people with diabetes, the threshold of lipid concentrations for the introduction of hypolipidaemic agents should be lower than in the general population. Fibrate drugs (for example, bezafibrate, gemfibrozil) appear to offer the most beneficial action in correction of the abnormal lipid profiles of Type 2 diabetes, particularly with respect to disturbed VLDL metabolism. Nicotinic acid derivatives (for example, acipimox) are useful second line or supplementary agents. Fish oils tend to decrease glucose tolerance, and are hence contraindicated, as are exchange resins as these tend to increase plasma triglyceride concentrations. The role of HMG CoA reductase inhibitors in diabetes has yet to be defined, but they appear promising where hypercholesterolaemia is accompanied by moderate hypertriglyceridaemia.

Skin Conditions in Diabetes

Diabetes is associated with a number of skin conditions, few of which will present diagnostic difficulties (Table 5.8). Injection site problems, and diabetic dermopathy, are discussed in Chapters 4 and 2, respectively. More generalized lipodystrophy should alert the observer to the possibility of a syndrome of insulin resistance, and similarly acanthosis nigricans to the possibility of insulin receptor abnormalities. Plasma insulin and C-peptide concentrations will be markedly raised in these conditions. Other rarities include the migratory necrotizing rash associated with a pancreatic glucagonoma (Chapter 6).

Skin abscesses and furunculosis will usually imply poor leucocyte function as a result of very poor metabolic control. In such patients marked glycosuria may also result in balanitis or vulval candidiasis. Intertrigo is common in obese diabetic patients. Foot infections are discussed in Chapter 2.

Necrobiosis lipoidica is a chronic disfiguring skin condition, usually affecting the skin over the shins, and occurring characteristically in broadly circular papular lesions, which enlarge and may ulcerate and fibrose. The plaques may appear before diabetes is diagnosed, and their aetiology is unclear. They are particularly associated with Type 1 diabetes and are more common in women. They are resistant to local therapy, but skin grafting is sometimes successful.

Table 5.8 Dermatological conditions found in people with diabetes

Infections
Pyogenic infections
Fungal infections
Vulval candidiasis
Balanitis
Intertrigo
Injection site problems
Lipoatrophy
Thickening
Lipohypertrophy
Allergic reactions
Reactions to spirit
Infection
Neuropathic/arterial problem
Pressure sores
Foot ulcers
Diabetes-associated conditions
Acanthosis nigricans
Haemochromatosis
Xanthoma and xanthalasma
Generalized lipodystrophy
Glucagonoma rash
Specific skin conditions
Necrobiosis lipoidica
Diabetic dermopathy
Granuloma annulare

Granuloma annulare is an uncommon condition, but seen more commonly in people with diabetes.

Infections and Diabetes

A number of infections are more common in people with diabetes (Table 5.9). Those associated with the renal tract or feet are discussed in Chapter 2. Infective problems usually reflect very poor metabolic control, with glycosylated haemoglobin concentrations above 6 SD from the normal mean. Indeed some of the rarer invasive fungal conditions are generally associated with extremely poor control and a degree of ketosis. It is well recognized that in these circumstances leucocyte function is depressed, but the precise metabolic cause of the impaired function is unclear.

Any invasive fungal condition should raise the suspicion of diabetes, particularly if no other reason is known for the patient to have poor immune responses. The classic association is with mucormycosis, but invasive pulmonary aspergillosis (secondary to tuberculous damage) is perhaps more common. In both cases attention should be given to classical management by surgery

Table 5.9 Infections particularly associated with diabetes

Skin Infected foot ulcers (neuropathic or arterial) Boils, furunculosis Injection site infections Intertrigo Balanitis Vulval irritation (candidal) Surgical wound infections Pressure sores
Urinary tract infections
Pulmonary Tuberculosis Invasive aspergillosis
Sinuses Mucormycosis
Soft tissues Cellulitis (legs) Fournier's gangrene Necrotizing fasciitis Other invasive fungal conditions

and chemotherapy, but at least as important is correction of the metabolic disturbance to restore white cell function.

Other recognized associations are with pulmonary tuberculosis, which may present with brittle diabetes and insulin resistance, and with invasive Pseudomonal otitis externa. Necrotizing fasciitis and Fournier's gangrene are also well described in association with diabetes. Surgical debridement, antibiotics and tight metabolic control may be life-saving in these conditions.

Further Reading

Crace, C.J. (1989). How does maternal diabetes disrupt embryonic and fetal development? *Diabetic Medicine* **6**, 387.

Hare, J.W. (ed.) (1989). *Diabetes Complicating Pregnancy*. Alan Liss, New York.

Baum, J.D. and Kinmonth, A-L. (eds), (1985). *Care of the Child with Diabetes*. Churchill Livingstone, Edinburgh.

Alberti, K.G.M.M. (1989). Diabetic emergencies. In *Diabetes. British Medical Bulletin*, volume **45 (1)** pp. 242–263. Edited by Leslie, R.D.G.

Alberti, K.G.M.M. and Marshall, S.M. (1988). Diabetes and surgery. In *Diabetes Annual 4*, pp. 248–271. Edited by Alberti, K.G.M.M. and Krall, L.P. Elsevier, Amsterdam.

Betteridge, D.J. (1989). Lipids, diabetes and vascular disease. *Diabetic Medicine* **3**, 195.

6

GUT ASSOCIATED PEPTIDE HORMONES

The APUD System and Multiple Endocrine Neoplasia

While the existence of some gut hormones (for example, secretin, gastrin, cholecystokinin, insulin) has been known for many decades, and while some of these peptides were known from their roles in gut physiology, it is only in recent years that the extent of the galaxy of gut and pancreatic peptides has been appreciated. For many of these peptides, however, their significance in gut physiology or in the regulation of metabolism or of feeding behaviour remains unclear, and in many the delineating line between a hormone and a neurotransmitter remains blurred. Indeed many are found both in the gut and the brain, and appear to exert their functions neither at a distance via the blood nor across a classical synapse, but rather locally by diffusion (so-called paracrine effects).

It was previously suggested that these peptides were secreted by cells that had an embryological origin in neural crest tissue. However, anatomical and grafting studies of embryos have now established that this cannot be the case, and their origin is now believed to be from budding of the endoderm.

The clinical significance of many of these peptides is generally limited to hormone secreting tumours, or less commonly hyperplasia. Deficiency syndromes are barely recognized or of any obvious clinical consequence, with the single overwhelming exception of insulin in diabetes mellitus. Indeed insulin also dwarfs other gut peptides in terms of the clinical resources devoted to the investigation and management of possible insulin-secreting tumours. By contrast, many gut hormones have never been described as major products of pancreatic or gut tumours (Table 6.1), and will not be further discussed here.

It has been fashionable to classify the cell types producing gut hormones as belonging to a single group on the basis of histochemical studies that demonstrate the universal presence of neurone-specific enolase, and leading to the terminology 'APUD cells' (Amine Precursor Uptake and/or Decarboxylation). The clinical rationale for this is helpful only in that it emphasizes that many tumours secrete more than one of the series of peptide hormones. In particular many endocrine tumours of the pancreas or gut secrete pancreatic polypeptide but because this hormone has no clinical effects even when present

160 Gut Associated Peptide Hormones

Table 6.1 Gut-associated peptides

Produced by tumours and causing symptoms Insulin Glucagon Somatostatin Gastrin Vasoactive intestinal peptide
Detected in tumours but of uncertain significance Peptide histidine isoleucine Motilin Neurotensin
Produced by many tumours but not causing symptoms Pancreatic polypeptide
Not secreted from tumours in significant amounts Secretin Cholecystokinin Gastric inhibitory peptide Bombesin Encephalins Endorphins
Secreted by gut–pancreas tumours, but not usually found there ACTH and ACTH-related Calcitonin Growth hormone releasing factors

in the circulation in very high concentrations, it is of only diagnostic significance. Furthermore, gut and pancreatic tumours can secrete clinically significant quantities of other hormones, including corticotrophin-related peptides.

Other major associations of APUD cell tumours are as part of the multiple endocrine adenoma syndromes (Table 6.2). The classical involvement here is of pancreatic endocrine tumours in multiple endocrine neoplasia Type 1 (MEN1, with pituitary adenomas and parathyroid adenoma or hyperplasia), an association particularly well described for gastrinomas. Carcinoid tumours may, however, occur both in MEN1 and MEN2 (the latter with medullary thyroid carcinoma, parathyroid hyperplasia and phaeochromocytoma), while confusingly patients with gastrinomas and MEN1 occasionally develop phaeochromocytomas. Clinically the issue can be further complicated by the occurrence of calcitonin-secreting pancreatic tumours.

Table 6.2 Syndromes of multiple endocrine neoplasia (MEN)

MEN 1	MEN 2A	MEN 2B

Parathyroid adenoma(ta)
Anterior pituitary adenoma
   (often chromophobe)
Pancreatic adenoma
	Medullary thyroid
	   carcinoma
	Phaeochromocytoma
	(Parathyroid adenoma)
		Medullary thyroid
		   carcinoma
		Phaeochromocytoma
		Mucosal abnormalities
		Marfanoid habitus

Both MEN1 and MEN2 appear to have dominant inheritance, and have been mapped to chromosomes 11 and 10. The finding of two tumours in any one patient is therefore an indication for regular family screening in particular for hypercalcaemia. If one of these tumours is of gut or pancreatic origin the possibility of adenomas of the other series should be considered.

As a result of these difficulties the most satisfactory classification of gut associated endocrine tumours, which in any case are most commonly found in the pancreas, is by the clinical syndrome they cause, usually but not always as a consequence of their major hormone product. Failure to secrete significant quantities of a systemically active hormone will result in a 'cold' endocrine tumour, which will become evident only through its mass or metastatic effects, and which may even then be difficult to identify histologically.

Insulin Hypersecretion

Introduction

Primary hypersecretion of insulin occurs in two clinical conditions, namely, nesidioblastosis and islet B-cell tumours, which are only likely to give problems of differential diagnosis in the young child. The major clinical manifestation of insulin hypersecretion, hypoglycaemia, can however cause significant diagnostic problems, either because it may be due to other metabolic disorders, or because the symptomatology may be similar to unrelated conditions. As a result relatively large numbers of patients undergo investigation for possible insulin hypersecretion, and most do not turn out to have significant pancreatic pathology. Fortunately improvements in radioimmunoassay techniques have significantly refined the diagnostic tools, while advances in imaging techniques have greatly improved the chances of localizing discrete pancreatic lesions.

Clinical Manifestations of Hypoglycaemia

The classical manifestations of hypoglycaemia are well recognized, and usually divided into those due to sympathetic arousal (for example, tremor, cold sweating, hunger, fear, palpitations) and those due to neuroglycopenia (for example, confusion, forgetfulness, disorientation, poor co-ordination). Headache on waking may be a useful pointer. Unfortunately many of these symptoms are both common and non-specific, and where they do occur in other conditions they are often recurrent and worrying to the patient. The symptoms can furthermore be modified by the presence of other conditions such as autonomic neuropathy and arteriosclerosis, or by therapeutic agents such as beta-adrenergic blockers. Hypoglycaemia can precipitate epilepsy in those with a latent EEG abnormality, and prolonged hypoglycaemia can itself cause organic brain damage.

As a result, the possible psychological and behavioural presentations of

Table 6.3 Conditions which may give symptoms or signs similar to those of hypoglycaemia

Imitating sympathetic arousal Anxiety Palpitations and tachycardia Sweating Hyperventilation Shaking Therapeutic or illicit drugs Functional disorders
Imitating neuroglycopenia Headache Confusion/coma Inco-ordination Weakness Epilepsy Transient ischaemic attacks Functional disorders Therapeutic or illicit drugs
In infants Any symptom or sign of being unwell

hypoglycaemia are enormous. Numerically the greatest diagnostic problems are in relation to anxiety syndromes, other neuroses and functional disorders (Table 6.3). Often a careful clinical history will demonstrate that the symptoms are either associated with circumstances likely to exacerbate psychiatric problems (in crowds, for example), or that they sometimes occur at times unlikely to be associated with hypoglycaemia (20–90 min after meals). Other conditions which can mimic hypoglycaemia, but which may be excluded by a careful history or examination, include dumping syndrome, hyperventilation and mitral valve prolapse.

Where hypoglycaemia cannot be excluded by clinical acumen, a provocation test may be necessary to establish the diagnosis. In many patients with islet B-cell tumours simple overnight fasting with measurement of pre-breakfast plasma glucose and insulin (or C-peptide, see below) will confirm the diagnosis. However, this cannot exclude the diagnosis in the many patients with suspect symptoms, and for these a prolonged (72 h) fast remains the most useful test, and one that often uncovers psychological as well as organic problems. Blood samples should be taken 12-hourly for glucose, insulin and C-peptide, and additionally in the event of symptoms. Diagnosis of inappropriate insulin secretion is made when insulin concentrations fail to suppress at a time when glucose concentrations are sub-normal.

Other Causes of Hypoglycaemia

Even when hypoglycaemia is established from blood glucose concentrations, other causes than inappropriate insulin secretion may need to be considered. In the neonate or infant these are mainly metabolic disorders (Table 6.4), but the possibility of high titres of maternal insulin antibodies, or surreptitious insulin or sulphonylurea administration should never be ignored.

Factitious hypoglycaemia is also not uncommon in the adult patient, a useful pointer often being access to medical supplies through hospital or pharmacy work, or a relative with diabetes. Hypoglycaemia induced by covert insulin injection can be distinguished from insulin hypersecretion by the measurement of C-peptide, the connecting peptide cleaved from proinsulin in the process of insulin secretion, and thus delivered in equimolar amounts into the circulation. Sulphonylureas will, however, promote secretion of both insulin and C-peptide, but can be excluded by 24-h urine toxicology screen.

A commoner diagnostic problem is reactive hypoglycaemia, which can be defined as recurrent symptoms in association with low plasma glucose concentrations (<2.5 mmol/l) occurring 2–3 h after meals, especially those containing large quantities of refined carbohydrates. Reactive hypoglycaemia is best diagnosed using a prolonged glucose tolerance test with half-hourly glucose and insulin measurements. In these circumstances insulin secretion is suppressed at the time of hypoglycaemia, and since the hormone has a short plasma half-life (5 min) this is quickly reflected in plasma concentrations. Reactive hypoglycaemia is further distinguished from insulin hypersecretion by the absence of fasting and pre-prandial hypoglycaemia, confirmed if necessary by prolonged fasting.

Table 6.4 Conditions to be considered in the differential diagnosis of confirmed hypoglycaemia

Reactive hypoglycaemia
Idiopathic
Alimentary tract dysfunction
Glucose intolerance
Sulphonylurea therapy
Counter-regulatory hormone deficiency

Primary metabolic disorders
Disorders of glycogen metabolism
Disturbances of gluconeogenesis
Liver failure
Galactosaemia, fructose intolerance
Leucine hypersensitivity

Pharmacological conditions
Insulin administration
Sulphonylurea therapy
Ethanol
Insulin antibodies

Islet B-cell abnormalities
Insulinoma
Islet cell hyperplasia
   Nesidioblastosis
   Maternal diabetes

Reactive hypoglycaemia may occur in association with dumping syndrome, or in its absence with forms of gastric surgery that can be associated with dumping syndrome. It is more common in patients with counter-regulatory hormone deficiencies, and will be exaggerated by meals in which a high percentage of calories are taken as refined carbohydrates.

Interesting but unusual causes of hypoglycaemia, which may be profound and difficult to manage, are mesotheliomas and sometimes carcinomas, particularly retroperitoneal, but not of pancreatic origin. These tumours do not secrete insulin, or insulin-like peptides cross-reacting in the insulin radio-immunoassay. The diagnosis should be suspected where significant fasting hypoglycaemia is associated with suppressed plasma insulin concentrations.

Other causes of hypoglycaemia are glucocorticoid or glucagon deficiency, acute liver failure and excess alcohol intake.

Provocation and Suppression Tests

The role and protocol of the 72-h fast are discussed above. It remains the provocation test of choice, being simple to interpret, useful in patients with functional problems, and long enough for there to be a good chance of intermittent symptoms occurring. Appropriate supervision to prevent access to food or drugs is required.

Other provocation tests use a sulphonylurea (tolbutamide 1 g IV), glucagon (1 mg IV), or a calcium infusion to stimulate insulin secretion, whose plasma concentrations are then measured. With tolbutamide or calcium late hypoglycaemia may also occur when insulin hypersecretion is present. All of these tests give clear results where a significantly increased mass of insulin-secreting tissue is present, but in these patients the diagnosis is anyway easily established by fasting. Discrimination by these tests is not good where the diagnosis is already uncertain.

Suppression tests involve making the patient hypoglycaemic, and demonstrating continuing unphysiological insulin secretion during this hypoglycaemia. They may also offer the possibility of comparison of true hypoglycaemic symptoms with the symptoms complained of by the patient. In order to distinguish endogenous insulin secretion from the insulin needed to obtain hypoglycaemia the test was at first performed using fish insulin injection, but more recently ordinary unmodified insulin has been injected, and endogenous secretion measured as C-peptide. The test is not easy to interpret in marginal cases. Endogenous insulin and C-peptide secretion will fall steadily over 30 min in the normal subject as blood glucose concentrations fall, but C-peptide has a long plasma half-life (30 min), thus making expert interpretation of the falling plasma concentration curve necessary. C-peptide clearance is renal, and the test cannot be used in patients with significant renal impairment.

Localization of Suspected Insulinomas (Fig. 6.1)

If inappropriate insulin secretion has been demonstrated in a patient beyond infancy, then it is overwhelmingly likely that there is a panceatic tumour, most likely an adenoma. Islet B-cell carcinomas are not uncommon, however, but extrapancreatic lesions producing significant amounts of insulin are rare, and islet B-cell hyperplasia has only questionably been described in adulthood. Investigations should therefore be directed to localizing the lesion within the pancreas, while excluding liver and lung metastases.

Pancreatic ultrasonography is an insensitive technique, but is cheap, useful when a lesion is identified, and is generally performed at the time of liver and porta hepatis scanning for metastases. Computerized tomography (CT), with and without contrast, will require multiple cuts at the level of the pancreas, as insulinomas are often at the limits of resolution of this technique. If a lesion is not identified then coeliac axis angiography should be performed, preferably in combination with CT.

Most lesions will be localized by these techniques, but a significant proportion are not. Magnetic resonance imaging may give better resolution than CT. Abdominal CT is, however, useful to exclude any larger extrapancreatic tumour. Endoscopic ultrasonography is available in some centres. Cannulation and contrast injection of the pancreatic duct is probably the next investigation of choice, but carries a significant risk of inducing acute pancreatitis. An

Ultrasonography (including liver and porta hepatis)
↓
Computerized tomography (with multiple cuts)
↓
Selective angiography (with computerized tomography)
↓
Endoscopic pancreatic duct radiography
↓
Endoscopic ultrasonography
↓
Transhepatic multiple venous sampling
↓
Laparotomy (with intraoperative ultrasonography)

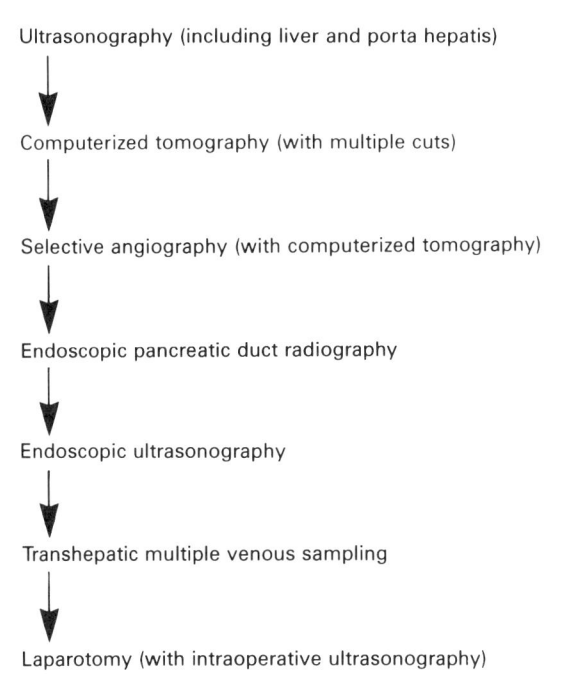

Fig. 6.1 Algorithm for localization of pancreatic endocrine tumours.

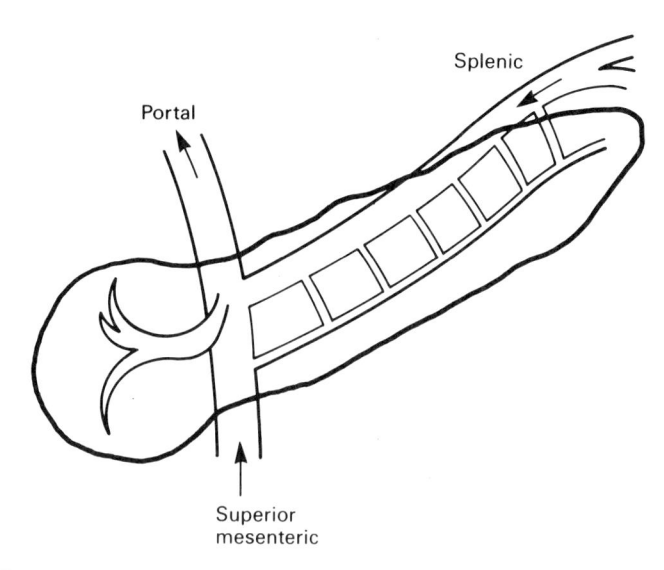

Fig. 6.2 The venous drainage of the pancreas into the splenic, superior mesenteric and portal veins, allows tumour localization by multiple sampling for the secreted peptide.

alternative is to cannulate the portal vein transhepatically, and perform multiple selective venous sampling for insulin from the portal, splenic and superior mesenteric veins (Fig. 6.2).

Failure to localize the lesion by these techniques should, after further review of the diagnosis, be followed by laparotomy if symptoms justify it. Intraoperative ultrasonography of the pancreas may then be useful.

Medical Management of Insulin Hypersecretion

Dietary measures are helpful in many patients, and are directed to ensuring as continuous a delivery of glucose into the circulation as possible, without periods of acute stimulation of islet B-cells. The diet should therefore be free of added mono- or disaccharides, but contain large amounts of complexed carbohydrate and fibre, taken as frequently as possible. Snacks may be necessary during the night. Viscous fibres which significantly delay intestinal absorption may be given in pharmacological forms, for example, as guar tablets.

Diazoxide is the most widely used hyperglycaemic agent, apparently working by both inhibition of insulin secretion and effects on glucose metabolism. In many patients with only mild degrees of hypoglycaemia, diazoxide can be very effective in the longer term, and may be the treatment of choice in the elderly. Fluid retention and hair growth may however limit treatment. Glucocorticoids in higher doses induce insulin resistance and may be useful in some patients, but glucagon therapy is limited to intravenous use and may induce further

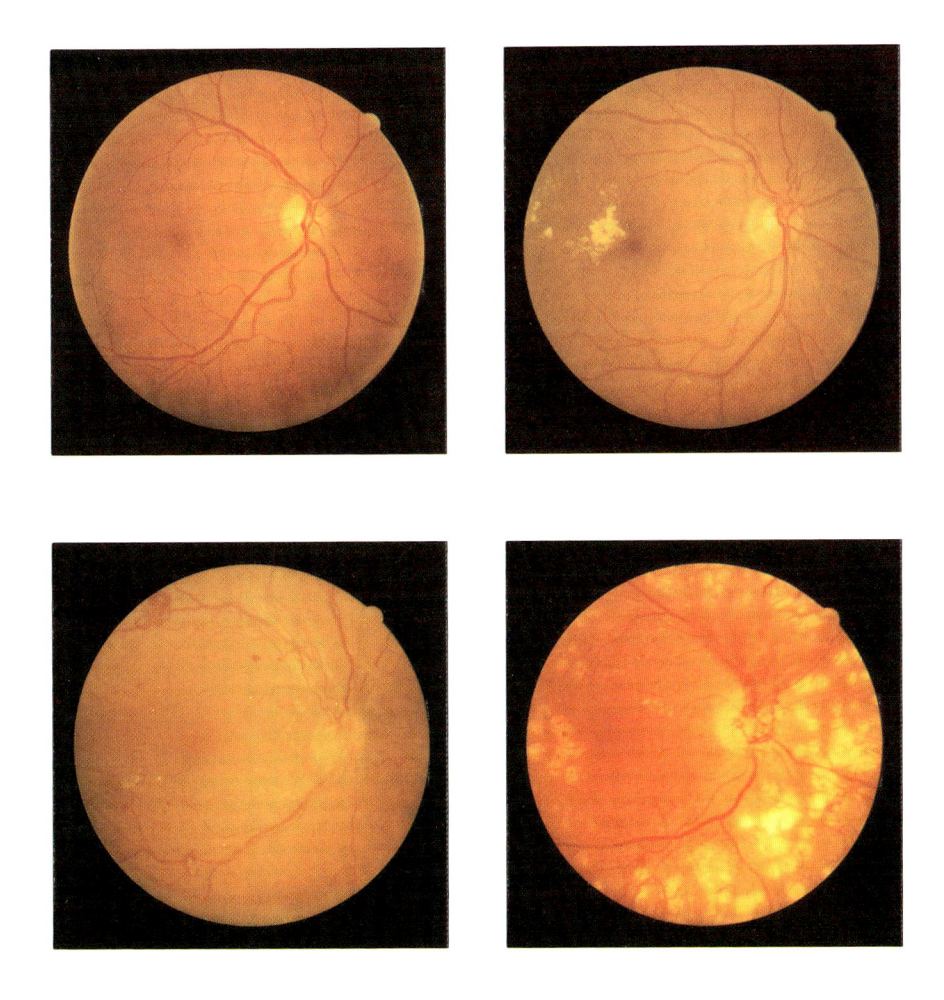

Fig. 2.2 Examples of diabetic retinopathy. *Top left:* Maculopathy with minimal retinopathy. Most of the retina appears normal. Careful inspection of the macular reveals a microaneurysm and a small hard exudate. Another microaneurysm is present above and to the right of the macula. Visual acuity had dropped one line over the last year. *Top Right:* Hard exudates in a typically circinate pattern, temporal to the macula, and threatening it. Plasma will be leaking from a single point in the centre of the ring. Visual acuity is as yet still normal. *Bottom left:* Proliferative retinopathy. New vessels are visible growing both upwards from the disk, and in the periphery (top left). Two areas of infarction surrounded by haemorrhage are seen bottom left, together with scattered microaneurysms and retinal haemorrhages. *Bottom right:* Laser photocoagulation scars are seen throughout the peripheral retina. Venous abnormalities, particularly microaneurysms, retinal haemorrhages, and new vessels are extensive. A leash of new vessels is growing upwards and forwards from the optic disk, and is hence out of focus.

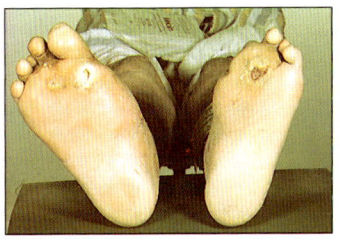

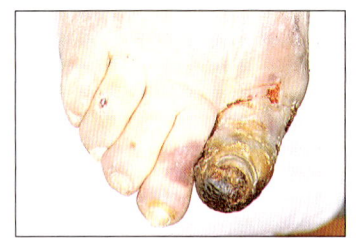

Fig. 2.3 Examples of neuropathic *(a)* and vascular ulceration *(b)*. Neuropathic ulcers are typically on the plantar sufaces of the foot, in a site of high pressure on standing or walking, and is often covered by callus. Removal of the pressure will usually result in quite rapid healing. Vascular ulceration typically occurs distally at the toes, and proceeds to ischaemia and mummification. Ulceration in areas of thin skin over the dorsal aspects of the toes or the sides of the feet is often mixed in aetiology, but will generally heal slowly provided infection is superficial.

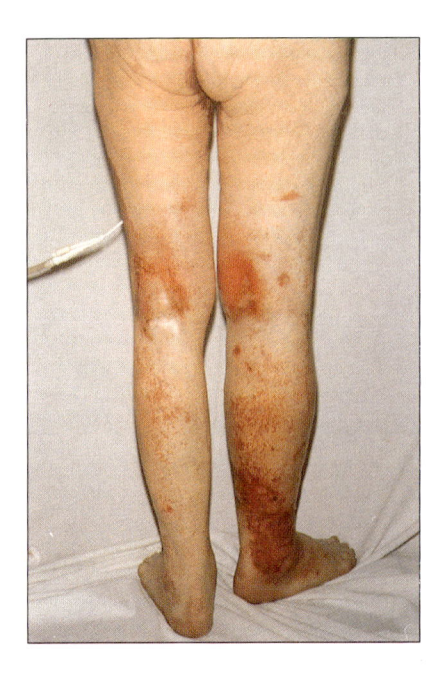

Fig. 6.3 A glucagonoma associated skin rash. Features of the rash are quite variable. Any erythematous or necrotizing rash between waist and knees should arouse suspicion in someone with diabetes, particularly if the rash is migratory.

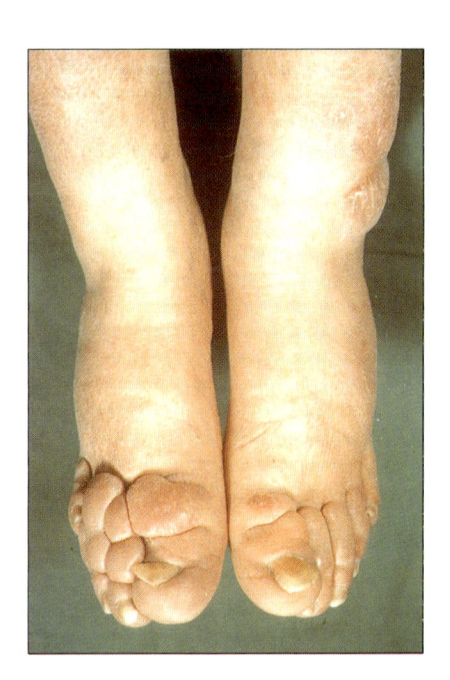

Fig. 8.12 Pretibial myxoedema..

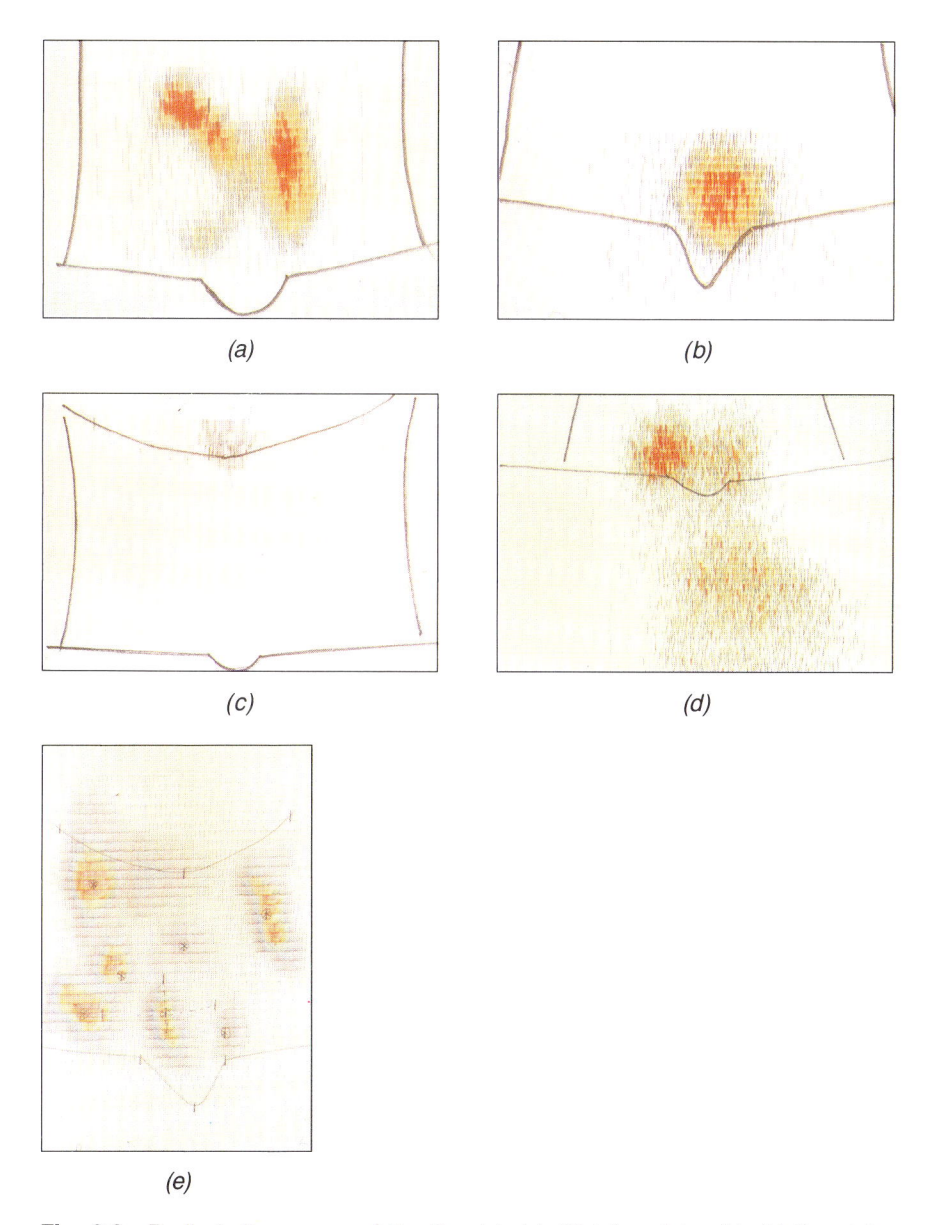

Fig. 8.9 Radio-iodine scans of the thyroid. *(a)* 'Cold' nodule. *(b)* 'Hot' nodule. *(c)* Ectopic tyroid tissue (lingual). *(d)* Multinodular goitre with retrosternal extension. *(e)* Metastatic thyroid carcinoma involving local lymph glands. Reproduced courtesy of the Department of Medical Physics, Newcastle General Hospital.

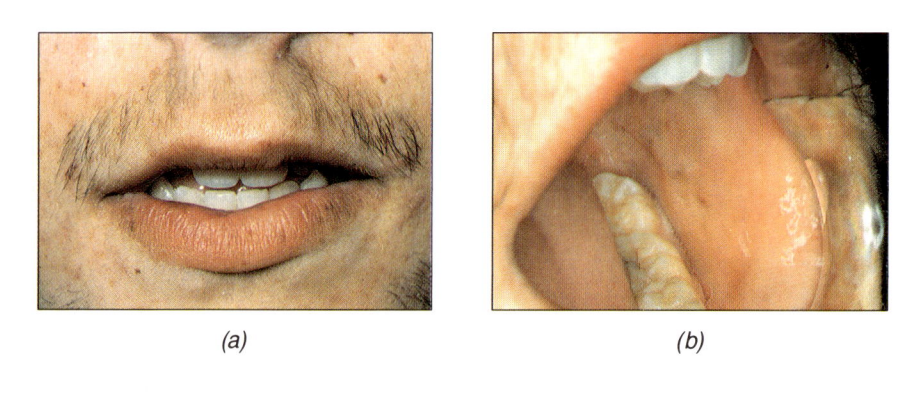

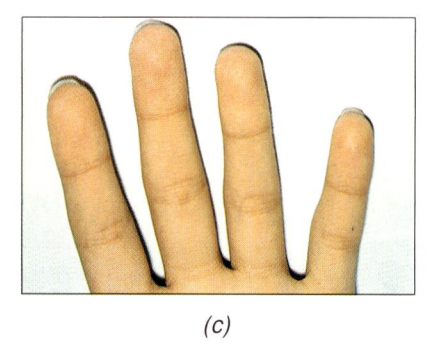

Fig. 9.4 Clinical features of Addison's disease. Increased pigmentation of *(a)* Lips and face. *(b)* Buccal mucosa. *(c)* Palmar creases.

insulin secretion. Experience with long-acting somatostatin analogues is limited as yet.

Islet B-cells in many species are unusually sensitive to the cytotoxic effects of the drug streptozotocin, which is however also rather nephrotoxic. To avoid this as far as possible it is given in repeated small doses, intravenously over several days, for example, as 500 mg/m^2 repeated five times, in the fluid replete patient. This is the therapy of choice in metastatic insulinoma, and may give beneficial results for many months. Experience with other cytotoxic agents is limited, and, apart from the combination of streptozotocin with 5-fluorouracil, their benefit is uncertain.

Nesidioblastosis

This condition, recognized in infancy up to about two years of age, is characterized by hypertrophy and increased number of pancreatic islets throughout the gland. Its cause is uncertain, but it has been suggested that it is secondary to deficiency of somatostatin production by islet D-cells. Because of the age of the patients clinical presentation may be non-specific, and possibly even as sudden infant death syndrome. The finding of hypoglycaemia in infancy leads to the difficult differential diagnosis of inherited metabolic disorders or insulinoma. Medical management of nesidioblastosis is as far as possible as for insulinoma, but the condition often requires radical pancreatic resection.

Abnormalities of Glucagon Secretion

Introduction

Glucagon is the second peptide, in terms of physiological and clinical significance, produced by the pancreatic islets. The islet A-cells which produce glucagon are situated around the periphery of the islet in a layer over the B-cells, but the significance of this is not known. Glucagon becomes important in the mobilization of liver glycogen with fasting and exercise, its secretion being chiefly controlled by catecholamines and the autonomic nervous system. Glucagon deficiency is, however, only recognized in patients with Type 1 diabetes mellitus of more than five years' duration, in whom the response to hypoglycaemia induced by injected insulin is often severely blunted. The clinical importance of glucagon is otherwise manifested only in the rare case of a pancreatic tumour, usually a carcinoma, producing large amounts of the hormone.

Clinical Features of Glucagonoma Syndrome

Glucagonomas are often clinically silent until well advanced, because the major action of the hormone in promoting hyperglycaemia is generally countered by increased insulin secretion. Glucose intolerance, and later diabetes, may therefore be slow to appear, and may not be marked even in patients with other evidence of the condition. The diabetes will, however, often progress to being insulin requiring.

The most characteristic lesion is a necrolytic migratory erythematous rash, classically described as being over the buttocks and perineum, less commonly on other parts of the legs or trunk, and sometimes associated with lesions elsewhere (Figure 6.3).

Other clinical features may include anaemia, mild tachycardia, glossitis, mild diarrhoea with hypokalaemia, and general malaise and weight loss. Venous thrombosis and consequent pulmonary embolism can be troublesome. Hypoaminoacidaemia is usual, and plasma pancreatic polypeptide concentrations will be raised in 50% of patients.

The diagnosis is made by radioimmunoassay of glucagon, which is usually markedly elevated by the time of clinical presentation.

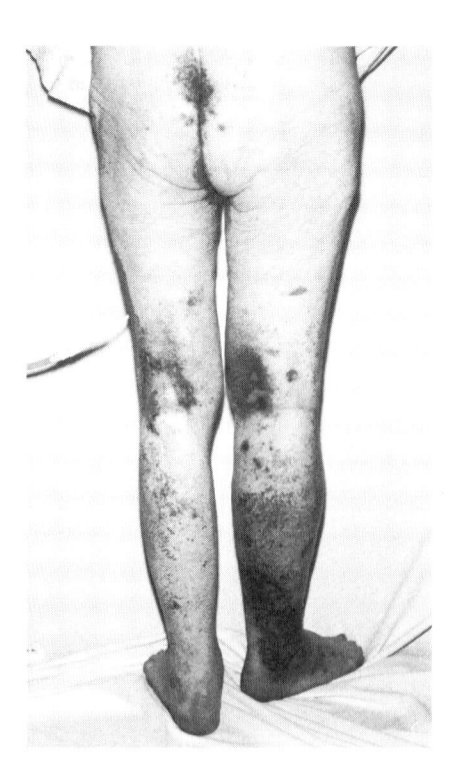

Fig. 6.3 A glucagoma associated skin rash. *See also* colour plate between pages 166 and 167. Features of the rash are quite variable. Any erythematous or necrotizing rash between waist and knees should arouse suspicion in someone with diabetes, particularly if the rash is migratory.

Localization of Glucagonoma

Localization of a glucagonoma should follow the guidelines given above for an insulinoma. As the lesions are usually more advanced, localization is however generally easier.

Management of Glucagonoma

Management will be surgical even if the lesion is believed to have metastasized beyond the pancreas, as the troublesome dermatological condition may then remit. The prognosis should, however, be guarded even in the absence of evidence of lymphatic or hepatic secondaries. Where hepatic secondaries are present they may respond to embolization. Somatostatin analogues may have a greater role in the management of inoperable glucagonoma than insulinoma. The tumours are less sensitive to streptozotocin, suggesting that local administration (coeliac axis) might be preferable, but with insulin-dependent diabetes as an inevitable consequence. The agent dimethyl-trianzenoimidazole-carboxamide (DTIC) has been reported to induce useful responses in some cases of pancreatic endocrine tumours, in particular glucagonoma.

Abnormalities of Somatostatin Secretion

Somatostatin is found in other parts of the body than the islet D-cells in which it is found in the pancreas, but tumours producing this small peptide hormone generally originate from the pancreas and gut. Medullary carcinoma of the thyroid can, however, also produce significant amounts of somatostatin. Somatostatin inhibits insulin and particularly glucagon secretion with a high potency, as well as other hormones, but its physiological significance is still not well understood. Islet D-cells form only a small proportion of islet mass, and somatostatin-secreting tumours are correspondingly rare.

Somatostatin deficiency has been suggested as a possible cause of the condition of insulin hypersecretion of infancy known as nesidioblastosis.

Somatostatin hypersecretion has been associated with mild diabetes mellitus, cholelithiasis, hypochlorhydria and steatorrhoea, but none of these are constant features. The condition is often diagnosed incidentally at cholecystectomy. General malaise, weight loss and anaemia may be present. Plasma somatostatin concentrations will be raised, but much of the hormone is often present as high molecular weight forms, believed to be inactive. The approach to tumour localization and management follow those suggested above for insulinoma, but the role of drug therapy has not been defined.

170   Gut Associated Peptide Hormones

The VIPoma Syndrome

The occurrence of episodic watery diarrhoea, a pancreatic tumour and hypochlorhydria, with high plasma vasoactive intestinal polypeptide concentrations is known as the VIPoma syndrome. In childhood the peptide may be secreted from a neuroblastoma to give the same syndrome. Co-secretion of pancreatic polypeptide is usual.

The syndrome is associated with profound electrolyte disturbance, in which life-threatening hypokalaemia occurs together with a metabolic acidosis secondary to bicarbonate loss. In earlier stages, however, gastric aspiration may be helpful in distinguishing the condition from Zollinger–Ellison syndrome (see below). Hyperglycaemia and hypercalcaemia are also common, although the extent to which the latter may be a manifestation of familial multiple endocrine adenomatosis Type 1 is unclear.

Localization and management are generally as for other endocrine pancreatic tumours. The lesion may be single and discrete, or multiple, or metastatic. Removal of tumour mass may in any case palliate the diarrhoea.

Medical treatment to control fluid and electrolyte abnormalities should be with the oral glucose–electrolyte formulae used for the management of infective diarrhoea, although specific therapy for hypokalaemia and acidosis may also be necessary. Amongst pharmacological agents only high doses of prednisolone have been shown to have a useful consistent effect on the diarrhoea. Cytotoxic drug therapy has generally followed the guidelines established for malignant insulinoma.

Gastrinoma (Zollinger–Ellison syndrome)

Introduction

The Zollinger–Ellison syndrome was first recognized as an association between chronic or recurrent peptic ulcer disease, often with complications, and the presence of a pancreatic tumour or tumours. The ability to measure gastrin allowed confirmation that these tumours secreted large amounts of the hormone, which is a physiological regulator of gastric hydrogen ion secretion in response to meals. Prior to gastrin assay the nature of the tumour was something of a puzzle as gastrin-secreting cells are not usually found in the pancreas, and at the time only insulin-producing endocrine tumours were known to occur in the gland. It has since become clear that only 85% of gastrinomas are located in the pancreas, most of the remainder being in the wall of the duodenum or stomach, although there are isolated reports of tumours in other sites.

Before the advent of H_2-antagonists recurrent peptic ulcer disease was troublesome and common, and a diagnosis of gastrinoma relevant as it suggested the need for total gastrectomy, and as a possible means of palliation. Gastrinomas are however uncommon, and the need for damaging gastric surgery is now absent. As yet there is little evidence of late diagnosis of malignant gastrinoma as a result of use of H_2-antagonists, but patients needing high doses for maintenance therapy should arouse clinical suspicion. Metastasis is common, and is generally to the liver.

A gastrinoma is the commonest pancreatic component of familial multiple endocrine neoplasia Type 1 (MEN 1), when the pancreatic tumours are often multiple. The parathyroid element is then generally manifested as hyperplasia of all four glands. Evidence of other endocrine tumours should be sought in all patients.

Clinical features

The cardinal feature is long-standing and often progressive peptic ulcer disease, asymptomatic patients only having been described on screening families with MEN1. Where gastric acid secretion is uncontrolled abdominal pain and diarrheoa may be a feature, but these will respond to H_2-antagonists. In contrast to VIPomas the diarrhoea is not associated with marked electrolyte disturbance. High rates of acid secretion are associated with a large stomach volume, and prominent gastric mucosal folds.

Co-secretion of pancreatic polypeptide can be a useful marker. Co-secretion of corticotrophin-like hormones, insulin and chorionic gonadotrophin have also been described. Hypercalcaemia should suggest the possibility of parathyroid hyperplasia.

Diagnosis

If a clearly elevated fasting plasma gastrin level can be measured on two occasions at times of high gastric acid secretion then the diagnosis is secure. Unfortunately moderate elevations of fasting plasma gastrin can occur in other conditions, particularly when gastric acid secretion is in some way inhibited (for example, pernicious anaemia, H_2-antagonists, post-vagotomy, atrophic gastritis). The assay is rather imprecise in some laboratories, and will need to measure the different molecular forms of gastrin. Furthermore, the certainty of fasting is not always obtained. Measurement of a basal gastric acid secretion rate above 15 mmol/h may be helpful, but is only usefully specific above 25 mmol/h. Detection of a rise in gastrin concentrations after injection of secretin, or an abnormal response to calcium infusion, is generally possible when gastrin levels are already diagnostically high, but often unhelpful in marginal cases.

Localization of gastrinomas

Localization of pancreatic tumours should follow the guidelines set out above for insulinomas. Endoscopy of the stomach and duodenum is, however, a useful early investigation, with careful inspection of the lining of both areas for sub-mucosal tumours.

Management of Gastrinomas

Single adenomas should be removed, but the possibility of multiple lesions or metastases is high. As resultant peptic ulcer disease can now be generally managed with drug therapy, the indication for debulking of the tumour has weakened. Hepatic secondaries may be susceptible to embolization, and there is some sensitivity to streptozotocin (see insulinomas). Total gastrectomy should no longer be necessary.

Carcinoid Syndrome

Introduction

Carcinoid tumours can arise in any tissue derived from the embryonic gut, and even very rarely the gonads. Tumours arising from the lung or thyroid are, however, much less common than those from the gut itself, where the majority are found in the terminal ileum and appendix. Many carcinoids of the appendix, and usually those of the colon and rectum, are devoid of significant secretory products, and may be detected only through mass effects or incidentally at autopsy.

Carcinoids are sometimes associated with gastrinomas and parathyroid hyperplasia in MEN1 but also occur together with the tumours of MEN2. Pancreatic carcinoid tumours may produce clinically significant amounts of corticotrophin-related hormones.

The major secretory product of these tumours is 5-hydroxytryptamine (serotonin, 5-HT), and although carcinoids are usually classified with endocrine tumours, their other products tend to be mast cell associated (histamine, kallekrein) rather than those of pancreatic endocrine tumours. Histochemistry may however, show the presence of pancreatic polypeptide and vasoactive intestinal polypeptide (VIP). 5-Hydroxytryptamine is avidly taken up by the liver, so that tumours of gut or pancreatic origin which have not metastasized to the liver are generally silent. The clinical course of these tumours is nevertheless slow, and even hepatic metastases are often amenable to surgical resection.

Clinical Features of Carcinoid Syndrome (Table 6.5)

The classical feature of carcinoid with liver metastases is flushing with hypotension, but the character and duration of the flushing are variable in nature and time, and to some extent dependent on the site of the primary lesion. The flush tends to be most prominent over the head and neck. With peripheral vasodilatation the patient may have an intense feeling of heat. The

Table 6.5 Clinical features of the carcinoid syndrome

Flush-associated symptoms and signs
Sensation of intense heat over the face
Systolic hypotension
Wheezing
Reflex adrenergic effects
    Tachycardia
    Palpitations
    Distress
Facial oedema
Lacrimation

Precipitants of flushing
Ethanol ingestion
Some foods
? Emotion

Other problems
Diarrhoea
Facial telangiectasia
Cardiac valvular problems
Abdominal/hepatic pain
Ectopic ACTH syndrome
Associated parathyroid (and other) tumours

concomitant fall in blood pressure may be associated with palpitations due to reflex tachycardia. Significant wheezing is reported by some patients. These disturbing sensations will often be exacerbated by a secondary adrenergic response and anxiety. Emotional stress and alcohol are reported as precipitating flushing.

Tumours of gastric origin may be more likely to produce skin wheals perhaps because of a greater tendency to produce histamine. Tumours of bronchial origin tend to cause less episodic symptoms.

A curiosity that is not uncommon is scarring of the valves of the right side of the heart, with consequent functional abnormalities that can be clinically significant if tricuspid incompetence and pulmonary stenosis occur together. Whatever agent is responsible for this is presumably removed by the lungs, since left-sided valvular problems may be found with bronchial carcinoids.

Carcinoids may cause mass effects including right hypochondrial pain from liver secondaries, and intestinal obstruction. Watery diarrhoea is a prominent symptom in some patients, but the extent to which this is due to secretion of a further peptide hormone such as motilin is unclear. Anorexia and consequent weight loss with associated problems such as anaemia occur with advanced disease.

Diagnosis of Carcinoid Syndrome

Most of the 5-HT is converted through monoamine oxidase to a hydroxyindole-acetaldehyde and thence to 5-hydroxyindole acetic acid (5-HIAA). This can be measured in 24-h urine collections, and be followed as a marker of progression of the condition. Intake of bananas (which contain 5-HT) and monoamine oxidase inhibitors will interfere with the test, while some phenothiazine metabolites interfere with the assay. Measurement of pancreatic polypeptide may be helpful, and plasma calcium should be checked. Assay of other plasma hormone concentrations (for example, calcitonin, motilin, ACTH, glucagon, insulin) may be contributory.

Ultrasonography and isotope scans may be useful in defining the number of hepatic metastases if surgery or embolization is contemplated. Liver biopsy with silver staining can be used to confirm the diagnosis. Radiological investigations and laparotomy may be needed to locate the primary lesion. In the absence of hepatic lesions a search for a bronchial, thyroid, gonadal or other tumour may lead to a curative procedure.

Management of Carcinoid Syndrome

Surgical and embolic procedures may be useful as described above. The role of cytotoxic therapy is uncertain, largely because the long course of the condition makes outcome difficult to measure. Some success has been claimed for mixtures of streptozotocin and 5-fluorouracil.

The role of somatostatin analogues is not established, but intravenous infusion of the native peptide may be helpful in carcinoid crises, together with high-dose steroids.

Symptomatic medical treatment may result in a better quality of life than cytotoxic therapy, with a life prognosis of some years. Symptoms believed to be due to 5HT may respond to cyproheptadine or, with caution, methysergide. Alpha-adrenergic blockers are also said to be helpful. Where histamine is believed to be a major problem then H_1-antagonists should be used. Loperamide may be helpful where diarrhoea is present, and fluid and electrolyte correction arranged as necessary.

Further Reading

Bloom, S.R. and Polak, J.M. (1980). VIPomas. In *Vasoactive Intestinal Peptides*, p. 457. Edited by Said, S.I. Raven Press, New York.

Larsson, L-I., Holst, J.J., Kuhl, C. *et al.* (1977). Pancreatic somatostatinoma: Clinical features and physiological implications. *Lancet* **i**, 666.

McCarthy, D.M. and Jensen, R.T. (1985). Zollinger–Ellison syndrome—current issues. In *Hormone Producing Tumors of the Gastrointestinal Tract*. Edited by Cohen, M. and Soloway, R.D. Churchill Livingstone, New York.

Mallinson, C.N., Bloom, S.R., Warin, A.P. *et al.* (1974). A glucagonoma syndrome. *Lancet* **ii**, 1.

Thakker, R.V. and Ponder, B.A.J. (1988). Multiple endocrine neoplasia. *Ballière's Clinics in Endocrinology and Metabolism* **2**, 1031.

7

THE HYPOTHALAMUS AND PITUITARY

A knowledge of the normal anatomy and physiology of the hypothalamus and pituitary and of the functional relationships with various target organs is essential to a proper understanding of the conditions of hormone excess or deficiency that occur in pathological states.

Development and Anatomy

The pituitary gland consists of anterior and posterior lobes which are of different embryonic origin. The anterior lobe develops from Rathke's pouch, an ectodermal diverticulum in the floor of the primitive oro-pharynx, whereas the posterior lobe derives from the neural tissue of the forebrain. Both parts of the future pituitary separate from their original sites of development and become juxtaposed, but the posterior lobe retains its neural connections with the hypothalamus whereas the anterior lobe is connected by a vascular network, the hypophyseal portal vessels, in the pituitary stalk (Fig. 7.1). In the adult the pituitary is situated at the base of the brain, protected by the sphenoid bone in which it is recessed. The pituitary fossa or sella turcica can be identified on a plain X-ray of the skull as an approximately spherical sac with an open neck, bounded by the anterior and posterior clinoid processes. Laterally the pituitary is bounded by the cavernous sinus on the lateral wall of which run the 3rd, 4th and 6th cranial nerves. Superiorly the fossa is roofed by the dura mater forming the diaphragma sella through which passes the pituitary stalk. The optic nerves cross at the optic chiasm just above the diaphragma sella and above this lies the hypothalamus and the floor of the third ventricle (Fig. 7.2).

Pressure Effects of Pituitary Tumours

Headache may be a feature of pituitary tumours even when they are not very large and the exact mechanism is not always clear. Stretching of the dura over the tumour may occur but this is usually associated with suprasellar extension. A large suprasellar extension will impinge on the optic chiasm causing

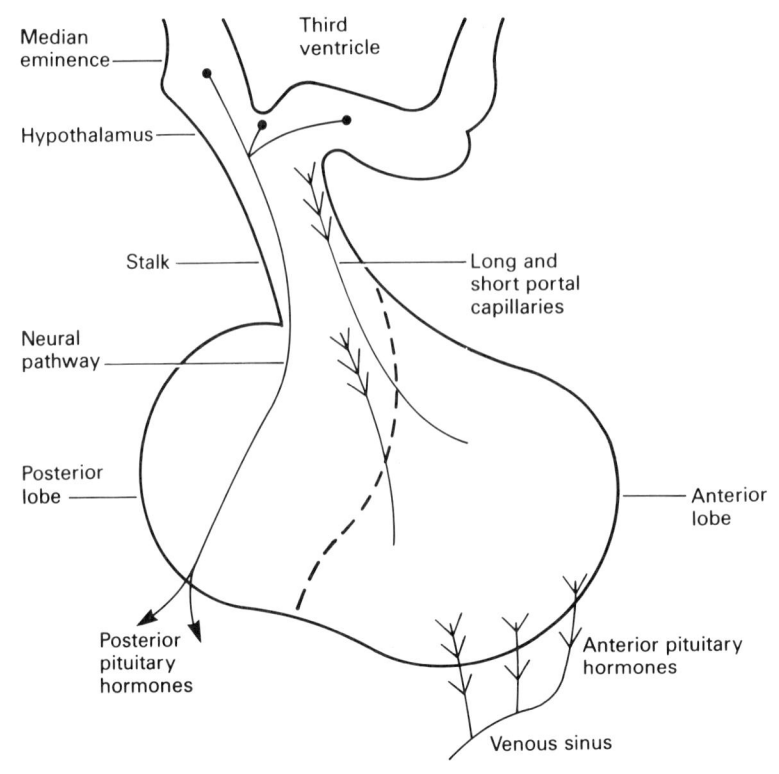

Fig. 7.1 Schematic representation of the anatomical relationship of the hypothalamus and pituitary.

compression of the medial nerve fibres where they cross to supply the medial aspects of the opposite retinae leading to bitemporal hemianopia (Fig. 7.3). The exact visual field defect will depend on the precise size and direction of growth of the tumour. Formal testing of the visual fields is undertaken using a Bjerrums screen. Long-standing pressure on the optic chiasm will result in optic atrophy and blindness which may not be reversible by surgical decompression. Rarely lateral extension of a pituitary tumour into the wall of the cavernous sinus may cause pressure on the 4th and 6th cranial nerves leading to oculomotor palsies. Downward extension of a tumour into the sphenoid sinus is quite common but has to be very extensive to cause CSF rhinorrhoea. Large tumours are commonly found in patients with acromegaly, with functionless pituitary tumours and with some prolactinomas, which present late in their natural history. They are uncommon in patients with Cushing's disease and others who present earlier.

Radiology of the Pituitary

Lateral X-ray of the skull may reveal ballooning of the fossa with erosion of the clinoid processes or of the floor of the fossa if the tumour extends downwards

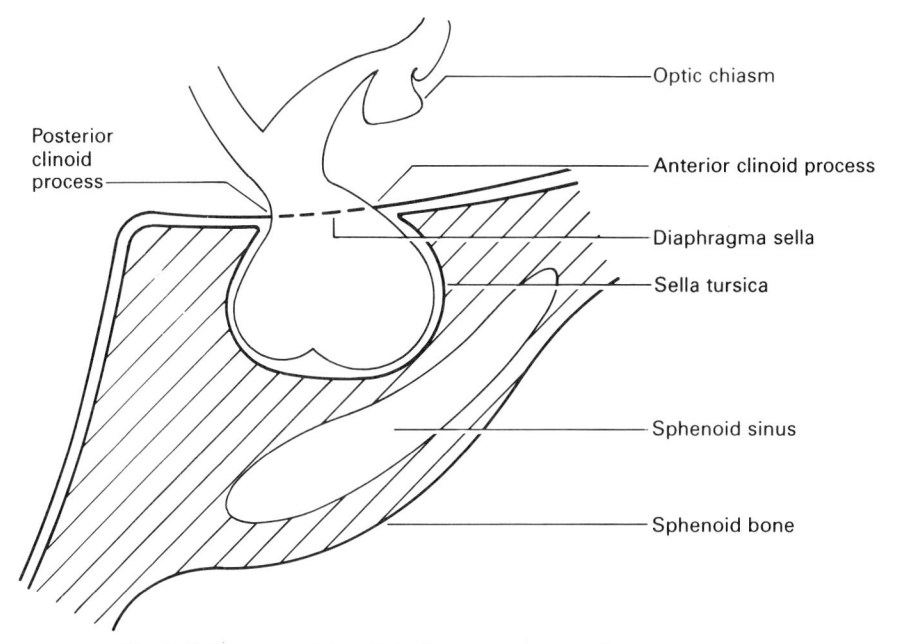

Fig. 7.2 Relationship of pituitary to surrounding structures.

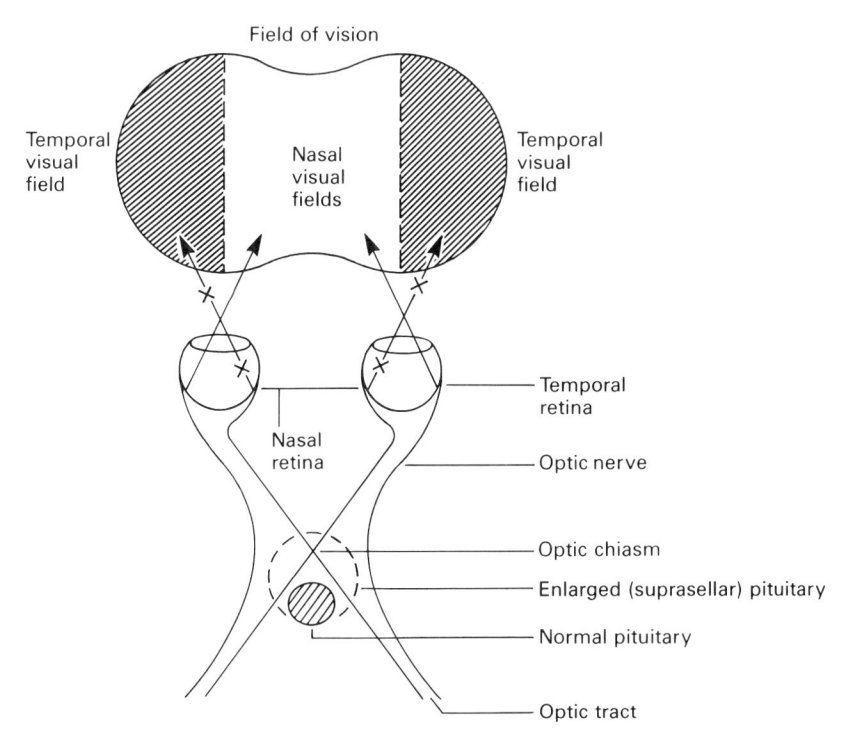

Fig. 7.3 Relationship of pituitary to optic chiasm showing bitemporal visual field defect resulting from a suprasellar enlargement of a pituitary tumour compressing the optic chiasm.

(a)

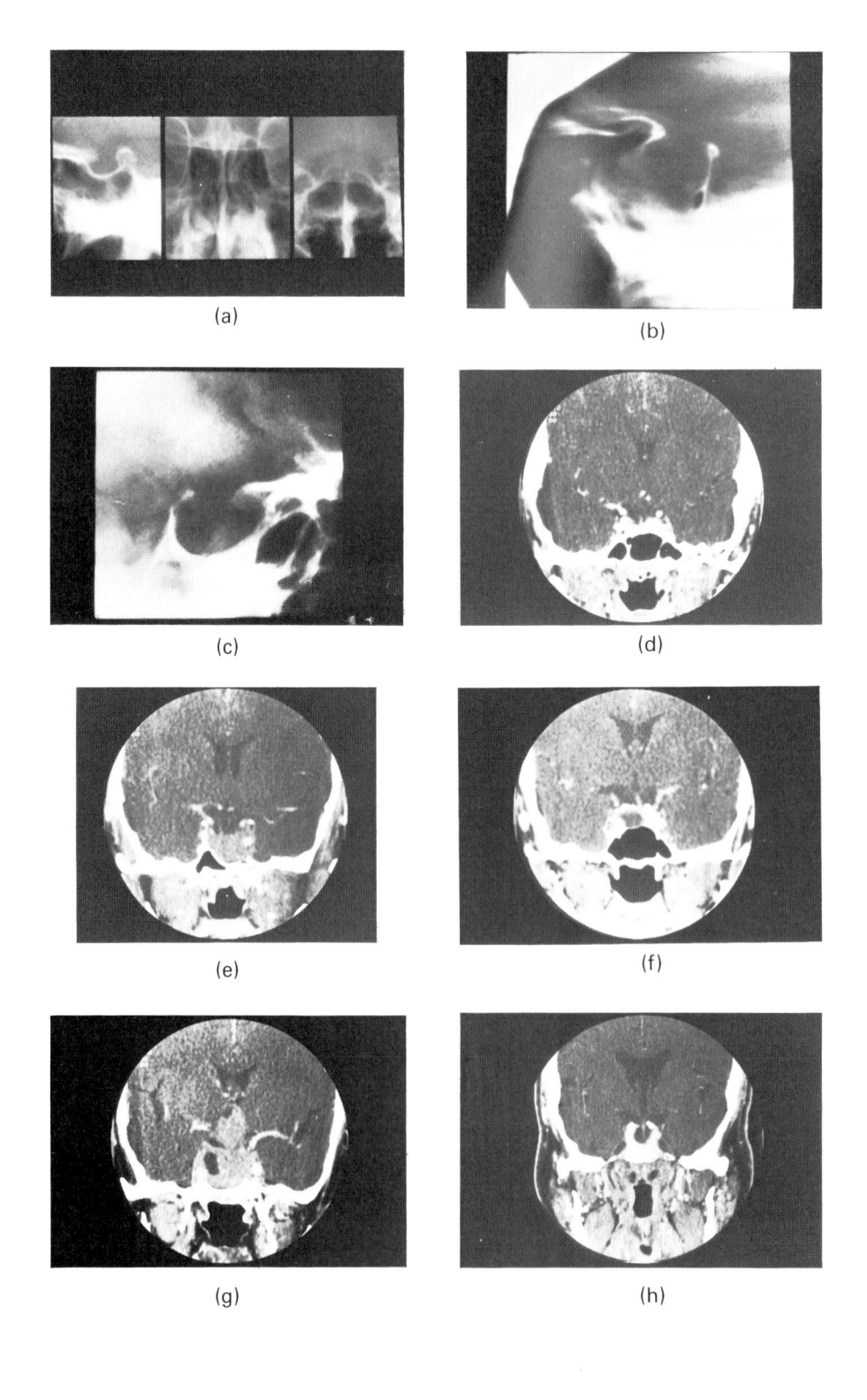

(b)

(c)

(d)

(e)

(f)

(g)

(h)

Fig. 7.4 Radiology of the pituitary fossa.
(a) Lateral, coronal and Town's view of the normal pituitary fossa
(b) Lateral view of enlarged fossa with eroded floor.
(c) Lateral view of pituitary with suprasellar calcification in a craniopharyngioma.
(d) A CT scan coronal view of a normal fossa.
(e) A CT scan showing an intrasellar tumour eroding the floor and lateral walls of the fossa.
(f) A CT scan showing a low density microadenoma within the fossa.
(g) A CT scan showing a large suprasellar extension.
(h) A CT scan showing an empty sella.

into the sphenoid bone. An anteroposterior view of the skull may also show lateral asymmetry with one side of the floor of the fossa more eroded than the other, which may result in the appearance of a double floor in the lateral view. A plain X-ray does not reveal the dimensions of the soft tissue of the tumour itself which can however be shown by a computerized tomography (CT) scan. The latter is necessary to reveal the extent of a suprasellar extension. A CT scan may also reveal a microadenoma of different density from the surrounding normal pituitary tissue within a normal sized fossa. Occasionally the scan reveals a so-called empty fossa in which the tumour is presumed to have infarcted or collapsed in on itself, leaving a rim of tissue round the edge (Fig. 7.4).

Physiology of Hypothalamic–Pituitary–Target Organ Relationships

The hypothalamus contains the intrinsic mechanisms which regulate the rhythms of pituitary hormone secretion, although these are modulated by neuronal impulses from the cerebral cortex and by the levels of other hormones in the peripheral circulation. The hypothalamus releases regulatory hormones which either stimulate or inhibit the anterior pituitary via the hypophyseal portal vessels in the pituitary stalk. Posterior pituitary hormones are synthesized in the hypothalamus and conveyed on carrier proteins down the neurones of the neurohypophyseal tract to be released into the circulation.

The anterior pituitary stores and releases trophic hormones into the circulation which then regulate the function of their respective target organs. The levels of circulating hormones from the target organs in turn feedback information to the pituitary and the hypothalamus to modulate the secretion of their respective regulatory hormones, forming a control loop. This loop may be negative feedback, i.e. inhibitory, or positive feedback, i.e. stimulatory (Fig. 7.5).

The regulatory hormones produced by the hypothalamus and the relevant pituitary hormones are shown in Table 7.1 and will be considered in turn.

180 The Hypothalamus and Pituitary

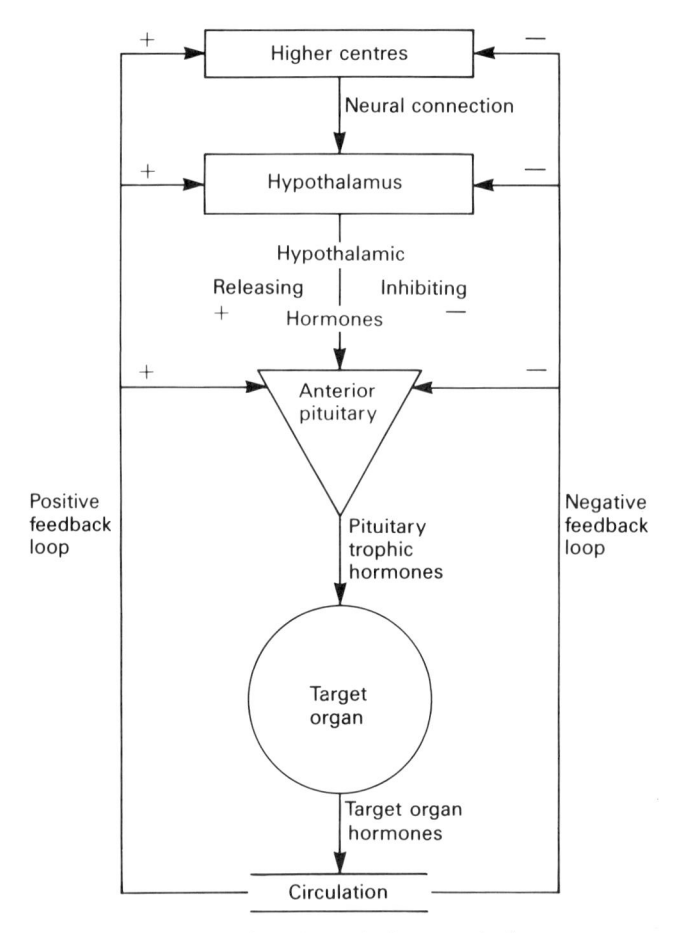

Fig. 7.5 Feedback regulation of the hypothalamus-pituitary-target organ axis.

The Hypothalamic–Pituitary–Thyroid Axis

Thyrotrophin releasing hormone (TRH) is a tripeptide stored and released by the hypothalamus which regulates the secretion of thyrotrophin (thyroid stimulating hormone, TSH) by the pituitary. Thyrotrophin releasing hormone has been synthesized and when given as a bolus injection of 200 µg to normal subjects it produces a rise in TSH which peaks at 20 min and then subsides, but is not completely back to baseline within 1 h (see Fig. 8.8 on page 218). Endogenous TRH is very difficult to measure in humans by current techniques. Thyroid stimulating hormone consists of alpha and beta subunits. The alpha unit is common to other glycoproteins (gonadotrophins and human chorionic gonadotrophin) and is biologically inert, but the beta subunit confers specific biological activity.

Thyroid stimulating hormone from the pituitary stimulates the release of the thyroid hormones thyroxine (T_4) and tri-iodothyronine (T_3) from the thyroid

Physiology of Hypothalamic–Pituitary–Target Organ Relationships 181

Table 7.1 Hypothalamic and pituitary regulatory hormones. Stimulatory (+), inhibitory (−).

Hypothalamus	Anterior pituitary	Target organ
Thyrotrophin releasing hormone (TRH) (+)	Thyroid stimulating hormone (TSH) (+)	Thyroid
Corticotrophin releasing hormone (CRH) (+)	Adrenocorticotrophic hormone ACTH (+)	Adrenal cortex
Growth hormone releasing hormone (GHRH) (+)	Growth hormone (GH) (+)	Peripheral tissues
Growth hormone release inhibiting hormone Somatostatin (GHRIH) (−)		
Gonadotrophin releasing hormone (GnRH) (+) (LH/FSH-RH)	Luteinizing hormone (LH) (+) Follicle stimulating hormone (FSH) (+)	Gonads
Dopamine (PIF) (−)	Prolactin (PRL) (+)	Breast

(see Chapter 8). T_4 and T_3 in the circulation have a negative feedback effect on the release of TSH by the pituitary and possibly on hypothalamic TRH. High levels of the thyroid hormones thus inhibit TSH secretion and low levels stimulate TSH production. If the hypothalamus is damaged failure of TRH production will result in low levels of TSH and consequent low levels of circulating thyroid hormones. The pituitary is nevertheless still capable of responding to exogenous TRH. If the pituitary is damaged, even though the hypothalamus is intact, it fails to respond to TRH and TSH levels and consequently T_4 and T_3 levels are again low. The damaged pituitary is incapable of responding to the low thyroid hormone levels.

In addition to the major stimulatory control by TRH secretion, TSH release is inhibited by somatostatin (see later) and also by dopamine, both of which are found in the hypothalamus. Dopaminergic agents such as bromocriptine therefore blunt TSH secretion and dopamine antagonists such as metoclopramide or domperidone enhance TSH release. Thyroid stimulating hormone secretion is also modified by oestrogens, which sensitize the pituitary response to TRH, and by pharmacological doses of steroids which blunt the TSH response to TRH (Fig. 7.6).

There is a small diurnal variation in serum TSH concentrations in normal subjects. Peak serum TSH concentrations occur between 2000 and 2400 h and the lowest values are found around midday. The amplitude of these changes is quite small and whilst they may be of physiological importance they are not of diagnostic significance in clinical practice in the timing of blood sampling.

The Hypothalamic–Pituitary–Adrenal Axis

Corticotrophin releasing hormone (CRH) is a peptide containing 41 aminoacids which has been synthesized relatively recently. Corticotrophin releasing hormone

182 The Hypothalamus and Pituitary

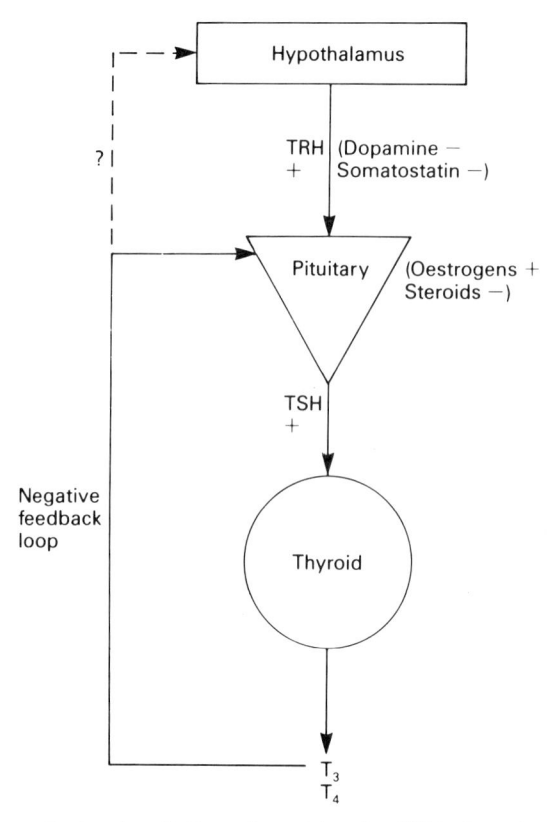

Fig. 7.6 The hypothalamic-pituitary-thyroid axis. TRH, thyrotrophin releasing hormone. TSH, thyroid stimulating hormone.

from the hypothalamus stimulates the pituitary to release peptides which belong to the pro-opiomelanocortin family. Pro-opiocortin is a large precursor glycoprotein from which a number of related peptides are derived which include adrenocorticotrophic hormone (ACTH), melanocyte stimulating hormones (MSH), beta and gamma lipotrophins, endorphins and met-encephalins (Fig. 7.7). These peptides share a number of aminoacid sequences in common although they have different functions. The endorphins (endogenous morphine) and met-encephalin relieve pain in humans. Adrenocorticotrophic hormone is a single chain polypeptide of 39 aminoacids which is produced by the pituitary and stimulates cortisol production by the adrenal cortex. It can also cause skin pigmentation such as seen in Addison's disease or the ectopic ACTH syndrome (see Chapter 9). Secretion of ACTH exhibits a diurnal rhythm with a peak in the morning between 0600 and 0900 h and a nadir at midnight, reflected by measurement of cortisol levels at these times. Secretion of ACTH responds to stress (for example, hypoglycaemia) which overrides the diurnal rhythm and feedback control. Circulating levels of cortisol exert a

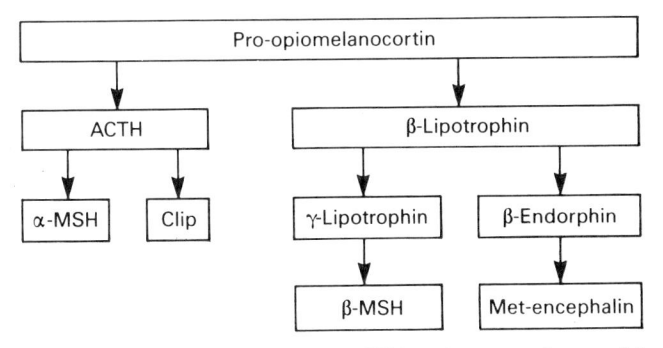

Fig. 7.7 Pro-opiomelanocortin family. ACTH, adrenocorticotrophin hormone. MSH, melanocyte stimulating hormone.

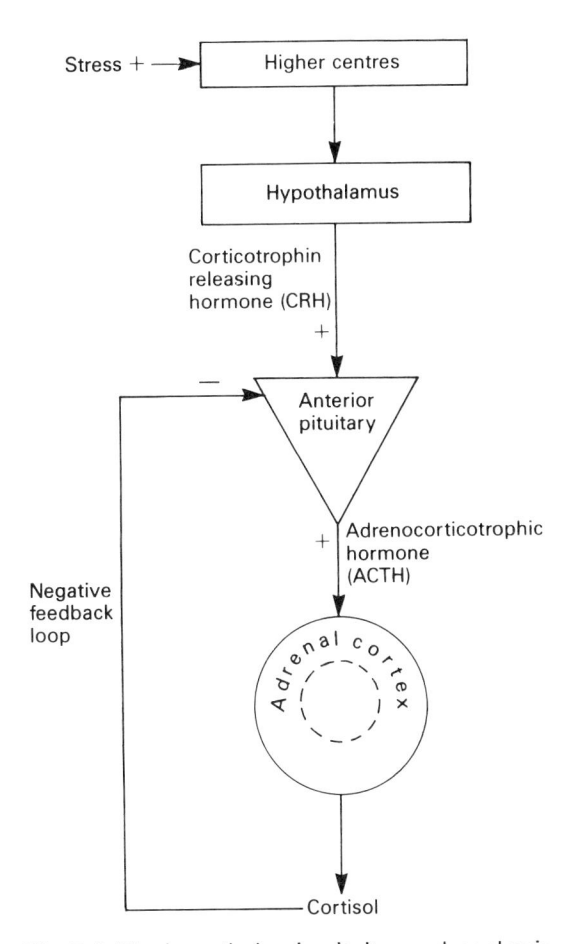

Fig. 7.8 The hypothalamic-pituitary-adrenal axis.

negative feedback control on ACTH secretion, with high cortisol levels suppressing and low cortisol levels stimulating ACTH production. Damage to the hypothalamus or pituitary results in low levels of ACTH and consequently low levels of cortisol, whereas damage to the adrenal cortex producing low levels of cortisol will result in high ACTH levels so long as the hypothalamus and pituitary are intact (Fig. 7.8).

The Hypothalamic–Pituitary–Growth Hormone Axis

Pituitary growth hormone production is regulated by both stimulatory and inhibitory hypothalamic factors. Growth hormone releasing hormone (GHRH) has been isolated from rare patients with pancreatic tumours causing acromegaly. The sequence of aminoacids in the GHRH from two of these tumours was almost the same, one containing 40 and the other 44 amino acids, of which the first 40 were common. Growth hormone releasing hormone releases growth hormone (GH) in normal humans. Growth hormone secretion is however inhibited by another hypothalamic hormone, somatostatin (growth hormone release inhibiting hormone, GHRIH). Somatostatin is a tetradecapeptide which is found in the hypothalamus, but is also found in pancreatic islet cells and other tissues (Chapter 6). It also inhibits insulin and glucagon secretion and other gastrointestinal hormones when administered in pharmacological doses and may have a more universal physiological role.

Growth hormone is a relatively large pituitary hormone which consists of 191 aminoacids. Growth hormone secretion is pulsatile with a periodicity of about 200 min regardless of growth rate. The amplitude of the pulses is a major factor in height development. In isolated GH deficiency, due to lack of GHRH there is negligible GH pulsation whereas in gigantism, both basal levels and the amplitude of GH pulsations are greatly increased. In between these extreme pathological examples the amplitude of GH pulsation in normal individuals varies widely, but higher GH pulses are found to occur in taller and lower amplitude pulses in shorter individuals during growth. There is also a diurnal rhythm of GH secretion with higher GH pulses in the first part of the night during the period of deep sleep. Growth hormone secretion is stimulated by stress, fasting, exercise, and by hypoglycaemia and certain aminoacid loads especially arginine. Conversely GH secretion is suppressed in normal individuals by a glucose load (to less than 4 mU/l (2 µg/l) and blunted by pharmacological doses of steroids (Fig. 7.9).

Growth hormone acts peripherally on many tissues and its effects are mediated by other growth factors in the serum and tissues. These intermediate polypeptide growth factors have been called somatomedins or sulphation factors and are produced in the liver and possibly other organs. The major somatomedin in adults is somatomedin C which is also known as insulin-like growth factor I because of its insulin-like properties including promotion of glucose uptake and oxidation by muscle and adipose cells. High levels of somatomedins are found in acromegaly and low levels in pituitary GH defic-

Physiology of Hypothalamic–Pituitary–Target Organ Relationships 185

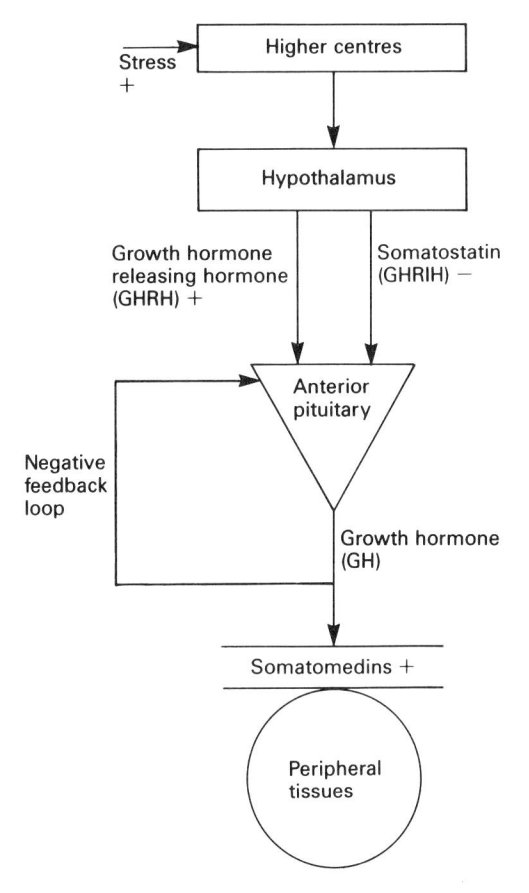

Fig. 7.9 The hypothalamic-pituitary-growth hormone axis.

iency. In a rare form of dwarfism, known as Laron dwarfism, somatomedin is absent and GH levels are high.

The Hypothalamic–Pituitary–Gonadal Axis

The hypothalamus produces a gonadotrophin releasing hormone (GnRH) which stimulates the release from the pituitary of both luteinizing hormone (LH) and follicle stimulating hormone (FSH), hence its alternative earlier name of LH/FSH-RH. Gonadotrophin releasing hormone is a tetradecapeptide which has been synthesized and is available for use as a provocative test of LH and FSH release and for therapeutic purposes. Secretion of GnRH is pulsatile and this is reflected by pulsatile secretion of LH and FSH. The pattern of GnRH pulsatility in men is less consistent in time and amplitude than in women in whom it varies according to the stage of the menstrual cycle. Pulses of GnRH are more frequent (approximately every 90 min) but of lower amplitude in the early follicular phase of the cycle than in the later luteal phase, when they occur with gradually decreasing frequency (every 2 to 4 h) but with greater amplitude. Administration of GnRH in pulses which mimic physiological changes can be used to induce ovulation in women lacking endogenous pulsation, but continuous administration of GnRH down-regulates the receptors and suppresses gonadotrophin production.

In males LH acts on the Leydig cells of the testis to produce testosterone which in turn has a negative feedback effect on LH release. Follicle stimulating hormone acts on the seminiferous tubules and is important for spermatogenesis. Secretion of FSH is selectively inhibited by a substance known as inhibin which is found in rete testis secretions and in follicular fluid in women. In females the modulation of gonadotrophin secretion is more complicated as

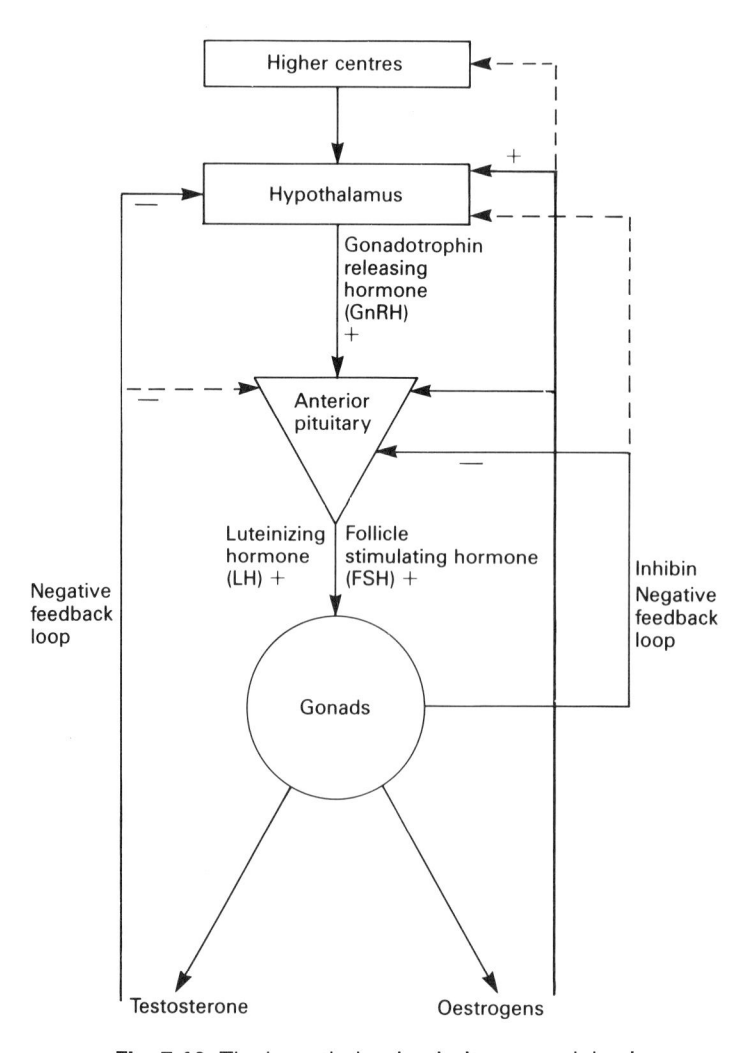

Fig. 7.10 The hypothalamic-pituitary-gondal axis.

Physiology of Hypothalamic–Pituitary–Target Organ Relationships 187

the sensitivity of the hypothalamus and pituitary to circulating gonadal hormone levels varies at different stages of the menstrual cycle. Follicle stimulating hormone is necessary for maturation of the follicles, as its name implies. Increasing oestrogen levels enhance LH secretion by positive feedback during the late follicular phase of the cycle. A rise in oestradiol levels always precedes the mid-cycle surge in LH secretion which occurs at the time of ovulation when the ovum is released from the ruptured follicle. Pulses of LH maintain progesterone production by the corpus luteum during the luteal phase of the cycle. If implantation does not occur the corpus luteum fails and menstruation occurs. The frequency of FSH pulsation then increases preparing the follicles for the next cycle.

Both LH and FSH are necessary for normal pubertal development and the maintenance of gonadal function in both sexes (see Chapter 10). Primary gonadal failure such as occurs naturally at the menopause results in low gonadal hormone levels and consequently high LH and FSH levels. Administration of oestrogens lowers gonadotrophin levels in post-menopausal women. Pharmacological doses of oestrogen and of progesterone prevent the mid-cycle surge of gonadotrophins, hence their use as oral contraceptives (Fig. 7.10).

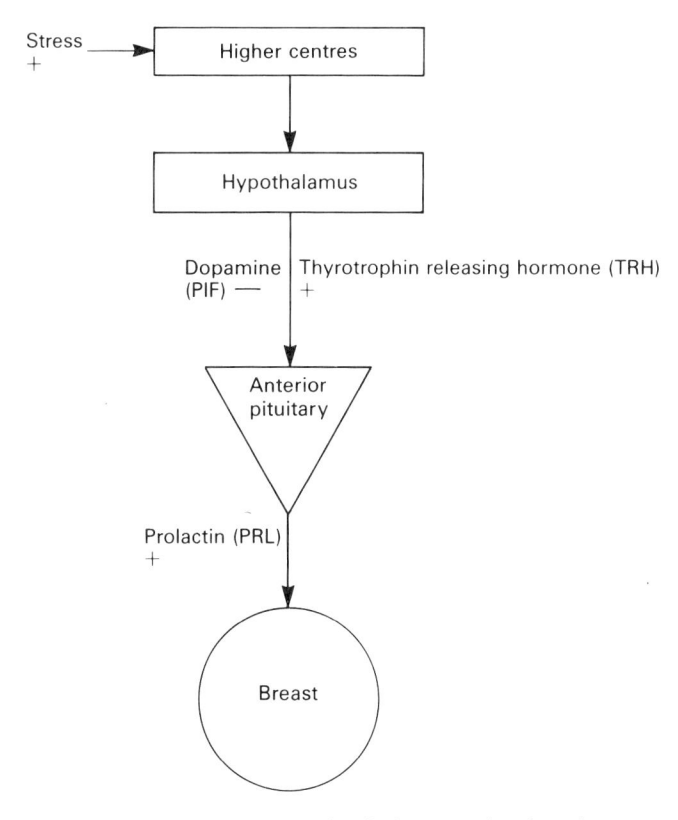

Fig. 7.11 The hypothalamic-pituitary-prolactin axis.

The Hypothalamic–Pituitary–Prolactin Axis

Prolactin (PRL) secretion from the pituitary is also pulsatile probably due to inherent pulsatility of the lactotroph in the pituitary. Unlike the other anterior pituitary hormones PRL is predominantly under the control of an inhibitory rather than a releasing factor. Dopamine is the major inhibitor of PRL secretion. Thyrotrophin releasing hormone provokes PRL as well as TSH release, but does not appear to be a major physiological regulator of PRL secretion. Levels of PRL rise in response to stress, as do GH and ACTH, whereas TSH levels do not rise (Fig. 7.11).

Prolactin as its name implies is necessary for lactation. Levels increase during pregnancy and are maintained by suckling. It may also have a wider physiological role but its exact function in the non-pregnant, non-lactating state in human beings is uncertain. In lower vertebrates PRL plays an important role in the regulation of fluid balance and growth.

Anterior Pituitary Disorders

Patients with pituitary disorders may present with one of the syndromes associated with hormone excess (Table 7.2) or because of partial or total failure of one or other or all of the pituitary hormones (Table 7.6,). They may also present because of the pressure effects of a large pituitary tumour causing a visual field defect, or an enlarged pituitary fossa may be seen on a skull X-ray taken for other reasons.

Acromegaly

Pathophysiology

Acromegaly is due to a tumour of the eosinophil cells of the anterior pituitary producing hypersecretion of GH, although it may be associated with chromophobe as well as chromophil adenomas as shown by immunocytological staining. Patients with acromegaly have persistently elevated GH levels and sleep pulsation is blunted. The GH concentrations are not suppressed in response to hyperglycaemia and this is used as a diagnostic test. Secretion of

Table 7.2 Conditions of hormone excess

Cushing's disease   (Chapter 9)
Acromegaly (Chapter 7)
Hyperprolactinaemia   (Chapter 7)
Thyroid stimulating hormone (TSH) secreting tumours (rare)   (Chapter 8)
Luteinizing hormone (LH) and follicle stimulating hormone (FSH) secreting tumours (rare)

GH is not, however, entirely autonomous in acromegaly as levels may rise even further in response to hypoglycaemic stress and are partially inhibited by infusion of somatostatin. L-dopa and the dopamine agonist bromocriptine also reduce GH secretion in some acromegalics. The pituitary somatotroph is also abnormal in acromegaly in that GH release occurs in response to the administration of TRH or GnRH which does not occur in normal individuals.

The peripheral effects of excess GH secretion include exaggerated protein anabolism, impaired glucose tolerance and increased fatty acid metabolism. Somatomedin levels are elevated in acromegaly but return to normal after successful treatment of the condition. Other hormonal changes may result from the expanding tumour compressing the remaining normal pituitary tissue. Gonadotrophin deficiency, ACTH deficiency and TSH deficiency occur in descending order of frequency and PRL levels are commonly raised.

Clinical features of acromegaly

Acromegaly was first described by Marie in 1886. Early recognition of acromegaly occurs only as a result of a high index of suspicion on the part of the family doctor, physician, surgeon or gynaecologist to whom the patient may present with an incidental or related complaint. Anyone with coarse features should be questioned about changes in their facial appearance, increasing shoe size and alterations to wedding rings. Examination of a series of old photographs of the patient can be helpful in revealing the developing coarsening of the facial features with thickening of the lips and nose, and frontal bossing. A change in bite due to increasing prognathism may be evident from dental records and a large tongue evident on inspection of the mouth. Heavy manual workers may have large stubby hands which resemble the spade-like hands seen in established acromegaly, but paraesthesiae are uncommon in the former whereas carpal tunnel syndrome or a previous operation for this condition is not uncommon in acromegalics. Women may present with secondary amenorrhoea or less commonly galactorrhoea, whereas men may present with loss of libido or potency. Headaches and increased sweating with coarse greasy skin are common findings. The insidious nature of the condition may not lead the patient to present until a visual field defect has occurred. Whilst symmetrical enlargement of the tumour may result in a bitemporal hemianopia, asymmetrical growth can produce a unilateral or partial quadrantic defect.

The common clinical features of acromegaly are listed in Table 7.3. A diastolic pressure of more than 100 mmHg is approximately twice as common in acromegalics as in age and sex matched controls. Cardiomegaly may develop even in the absence of hypertension and lead to cardiac failure. Clinical or biochemical diabetes mellitus occurs in approximately 25% of acromegalics but retinopathy is surprisingly uncommon given the postulated role of GH in the development of this condition in non-acromegalic diabetic patients. Osteoarthropathy and myopathy can be severely disabling in advanced acromegaly.

Table 7.3 Clinical features of acromegaly

Site/condition	Feature
Face	Coarse thick lips, tongue and nose
Hands	Large spade-like hands, Carpal tunnel syndrome
Feet	Increasing shoe size
Skin	Thick, greasy, increased sweating
Heart	Hypertension, cardiomyopathy
Muscle	Myopathy
Thyroid	Goitre, increased incidence of thyrotoxicosis
Diabetes mellitus	Clinical (10%), biochemical (25%)
Joints	Osteoarthropathy
Central nervous system	Headache, visual field defects
Other pituitary functions	Diminished libido, secondary amenorrhoea
	Diminished cortisol
	Increased prolactin, galactorrhoea

Gigantism

Excess GH production before puberty results in increase in the length as well as the breadth of bones. Thus in the early stages changes in facial features, hands and feet are less obvious because they are more in proportion than in acromegaly. Patients become disproportionately tall and greatly exceed the 97th centile for height and weight. Once the epiphyses have fused the growth in height ceases but the thickness of bone and soft tissues continues to increase and more typical acromegalic features develop. Other features of gigantism are similar to those already outlined above for acromegaly.

Diagnostic tests

When the diagnosis of acromegaly or gigantism is suspected it can easily be confirmed or refuted by estimation of GH levels during a glucose tolerance test (GTT). A single random GH of less than 1 mU/l or 0.5 µg/l excludes the diagnosis, but as GH responds to stress, and even venepuncture or the surrounding circumstances may be sufficiently stressful, a random GH estimation is likely to produce a falsely positive result. A GTT should be performed with the patient fasting and resting with an indwelling venous cannula inserted an hour prior to the test. Blood samples are taken for glucose and GH basally and at 30-min intervals for 150 min after oral administration of a standard glucose load. In normal individuals GH levels fall to less than 4 mU/l whereas in acromegaly GH levels are elevated and fail to suppress and may show a paradoxical rise. Levels of GH do not correlate very closely with the severity of the clinical features. Mean GH levels may be little more than 10 mU/l in patients with obvious acromegaly or > 100 mU/l in patients in whom the diagnosis was in doubt. There is a lack of standardization in the way that GH

Table 7.4 Investigations of acromegaly

Investigation
Growth hormone levels during a glucose tolerance test to confirm/refute diagnosis
Remaining pituitary function: Basal 0900 h cortisol, cortisol response to ITT, fT_4, TSH, TRH test, LH, FSH, testosterone ($\male$), prolactin
X-rays to show radiological heel pad thickness and tufting of terminal phalanges in the hards
Lateral skull X-ray to show enlargement of pituitary fossa
Computerized tomography scan to show soft contours of a tumour
Visual fields using Bjerrum's screen

data are handled, some authorities preferring to take the mean GH values obtained during a GTT and others the mean of GH samples obtained either fasting or throughout the day, which can make comparison of the outcome of different treatments from different centres difficult.

The full investigation of a patient with acromegaly includes clinical and biochemical assessment not only of GH secretion but also of the remaining pituitary function (see hypopituitarism below), and assessment of the tumour size and possible pressure effects. A plain X-ray of the skull, anteroposterior and lateral views, is likely to show an abnormal pituitary fossa because so many patients present late in the natural history of the condition. A normal skull X-ray does not, however, exclude a tumour, the soft contours of which are usually revealed by a CT scan. Radiological heel pad thickness greater than 25 mm is usually abnormal but is not invariably found, and X-rays of the hands may show tufting of the terminal phalanges as well as cortical and soft tissue thickening. A summary of the investigations of acromegaly is shown in Table 7.4.

Treatment

Untreated acromegalics have a reduced life expectancy and an increased risk of death from cardiovascular, cerebrovascular and respiratory diseases as well as suffering considerable disfigurement and disability. Successful treatment leads to a reduction of the soft tissue changes and correction of some of the metabolic features such as diabetes mellitus, although the bone changes are less reversible. Early treatment can prevent complications such as cardiomyopathy, osteoarthrosis and visual field defects, which once established may be irreversible. The morbidity as well as the effectiveness of treatment must also be taken into account in advising a patient of the appropriate method of treatment. The ideal treatment would safely and effectively remove all tumour tissue with remission of the clinical and biochemical evidence of GH excess whilst preserving or restoring normal pituitary function. The choice of treatment lies between surgery, radiation and medication.

Surgical treatment

Trans-sphenoidal hypophysectomy   The trans-sphenoidal approach under direct vision offers the best chance of selective removal of a discrete adenoma or of a tumour which is largely confined to the pituitary fossa. In many cases normal pituitary tissue can be left *in situ*. Applied to suitable patients this technique achieves a cure in approximately 75% of cases. About 20% regain gonadotrophin function, but approximately 50% remain or become deficient in one or several trophic hormones. The results of trans-sphenoidal surgery can be assessed within a few weeks of treatment.

Trans-frontal surgery   This approach provides limited access to the deeper parts of the pituitary fossa and it is not usually possible to remove all of a tumour by this route so that it seldom results in a cure of the endocrinopathy. It is the appropriate approach for removal of large suprasellar extensions and is most commonly used when there is a visual field defect where the primary objective is relief of pressure on the optic chiasm. The extent of recovery of the visual field defect is variable because it largely depends on the duration of pressure on the optic chiasm. The persistent endocrinopathy can be treated by combined therapy with trans-sphenoidal surgery or radiation or bromocriptine.

Radiation

External radiation offers the advantage of a non-invasive approach, but it is only suitable for tumours confined to the fossa. The maximum dose of radiation that can be given without risk of damage to the surrounding brain tissue is 4000 to 5000 cGy and it is slow to take effect. Claims have been made for 50% cure after two years and up to 80% after five years. Few patients who are not already deficient in other pituitary hormones require replacement therapy but equally few patients recover spontaneously from gonadotrophin deficiency and hypopituitarism can develop later insidiously. Larger doses of radiation have been administered using a proton beam which utilizes the Bragg peak effect but the overall results have not been any better than by conventional radiotherapy, and the complications, which include ocular muscle palsies, visual field damage and seizures have been greater.

Yttrium-90 implantation by the trans-sphenoidal route under radiological guidance allows the placement of radioactive seeds directly into the tumour and delivers 50 000 to 100 000 cGy to the tumour tissue. Improvement occurs in up to two-thirds of patients although GH levels often remain above normal. Deficiency of anterior pituitary hormones occurs in about a third of patients and complications which can occur include CSF rhinorrhoea, visual loss or ocular paresis and diabetes insipidus.

Medical treatment

Bromocriptine, a semi-synthetic ergot alkaloid which is a dopamine agonist, causes a fall in GH levels in the majority of acromegalics but seldom to the normal range even in doses of up to 20 mg/day. It leads to some improvement of the soft tissue features of the condition and may shrink the tumour. In some patients this makes a large tumour more amenable to surgery by the transsphenoidal rather than the trans-frontal route. Bromocriptine suppresses PRL more effectively than GH (see section on hyperprolactinaemia) and has the least morbidity, but the effects rapidly escape if the drug is discontinued and it cannot be regarded as curative. It may be a useful adjunct to other therapies, for example, pending the effect of radiation or after only partially effective surgery.

Long-acting somatostatin analogues, which can be given subcutaneously, have been developed recently and may have a therapeutic role in acromegaly. It remains to be seen whether they are truly selective in their actions or have unacceptable suppressive effects on insulin, glucagon and other hormones which limited the practical application of the original somatostatin which also had to be given intravenously.

It can be seen that no treatment meets the ideal aims and the choice of the most suitable treatment for an individual patient will depend on age and general health, the size of the tumour, the severity of the acromegaly and its complications, and the acceptability of the risk of potential side-effects of the treatment.

Hyperprolactinaemia

The control of prolactin secretion has been outlined earlier in this chapter. It is important to remember that prolactin differs from the other anterior pituitary hormones in being controlled primarily by an inhibitory factor, dopamine, rather than a stimulating factor. Thus lack of the inhibitor from whatever cause results in increased prolactin secretion. Raised prolactin levels may be due to physiological, pharmacological or pathological causes (Table 7.5). Apart from obvious physiological causes such as pregnancy and lactation, PRL levels rise in response to stress, so that it is important that the patient is relaxed and resting when samples are taken for PRL estimation or modest physiological elevations may be misinterpreted as due to pathological causes. A proper history of the patient's recent medication should exclude the drugs likeliest to cause hyperprolactinaemia such as phenothiazines or tricyclic antidepressants. The commonest pathological cause is a pituitary tumour secreting PRL which may be a macroadenoma (large enough to distort the pituitary and evident on a CT scan if not on plain X-ray of the skull) or a microadenoma (which may not be demonstrable on CT scan but found only on direct vision at surgery). It may not be possible to distinguish clinically between a microadenoma and hyperplasia of the lactotrophs. Hyperprolactinaemia may also be present with other pituitary tumours such as Cushing's disease or acromegaly, or follow damage to the pituitary by surgery, radiation or trauma causing section of the pituitary stalk.

Table 7.5 Causes of hyperprolactinaemia

Physiological
Stress
Sleep
Pregnancy
Suckling
Exercise

Pharmacological
Dopamine depleting agents
  Reserpine
  α-Methyldopa
Dopamine receptor blockers
  Tricyclic antidepressants
  Phenothiazines
  Butyrophenones
  Metoclopramide
  Sulpiride
Direct release
  TRH

Pathological
Idiopathic
Prolactinoma
Other pituitary tumours
  Chromophobe
  Acromegaly
  Cushing's disease
Post-hypophysectomy
Pituitary stalk section
Pituitary irradiation
Other conditions
  Primary hypothyroidism
  Chronic renal failure
  Carcinoid syndrome

Clinical features

Presenting features of hyperprolactinaemia include amenorrhoea, oligomenorrhoea or irregular periods and galactorrhoea in women, although less than half of all patients with raised prolactin levels have galactorrhoea and vice-versa. Galactorrhoea is even less common in men in whom the presenting feature is more commonly impotence. Prolactin should be measured in the investigation of all cases of infertility and should also be part of the assessment of anyone suspected of having pituitary tumour or hypothalamic disease. Patients with raised prolactin levels may not exhibit any abnormal physical signs at all whereas others may present with visual field defects and other pressure features of a large pituitary tumour.

Laboratory investigations

A random prolactin level of less than 400 mU/l almost certainly excludes hyperprolactinaemia, but patients are often stressed by the circumstances of a clinic visit and values between 400 and 1000 mU/l or even higher may be due to stress or to an underlying pathological state. Values of several thousand mU/l are usually pathological but where there is doubt about borderline values it is advisable to arrange for samples to be taken with the patient resting and via an indwelling cannula at hourly intervals for three hours to establish proper baseline levels. Remaining pituitary function should also be assessed (see section on pituitary failure). Basal testosterone levels in men and oestrodiol levels in women and gonadotrophin levels in both sexes are likely to be low but are not inevitably reduced. In severe hyperprolactinaemia particularly when associated with a large pituitary tumour other pituitary functions including ACTH, GH and TSH reserve are also likely to be impaired but can recover after suppression of prolactin.

A plain skull X-ray may reveal enlargement of the pituitary fossa but it is often normal. A CT scan will reveal either a modest adenoma or an empty sella in a proportion of patients with normal skull X-ray, but it is frequently also normal. The problem then lies in distinguishing between diffuse hyperplasia and a microadenoma which may have therapeutic importance. Demonstration of autonomy is taken as evidence in favour of a tumour rather than hyperplasia. Failure of PRL to respond to TRH or to metoclopramide has been used to distinguish tumours from hyperplasia, but such tests have not been found to discriminate as well as at first claimed.

Management of prolactinoma

Treatment of hyperprolactinaemia can be medical or surgical or by irradiation, although the latter is the least effective. The choice of treatment depends on the size and position of the tumour, the age and sex of the patient and the priorities for the patient.

Medical treatment with bromocriptine is highly effective in most cases provided it as well tolerated. Bromocriptine should be started gradually by taking a small dose of 2.5 mg with food or milk before retiring to bed, to minimize gastrointestinal upsets which are quite common initially. The dose can be increased after a week or two to 2.5 mg twice daily and then three times a day if necessary. Doses higher than 5 mg three times daily are more commonly associated with digital ischaemia (bromocriptine is a derivative of an ergot alkaloid). Successful treatment with bromocriptine not only suppresses PRL but restores or maintains normal remaining pituitary function and often shrinks the tumour. Some large tumours may not respond to medical treatment and some patients cannot tolerate any dose of bromocriptine. Prolactin levels rise rapidly when bromocriptine is discontinued.

Surgical treatment is either by trans-frontal hypophysectomy for large tumours with suprasellar extension which have not shrunk with medical treatment, or by the trans-sphenoidal route for tumours largely confined to the pituitary fossa. A trial of bromocriptine is worthwhile even with very large tumours as it may be possible to shrink the tumour, if not completely, at least to a size that would permit effective removal by the trans-sphenoidal rather than trans-frontal route. The likelihood of hypopituitarism following surgery increases with the size of the tumour.

Selective removal of a microadenoma by trans-sphenoidal surgery offers the best chance of a cure with maintenance of normal pituitary function. If at surgery a discrete lesion is not seen then the surgeon is faced with the dilemma of removing the likeliest part or all of the pituitary. The possible risk and consequences of hypopituitarism following surgery must be understood by the patient and all concerned before the decision to operate is made.

External radiation is sometimes given as a supplement to surgery after incomplete removal, such as is inevitable after a trans-frontal approach, in the hope of preventing recurrence or further expansion of the tumour. Such treatment is seldom effective in reducing PRL levels *per se* although it may be a few years before the effects can be judged. Bromocriptine may need to be continued post-operatively to control persistent hyperprolactinaemia and stopped at intervals to reassess the effect of the original treatment.

The natural history of untreated prolactinoma is not yet fully known. Patients presenting with a large pituitary tumour are assumed to have had the lesion for a considerable time but this may not be true. Other patients who have been found incidentally to have persistently high PRL levels but not been treated, because they have been asymptomatic, have been followed up for several years without progression of either the PRL levels or the size of the tumour. It follows therefore that a patient who is otherwise well and the rest of whose pituitary function is normal, particularly in the older age group, does not necessarily need any treatment although continued follow up is advisable. The choice in a younger patient may be more difficult, particularly if fertility, rather than simply suppression of galactorrhoea or restoration of libido or periods is the prime objective. Whilst selective trans-sphenoidal microadenomectomy offers the ideal cure there is a risk of hypopituitarism that is greater than with medical treatment. It may be more appropriate in this circumstance to suppress PRL with bromocriptine to restore normal gonadal function and hopefully for pregnancy to be achieved. Bromocriptine has not been shown to have any teratogenic effects and can be continued during the pregnancy although it is conventional for it to be discontinued once the pregnancy is successfully established. Pituitary tumours may, however, be expected to enlarge during pregnancy and if there is any suspicion of suprasellar extension bromocriptine would need to be reintroduced or surgery performed. If the patient has already completed a family and the risk of hypopituitarism is relatively less important then surgical treatment may be the first choice with subsequent medical treatment if surgery has not effectively cured the problem.

Anterior Pituitary Failure

Pituitary tumours are the commonest cause of anterior pituitary failure but this may also occur secondary to hypothalamic disease or as a result of more widespread systemic disease (Table 7.6).

The commonest pituitary tumours are chromophobe (usually non-functioning) adenomas and prolactinomas, whereas acromegaly and Cushing's disease are relatively uncommon. It is important to remember that hypersecreting tumours are often associated with deficiencies of other anterior pituitary hormones. Infarction of a pituitary following severe post-partum haemorrhage (Sheehan's syndrome) is fortunately rare nowadays but acute pituitary insufficiency may follow haemorrhage into or infarction of a pituitary tumour. Hypopituitarism may also result from treatment of a pituitary tumour by surgery or radiation.

Craniopharyngioma is a congenital abnormality, although it can present at any age, which involves the hypothalamus as well as the pituitary, and is probably best regarded as a primary hypothalamic disorder.

Isolated gonadotrophin releasing hormone (GnRH) deficiency is a rare congenital abnormality leading to lack of secondary sexual development, whereas loss of gonadotrophin function is a common presentation of many pituitary tumours and is often found in a wide variety of severe systemic diseases. Space occupying lesions involving the hypothalamus or pituitary other than primary pituitary tumours are relatively uncommon but can rarely be due to metastatic carcinoma usually from the bronchus or breast, or

Table 7.6 Causes of anterior pituitary failure

Hypothalamic	Pituitary

Craniopharyngioma
Primary tumours
Isolated gonadotrophin releasing
   hormone (GnRH) deficiency
Isolated GHRF deficiency
	Primary tumours
	   Chromophobe
	   Prolactinoma
	   Acromegaly
	   Cushing's disease

Secondary tumours
   Sarcoidosis
   Histiocytosis-X
   Tuberculosis
   Lymphoma
   Metastatic carcinoma
 	
Functional
   Anorexia nervosa
   Starvation
	Secondary tumours
	   Sarcoidosis
	   Tuberculosis
	   Lymphoma
	   Metastatic carcinoma
	
	Tertiary tumours
	   Feedback tumours: TSH
	                               ? LH FSH
	Post-partum necrosis, haemorrhage
	Trauma
	Autoimmune
	Irradiation

granulomas such as tuberculosis, sarcoidosis, lymphoma or the even rarer histiocytosis. Feedback tumours consequent upon long standing untreated primary target organ failure with stimulation of the relevant pituitary hormone leading to hyperplasia and enlargement of the pituitary are very infrequent but may occur, for example, in untreated hypothyroidism, particularly in areas of endemic cretinism (Chapter 8).

Isolated GH deficiency due to congenital lack of the hypothalamic GH releasing hormone (GHRH) is a relatively uncommon cause of failure to grow but GH secretion may be impaired in a variety of conditions. Other endocrine causes of short stature include craniopharyngioma, pituitary tumours, failure of peripheral tissue reponse to GH (for example, Laron dwarfism, pseudo-hypoparathyroidism, hypogonadism, hypothyroidism and androgen/oestrogen excess (precocious puberty; see Chapter 10).

The clinical assessment of suspected pituitary failure

Pituitary failure may present acutely due to sudden haemorrhage into or infarction of a pituitary tumour (pituitary apoplexy, mimicking a subarachnoid haemorrhage), but this is uncommon. It is more likely to present with chronic insidious symptoms of deficiency of one of the pituitary hormones or to be found in association with more readily recognizable conditions of hypersecretion of pituitary hormones such as acromegaly, hyperprolactinaemia or Cushing's disease. Pituitary tumours may also present because of pressure effects which include headache, although this is a relatively uncommon feature even in patients with large tumours, and visual field defects, particularly bitemporal hemianopia (Fig. 7.3), and such patients are commonly found to be suffering from pituitary deficiencies. It is essential to assess all aspects of pituitary function in a patient suspected of failure of any of the pituitary hormones. It is generally believed that in patients with pituitary tumours gonadotrophin function is lost early whereas GH and TSH reserve are lost relatively late, but this may depend on the age of the patient. The presentation of pituitary failure is greatly influenced by age. Thus, pre-puberty the commonest presentation is failure to grow, around the expected age of puberty it is likely to be failure of secondary sexual development, and in adults it may be loss of sexual function or any of the features elaborated in this chapter.

ACTH deficiency
Loss of ACTH reserve is the most serious deficiency because it can be life-threatening. It may occur acutely as part of the syndrome of pituitary apoplexy (see above) with sudden collapse of the patient due to acute cortisol insufficiency. More commonly a patient has adequate basal cortisol production but may not have an adequate ACTH reserve to be able to respond to stress such as infection or surgery. The symptoms of chronic cortisol insufficiency are non-specific and include anorexia, general malaise and lassitude. Postural hypotension is a feature of more severe cortisol deficiency.

Gonadotrophin deficiency
Isolated GnRH deficiency is associated with anosmia and other congenital midline deficiencies such as cleft palate and presents with failure of development of secondary sexual characteristics (Kallman's syndrome). Assessment of sexual function includes a record of pubertal development (see Chapter 10). In women the age of the menarche and an accurate record of the subsequent menstrual history as far as possible, including pregnancies and possible complications such as post-partum haemorrhage, and when menstruation ceased should be noted. In men the age of puberty, shaving habits, the ability to have morning erections and intercourse should be recorded. In both sexes libido and frequency of intercourse or the lack of it should be noted. The examination should pay particular attention to the overall appearance in relation to the patient's age, the texture of the skin which may be soft and hairless, and the degree of development of the secondary sexual characteristics. The distribution of the body hair, the size of the breasts, which should also be examined for galactorrhoea, and the anatomy of the external genitalia should be recorded. The position, size and consistency of the testes are important as they are usually small and soft in hypopituitarism.

Prolactin excess
A history of inappropriate lactation should be sought but galactorrhoea is not invariably present in women and seldom in men who may nevertheless be shown subsequently to have a raised PRL level. Women may present with oligomenorrhoea or amenorrhoea, and men with loss of libido or failure of erections.

TSH deficiency
Clinical evidence of hypothyroidism due to TSH deficiency is seldom as obvious as in primary hypothyroidism (see Chapter 8) and is not usually an isolated feature of pituitary failure. A history of increased sensitivity to cold, constipation and slowing of mental and physical activities should be sought, but are very non-specific findings. The examination may reveal puffiness of the face, thickening of the skin and delayed relaxation of the tendon reflexes but these features are often absent as other pituitary hormone deficiencies tend to predominate and TSH deficiency is a relatively late feature of pituitary failure.

GH deficiency
The role of GH in adults is not known and it does not appear to be important in practical terms. In children, however, lack of GHRH or impairment of GH secretion from whatever cause (Table 7.7) will lead to impaired growth. In infants the length of the upper segment of the body (from the top of the symphysis pubis to the crown) exceeds that of the lower segment (from the symphysis pubis to the floor) but subsequently the lower limbs grow more rapidly than the trunk until in adulthood both segments are of equal length. In normal adults the span of the outstretched arms is similar to the height.

Table 7.7 Causes of short stature

Primary	Secondary
Skeletal syndromes	Intrauterine growth retardation
Achondroplasia	Infections
Dyschondro osteosis	Maternal disease
Multiple epiphyseal dysplasia	Placental insufficiency
Fibrous dysplasia	Psychosocial deprivation
Chromosomal abnormalities	Malnutrition
Down's syndrome	Malabsorption
Turner's syndrome	Coeliac disease
In-born errors of metabolism	Cystic fibrosis
Glycogen storage disease	Inflammatory bowel disease
Mucopolysaccharidoses	Chronic renal disease
Genetic short stature	Cyanotic congenital heart disease
Constitutional	Asthma
	Steroid therapy
	Endocrine
	Craniopharyngioma
	Pituitary tumours
	Hypogonadism
	Hypothyroidism
	Pseudohypoparathyroidism
	Isolated GHRH deficiency
	Precocious puberty

Impairment of growth will thus usually be reflected by retention of a higher ratio of upper to lower segment than is appropriate for the chronological age. Bone age can be determined radiologically by the degree of fusion of the various epiphyses of the hands and wrists which can be compared with tables of standard deviations for normal healthy children of different ages, and by the degree of development of primary and secondary dentition.

The distribution of heights in any population shows a normal Gaussian curve. The height of an individual in that population is largely genetically determined and is related to the parental heights. Whilst men are on average some 13 cm taller than women there is wide individual variation. It is important to understand the expectations of an individual child and his or her parents in the context of the family and of the society in which they live. Centile charts for height and weight related to chronological age are invaluable for placing the child in the context of his or her peer group. Careful serial measurements of height and weight at intervals of six months or annually also help to determine whether growth is continuing along the expected line of development. In the individual, however, the annual rate of growth, particularly when it is related to the stage of development, may be a more useful guide to what further progress may be expected. Growth velocity declines from birth until the surge related to puberty after which it declines further and soon ceases. A delay in puberty is likely to result temporarily in relative shortness of stature given the variable age at which puberty occurs in the individual. Height below the third centile warrants investigation but more importantly a decline in the rate of growth from a higher centile requires assessment before the height has fallen too far behind.

Laboratory investigation of anterior pituitary failure

Basal and provocative tests of pituitary reserve are summarized in Table 7.8.

In a patient with frank clinical pan-hypopituitarism it may be sufficient to confirm the diagnosis by demonstrating that the basal levels of the pituitary hormones or those of their target organs are low. Many patients, however, have adequate basal hormone levels and the pituitary deficiency is revealed only by provocative tests of pituitary reserve.

Adrenocorticotrophic hormone
A low 0900 h plasma cortisol (<150 nmol/l) indicates an inadequate output, but a normal cortisol level does not exclude ACTH impairment. An insulin-induced hypoglycaemic stress test (so called insulin tolerance test, ITT) is necessary to demonstrate whether or not the hypothalamo–pituitary–adrenal axis is intact. Insulin is given as an intravenous bolus in a dose of 0.1 U/kg body weight, i.e. 7 units for a 70 kg patient to render the patient symptomatically hypoglycaemic with a blood glucose of <2.0 mmol/l. Alternatively, the insulin can be given as a rapid infusion until the same point is reached which has the advantage that infusion can then be stopped. Blood samples are taken basally and at the nadir of the blood glucose, and at 30-min intervals thereafter for 90 min for cortisol. The GH response can be measured at the same time. This test is safe as long as it is conducted under continuous careful supervision with hydrocortisone and glucose drawn up ready for immediate intravenous use if it is needed to abort the test. A rise in plasma cortisol to 500 nmol/l is regarded as an adequate response to hypoglycaemic stress.

Table 7.8 Basal and provocative tests of pituitary function

Axis	Basal test	Provocative test
Adrenocorticotrophic hormone (ACTH)	0900 h cortisol	Insulin tolerance test (ITT) Corticotrophin releasing hormone (CRH)
Growth hormone (GH)	(Serial samples)	ITT
Gonadotrophin	Luteinizing hormone (LH) Follicular stimulating hormone (FSH) Testosterone Oestrodiol	Gonadotrophin releasing hormone (GnRH)
Prolactin (PRL)	Resting PRL	(Thyrotrophin releasing hormone, TRH)
Thyroid stimulating hormone (TSH)	fT_4 TSH	TRH

The corticotrophin releasing hormone (CRH) test is not yet routinely practicable but may become so when the material becomes more widely available. A bolus of CRH, 100 µg, produces a rise in ACTH and hence of cortisol within 30 min which plateaus after 60 min in normal subjects. This test demonstrates whether or not the pituitary–adrenal components of the axis are intact but this is not the same information as provided by the ITT which stresses the whole hypothalamic–pituitary–adrenal axis. Similarly, the synacthen test (Chapter 9) only tests the ability of the adrenal to respond to ACTH and is of limited value in the assessment of pituitary function other than to establish that the adrenal is capable of a response before testing the rest of the axis with an ITT.

Growth hormone
Provocative tests of GH secretion, such as the insulin-induced hypoglycaemic stress test, produce a rise in GH secretion to 20 mU/l or more in normal individuals. Failure to produce any significant GH response to hypoglycaemia will identify severely GH deficient individuals but moderately impaired GH production may not be recognized by this or other provocative tests. A midnight blood sample for GH may coincide with a spontaneous GH peak and a value of 20 mU/l or more would reassure that there was no GH deficiency. However, even such a timed sample might miss a GH pulse and a random sample cannot be used to confirm GH deficiency. The definition of GH deficiency is not easy since it is seldom absolute, and serial sampling at close intervals over several hours to pick up the pattern and amplitude of GH secretion may be necessary.

A random GH measurement is of little value since the usual assays are not sufficiently sensitive to distinguish low from normal levels. Secretion of GH is best assessed by its response to an ITT (see above). An alternative, but less reliable, way of demonstrating that GH secretion is adequate is to measure the GH response after a standard aminoacid load, such as can be provided reasonably palatably by 20 g of Bovril. The latter test is sometimes preferred to an ITT in young children but is not as consistent or reproducible as the results of an ITT. A value of 20 mU/l GH in response to stress is deemed adequate evidence of a normal GH reserve.

Luteinizing hormone and follicle stimulating hormone
Basal LH and FSH should be low or undetectable in patients with impaired sexual function due to a hypothalamic or pituitary lesion. The main value of measuring LH and FSH is to exclude primary gonadal failure when LH and FSH levels are high. The GnRH test has proved disappointing in clinical practice because a wide variety of responses have been observed in normal subjects and in patients with impaired sexual function and proven pituitary tumours. Theoretically, no LH or FSH response would be expected with a pituitary lesion, but often a rise of LH or, to a lesser extent, of FSH is observed. Thus an absent response is consistent with pituitary failure but a small rise in either gonadotrophin does not exclude the diagnosis of impaired gonado-

trophin function. The hypothalamic–pituitary–gonadal axis is very sensitive to minor alterations of gonadal steroids. In practice the GnRH test adds very little to the information provided by measurement of basal circulating testosterone or oestrogens, LH and FSH.

Prolactin
Basal PRL levels must be measured with the patient at rest. Stress so readily causes PRL to rise that even a venepuncture or the anxiety of coming to hospital may make it difficult to interpret the result of a random test. Values <450 mU/l are regarded as normal and results >1000 mU/l are usually abnormal, but borderline results should be reassessed with the patient recumbent and an indwelling venous cannula inserted an hour before sampling, which should be repeated at hourly intervals for three hours. As the purpose is to show whether or not PRL levels are elevated, rather than depressed as with the other pituitary hormones, there is little point in undertaking any provocative test of PRL secretion although PRL does respond to TRH.

Thyroid stimulating hormone
TSH assays are now sufficiently sensitive to distinguish low from normal values which was not the case with previous assays. A low TSH, using a sensitive assay, together with low free thyroxine supports the diagnosis of secondary hypothyroidism and may obviate the need for a TRH test. A flat TSH response to TRH is consistent with the diagnosis of secondary hypothyroidism. In practice modest rises in TSH after TRH are commonly seen in patients with borderline low thyroxine levels and proven pituitary lesions, and the TRH test has not turned out to be as good a discriminator of pituitary hypothyroidism as might have been expected.

Treatment of pituitary failure

Functionless pituitary tumours
Many so-called 'functionless' pituitary tumours turned out to be PRL secreting with the advent of a PRL assay, but the term is still used for tumours, usually chromophobe adenomas, which do not produce hypersecretion of any hormones. The treatment of such tumours depends on their size and the age and condition of the patient. A large suprasellar tumour, causing a visual field defect, will need surgical decompression usually by the trans-frontal route. A moderately large tumour with no or only slight suprasellar extension may be removed by the trans-sphenoidal route. A modestly enlarged tumour largely confined to the pituitary fossa may not require surgical treatment at all, particularly in an older patient, but it is common to irradiate such tumours to prevent further growth.

Replacement therapy in hypopituitarism
Patients with inadequate cortisol reserve require replacement treatment with

oral hydrocortisone, 20 mg in the morning and 10 mg at night, for routine maintenance purposes, or alternatively with prednisolone, 5 mg in the morning and 2.5 mg at night, as mineralocorticoid function is usually adequate in secondary as opposed to primary adrenal insufficiency. Patients should carry a steroid card at all times to identify that they are on steroids and be advised to at least double their maintenance dose if they suffer any intercurrent illness or undue stress. If this is not sufficient to relieve any malaise immediately, or they cannot maintain therapy because of vomiting, they should seek prompt medical attention. Severe stress or a surgical procedure will require cover with intravenous hydrocortisone, initially 100 mg IV, repeated six hourly or given as a continuous infusion. The dose can be gradually reduced over succeeding days as the patient recovers until oral therapy can be given and the dose further reduced to maintenance levels.

Deficiency of GH does not require treatment in an adult but synthetic GH may be needed in carefully selected children with proven lack of growth due to GH deficiency whose long bone epiphyses have not fused. Such treatment is expensive and requires close supervision. It should not be given except under specialist direction. Biosynthetic human GH (somatropin) is produced using recombinant DNA technology and is identical in structure to human GH. It can be given either subcutaneously or intramuscularly in divided doses to a total of 0.5–0.7 U/kg/week. The optimum treatment regime should be determined for each patient in order to produce the desired increase in growth velocity.

Many of the causes of GH deficiency are not due to lack of GH but to impairment of hypothalamic GHRH secretion. Synthetic GHRH is not yet routinely available but has been used in therapeutic trials by intermittent injection to mimic the endogenous pulsation of GHRH and hence of GH. Growth hormone releasing hormone in a dose of 500 µg/day should produce a peak GH response of >30 mU/l. Some non-responders to GHRH may still respond to GH therapy.

Deficiency of TSH with resultant secondary hypothyroidism is readily corrected by replacement thyroxine in a dose of 100 to 150 µg daily. The dose should be sufficient to render the patient euthyroid clinically and to restore the patient's free thyroxine to normal. Thyroxine therapy should not be commenced before any cortisol deficiency has been corrected.

Gonadotrophin deficiency with resultant secondary hypogonadism requires treatment not only to restore adequate gonadal hormone levels but also to prevent premature osteoporosis. Testosterone can be given either orally as Restandol, 40–120 mg daily, or, if compliance is difficult or adequate testosterone levels are not achieved, by monthly injections of testosterone proprionate (Sustanon, 250 or 500 mg intramuscularly). Cyclical replacement therapy with combined oestrogen/progestogen or low dose oestrogen only pill is suitable for women of reproductive years. Such treatment will not of course restore fertility in either sex. Fertility may be restored by treatment with gonadotropins (Chapter 10).

Replacement therapy for hypopituitarism is summarized in Table 7.9.

Table 7.9 Replacement therapy for hypopituitarism

Axis	Replacement therapy
Adrenocorticotrophin hormone (ACTH)	Hydrocortisone, 20 mg a.m., 10 mg p.m. or Prednisolone 5 mg a.m., 2.5 mg p.m.
Growth hormone (GH)	Somatropin in children (see text)
Luteinizing hormone (LH), Follicle stimulating hormone (FSH)	Testosterone in males, Oral Restandol Sustanon, IM Oestrogen/progestogen in females or Low dose oestrogen (see text) Fertility drugs (see Chapter 10)
Thyroid stimulating hormone (TSH)	Thyroxine, 100–150 µg daily

The Neurohypophysis (Posterior Pituitary)

The neurohypophysis consists of the median eminence, the infundibular stem and the infundibular process. Impulses from higher centres reach the supraoptic and paraventricular nuclei which synthesize oxytocin and vasopressin stored as neurophysins in the form of granules which pass down the axons to be released directly into the capillary circulation (Fig. 7.12). Arginine vasopressin (AVP), otherwise known as the anti-diuretic hormone (ADH), acts on the distal part of the renal tubules to promote the reabsorption of water. Release of vasopressin results from a rise in plasma osmolarity or a fall in plasma volume signalled via osmoreceptors in the area supplied by the internal carotid artery, and volume receptors whose location is not certain. Stress, nicotine and opiates all stimulate vasopressin release. Vasopressin is inhibited by drinking which depends on having an intact thirst centre in the hypothalamus. The plasma osmolarity is normally maintained within narrow limits and thirst is perceived when osmolarity exceeds a given threshold, usually around 295 mosmol/l.

Oxytocin acts on the uterus and plays a role in parturition but its exact function is uncertain in normal humans. It is also present in follicular fluid and may have a role in the mechanism of contraction of Fallopian tubes during ovulation.

Diabetes Insipidus

Lack of the anti-diuretic hormone, AVP, results in polyuria and polydipsia. Other causes of polyuria such as diabetes mellitus, hypercalcaemia and renal failure can be readily excluded by simple blood tests. The main differential diagnosis lies between cranial and nephrogenic diabetes insipidus, and compulsive water drinking of psychogenic origin. The causes of diabetes insipidus are shown in Table 7.10.

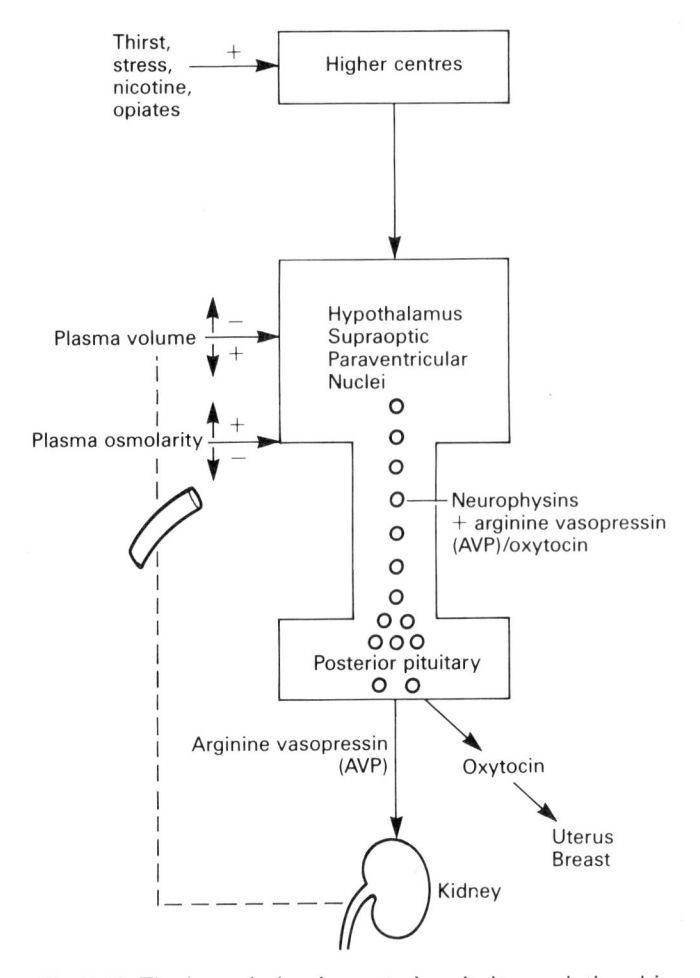

Fig. 7.12 The hypothalamic-posterior pituitary relationship.

The patient with thirst and polyuria who has a high plasma osmolarity (>300 mosmol/l) and a large urine volume of low osmolarity, less than that of plasma, almost certainly has diabetes insipidus and it may be dangerous and unnecessary to proceed to a water deprivation test. Many patients, however, with modest diabetes insipidus maintain normal plasma osmolarity and electrolytes although they have a high daily fluid input and output, provided that they have an appropriate thirst response. To establish the diagnosis in such patients it is necessary to show that they are unable to produce AVP in response to water deprivation or a saline load. The assay of AVP is technically difficult and not routinely available in many centres. The response of AVP to a hypertonic saline load (850 mmol) in normal subjects and the lack of such a response in a patient with diabetes insipidus is shown in Fig. 7.13.

The water deprivation test requires the patient to be denied access to fluids

Table 7.10 Causes of diabetes insipidus (DI)

Cranial	Nephrogenic
Familial (dominant or recessive)	Familial (sex-linked recessive)
Idiopathic	Metabolic
Trauma	Hypercalcaemia
Head injury	Hypokalaemia
Craniotomy	Poisons
Pituitary stalk section	Lithium
Tumours	Analgesics
Craniopharyngioma	Tubular nephritis
Large pituitary tumours	Interstitial nephritis
Metastases	Amyloid
Granuloma	
Sarcoidosis	
Histiocytosis-X	
Infections	
Encephalitis	
Meningitis	
Vascular	
Aneurysms	
Sickle cell anaemia	

for at least six hours and measurement of plasma and urine osmolarities made at hourly intervals. The patient should be weighed at the beginning of the test and at regular intervals and the test should be stopped if the weight falls by >3%. It is notoriously difficult to ensure that the test is properly conducted, particularly in a patient suspected of compulsive water drinking who may make surreptitious efforts to gain access to fluids. In the patient with true diabetes insipidus the plasma osmolarity rises above 300 mosmol/l and the urine osmolarity fails to reach twice that of the plasma. The patient with cranial diabetes insipidus will respond to exogenous AVP given in the form of desamino-dys-d-arginine vasopressin (DDAVP) whereas nephrogenic diabetes insipidus does not respond because such patients do not lack AVP but suffer from end-organ resistance to the hormone. The compulsive water drinker may suffer from an altered thirst threshold and the plasma osmolarity is often low and does not rise above normal levels in response to water deprivation.

Treatment of cranial diabetes insipidus is with DDAVP which is absorbed by nasal inhalation in a dose of 5 to 10 μg once or twice a day. The dose is adjusted to maintain a fluid balance of less than 2 l/day with normal plasma osmolarity. Excess treatment will cause fluid retention and haemodilution.

Inappropriate Anti-Diuretic Hormone Secretion

Inappropriate ADH secretion is usually due to ectopic production of the hormone by tumours, typically an oat-cell carcinoma of the bronchus, but it

208 The Hypothalamus and Pituitary

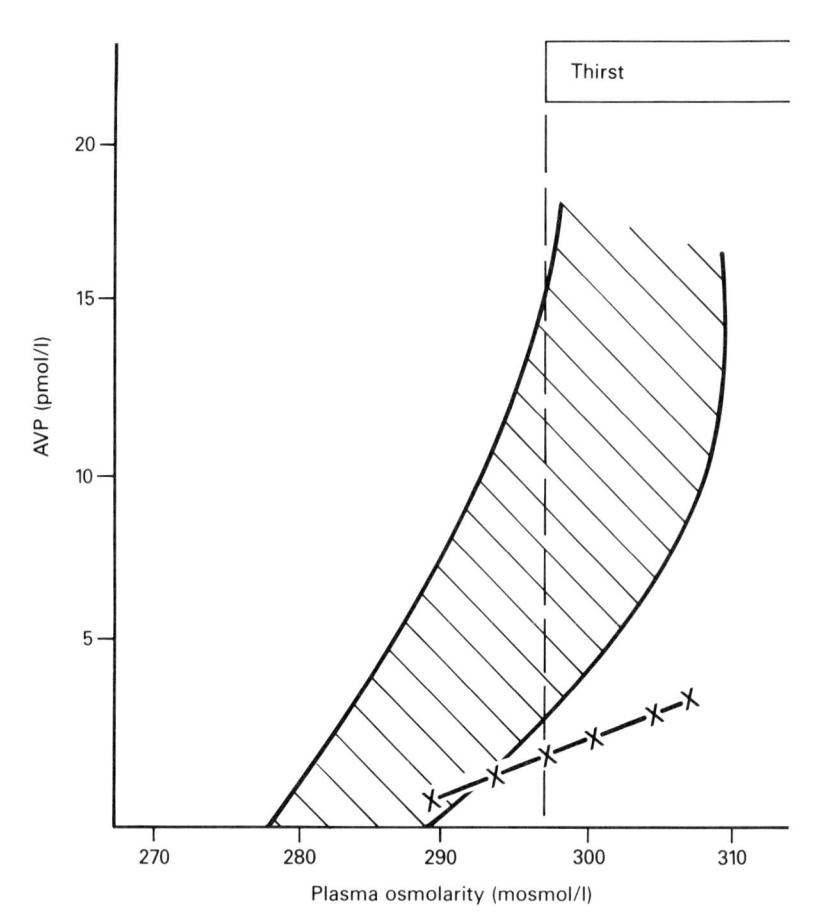

Fig. 7.13 Relationship between arginine vasopressin (AVP) and plasma osmolarity. The shaded area shows the normal response to a saline load. The line (X—X) shows a low response in cranial diabetes insipidus.

Table 7.11 Causes of inappropriate anti-diuretic hormone secretion

Malignancy	Oatcell carcinoma of bronchus
	Carcinomas of gastrointestinal tract, pancreas or prostate
	Lymphoma
Neurological	Meningitis
	Encephalitis
	Brain tumour
	Head injury
Respiratory	Chronic suppurative disorders
	Empyema
	Cystic fibrosis
	Pneumonia
Drugs	Chlorpropamide
	Lithium

may be due to other causes including head injury (Table 7.11). The patient may present with a confusional state, or the condition may be suspected from a low plasma urea and electrolytes in the absence of other causes such as diuretic therapy. Such patients seldom exhibit peripheral oedema and the primary tumour may not be obvious. The plasma osmolarity is low but the urine osmolarity is usually increased relative to the plasma. Treatment is by restriction of fluid input to 500 ml/day where practicable, although salt-retaining drugs such as the long-acting tetracycline demeclocycline may be of use in patients who cannot be fluid restricted. A hypertonic saline load is rapidly excreted and is of little use except in an emergency where a patient might fit because of the severity of the condition. Removal of the primary tumour, if located and surgery if practicable, will correct the inappropriate ADH secretion.

Further Reading

Baylis, P.H. (1987). The posterior pituitary. In Clinical Endocrinology London, p. 5.2. Edited by Besser, G.H. and Cudworth, A.G. Chapman and Hall, London.
Baylis, P.H. (1989). Regulation of vasopressin secretion. Ballière's Clinics in Endocrinology and Metabolism, **3**, 313–330. Edited by Baylis, P.H. Ballière Tindall, London.
Brook, C. G. D. (1988). Treatment of growth deficiency. *Clinical Endocrinology* **30**, 197.
Hall, R. and Besser, M. (eds) (1989) *Fundamentals of Clinical Endocrinology*, 4th edition. Churchill Livingstone Edinburgh.
Ho, K.Y., Evans, W.S. and Thorner, M.O. (1985). Diseases of prolactin and growth hormone secretion. Clinics in Endocrinology and Metabolism, **14**, 1–32.
Lawton, N.F. (1987). Prolactinomas: medical or surgical treatment. *Quarterly Journal of Medicine* **64**, 557.
Linton, E.A. and Lowry, P.J. (1989). Corticotrophin releasing factor in man and its measurement: a review. *Clinical Endocrinology* **31**, 225.
Nabarro, J.D.N. (1987). Acromegaly. *Clinical Endocrinology* **26**, 481.
Reichlin, S. (1987). Neuro endocrine control of pituitary function. In Clinical Endocrinology, p. 1.2. Edited by Besser, G.M. and Cudworth, A.G. Chapman and Hall, London.
Tanner, J.M. and Whitehouse, R.H. (1976). Clinical longitudinal standards for height, weight, height velocity, weight velocity and stages of puberty. *Archives of Diseases in Childhood* **51**, 170.
Van Couter, E. (1989). Physiology and pathology of circadian rhythms. In *Recent Advances in Endocrinology and Metabolism*, No. 3, pp. 109–134. Edited by Edwards, C.R.W. and Lincoln, D.W. Churchill Livingstone, Edinburgh.

8

THE THYROID

Development and Anatomy

The thyroid develops from a pouch in the floor of the primitive pharynx between the first and second branchial arches in the first month of fetal life. As the fetus grows the pouch separates and migrates caudally, and come to lie in the anterior part of the neck. The line of its descent is marked by the thyroglossal duct which originates in the midline at the junction of the anterior two-thirds and posterior one-third of the tongue, the foramen caecum, and subsequently becomes obliterated. Fragments of the duct can persist either as islets of functioning thyroid tissue such as a lingual thyroid or pyramidal lobe or as non-functioning thyroglassal cysts. The fetal thyroid starts to function between the 8th and 12th weeks of fetal life at the same time as the fetal pituitary gland starts to produce thyrotrophin. Failure of development of the fetal thyroid results in congenital hypothyroidism (Fig. 8.1).

The adult thyroid consists of two conical lobes joined by a central band, the isthmus, lying anterior to the trachea. The isthmus covers the second and third tracheal rings and the lateral lobes are usually about 4 cm long and taper upwards. The gland may be palpated by standing behind the patient and curling the tips of the middle three fingers round the anterior border of the sternomastoid muscles just above the sternal notch so that they rest lightly on the trachea. The gland moves with the trachea on swallowing. A normal gland may nevertheless not be palpable in 75% of men and 50% of women depending on their build and the bulk of their necks. Estimates of the size of the gland by weight or volume on clinical examination are notoriously inaccurate. World Health Organization criteria define a goitre as a thyroid whose lateral lobes have a volume greater than that of the terminal phalanx of the thumb of the person being examined. A thyroid that is visible as well as palpable is almost always regarded as enlarged (Fig. 8.2).

The functioning unit of the thyroid is the follicle, and the gland consists of numerous such follicles of varying sizes separated by connective tissue. The parafollicular C-cells found embedded in the connective tissue are of separate origin from the thyroid and secrete calcitonin. Each thyroid follicle is spherical and consists of a lining of epithelial cells surrounding a central space filled with fluid known as colloid. The base of each follicular cell lies adjacent to a capillary

Development and Anatomy 211

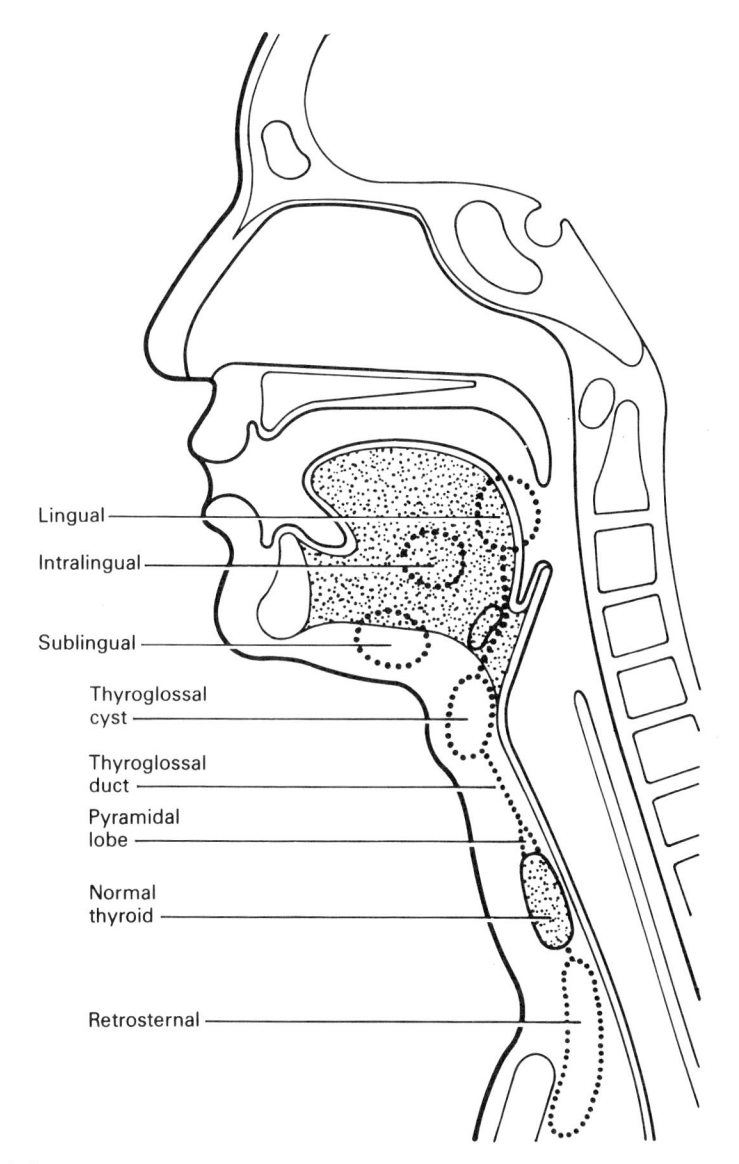

Fig. 8.1 Sites of normal and ectopic thyroid tissue along the line of the thyroglossal duct.

and the apex of the cell consists of microvilli pointing into the colloid. The nucleus is close to the base of the cell. The size of the cells depends on the activity of the follicle and in general the height of the cells is inversely related to the amount of colloid (Fig. 8.3).

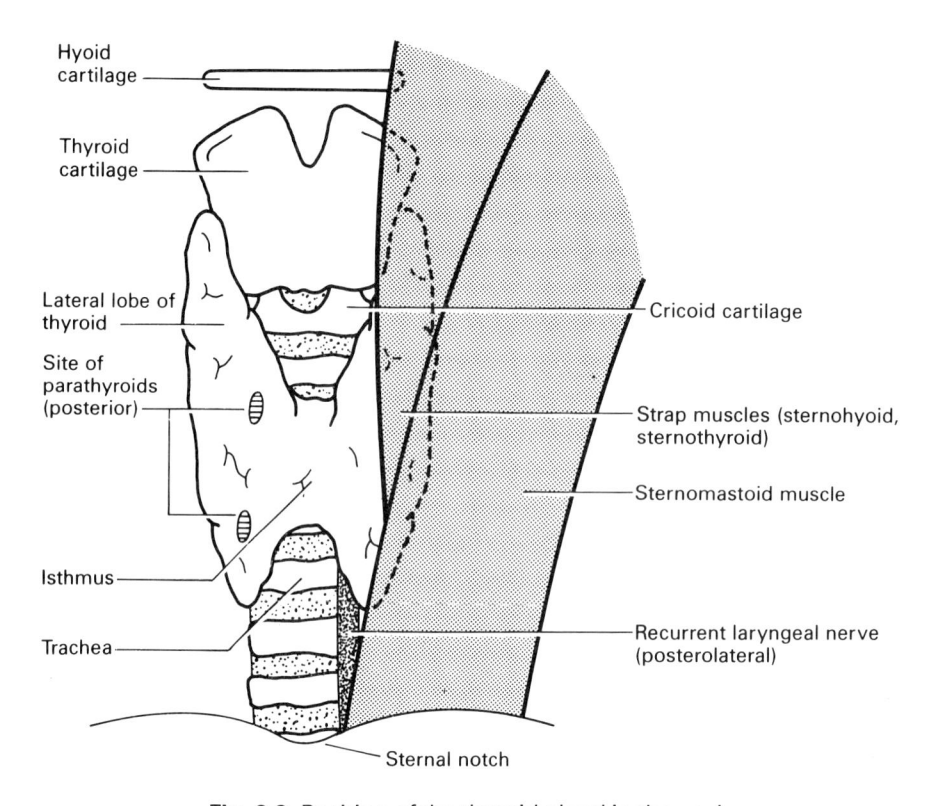

Fig. 8.2 Position of the thyroid gland in the neck.

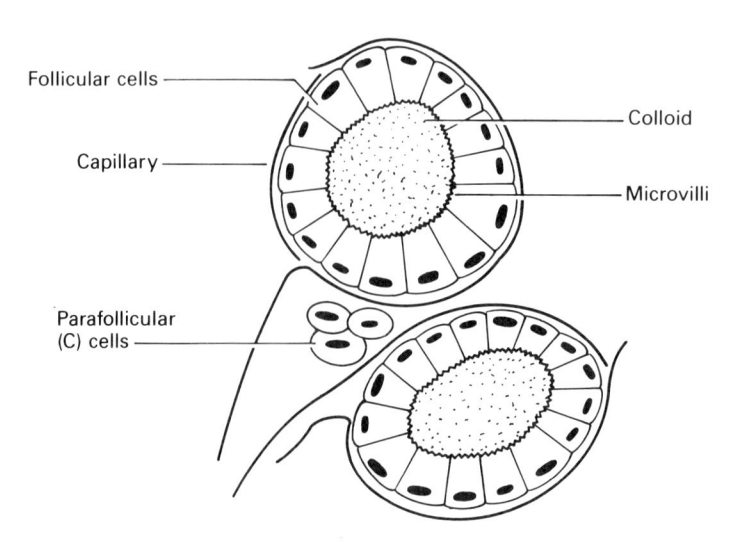

Fig. 8.3 Thyroid follicles and parafollicular (C) cells.

Physiology

Thyroid hormone synthesis and release

The thyroid produces two major hormones, thyroxine (T_4) which may be regarded as a pro-hormone and tri-iodothyronine (T_3) which is the active principle. Both hormones are produced within the thyroid follicle and are released into the circulation. Tri-iodothyronine is also produced by conversion from T_4 taken up by other cells of the body, particularly in the liver and kidneys.

The various steps in the formation and release of the thyroid hormones are shown in Fig. 8.4. Failure of any one of these steps due to absence of the appropriate enzyme will result in hypothyroidism and usually also a goitre. Such defects are uncommon but should be considered in the investigation of childhood and familial goitres. Disorders of thyroid hormonogenesis are usually inherited as autosomal recessives.

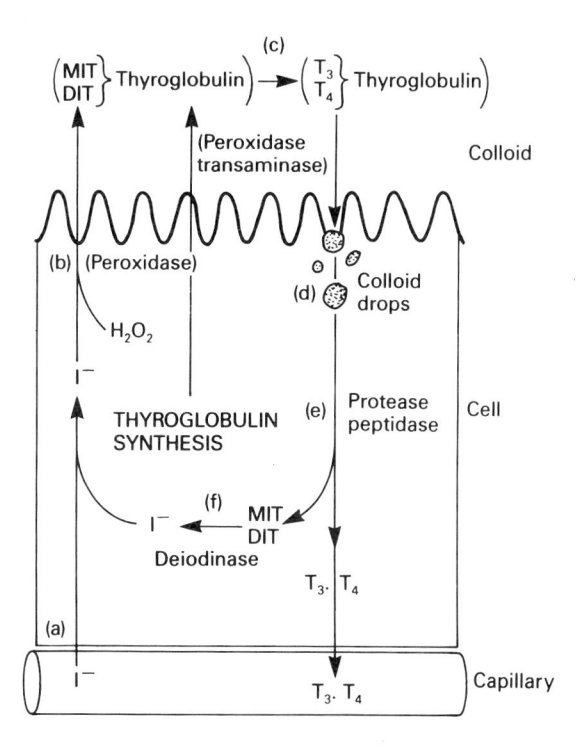

Fig. 8.4 Schematic representation of a thyroid cell showing steps in thyroid hormone synthesis and release. (a) Iodide transport. (b) Oxidation. (c) Coupling. (d) Colloid resorption. (e) Proteolysis. (f) Deiodination. MIT, mono-iodotyrosines. DIT, di-iodotyrosines. T4, thyroxine. T3, tri-iodothyronine.

214   The Thyroid

The steps of thyroid hormone synthesis and release are as follows:

Step a   Iodine in the diet, in drinking water and food such as fish or iodized bread or salt, is absorbed from the gut. Inorganic iodide (I^-) in the circulation is trapped in the thyroid by active transport across the follicular cell membrane. An iodide trapping defect will be revealed by a very low radio-iodine uptake.

Step b   Iodide is rapidly transferred across the cell and into the colloid lumen during which process it is oxidized by peroxidase and linked to tyrosine molecules to form mono-iodotyrosines (MIT) and di-iodotyrosines (DIT). Tyrosines are contained within thyroglobulin which is a large protein synthesized within the cell and secreted into the colloid.

Step c   MIT and DIT are then coupled by further enzyme action (transaminase and peroxidase) to form T_4 and T_3 still linked to thyroglobulin within the colloid lumen. Steps b and c form the process of the organification of iodide. Defects of organification may be revealed by the perchlorate discharge test: isotope-labelled iodide accumulates in the cell because it is not incorporated into tyrosine and treatment with perchlorate rapidly discharges any radio-idodide left in the form of iodide which is normally a negligible fraction of the total radio-iodine accumulating in the labelling process.

Step d T_4 and T_3 linked to thyroglobulin are reabsorbed into the follicular cells in the form of colloid droplets by a process of endocytosis.

Step e T_4 and T_3 are then separated from thyroglobulin by proteases contained within lysosomes.

Step f   Any uncoupled MIT and DIT are further deiodinated to release tyrosine and iodide which may be recycled. T_4 and T_3 are secreted into the circulation.
Figure 8.5 shows the structures of iodotyrosines and iodothyronines.

Circulating Thyroid Hormones

Thyroxine and T_3 are largely bound to plasma proteins, mainly thyroxine-binding globulin (TBG) and albumin. Thyroxine-binding globulin has a much greater affinity for T_4 than T_3. Albumin has a much lower affinity than TBG for both thyroid hormones but binds a significant proportion of the hormones because it is present in greater quantities. Conditions which affect the quantity of circulating binding proteins will influence the measurement of total circulating thyroid hormones. Thus pregnancy or oestrogen-containing oral contraceptive drugs which increase protein binding cause an increase in total T_4 and total T_3, whereas low protein states, for example, nephrotic syndrome, liver disease or malnutrition, lead to low total thyroid hormone levels. Rarely TBG deficiency can be inherited as an X-linked recessive or autosomal dominant and TBG excess as a probable X-linked dominant. Occasionally abnormal albu-

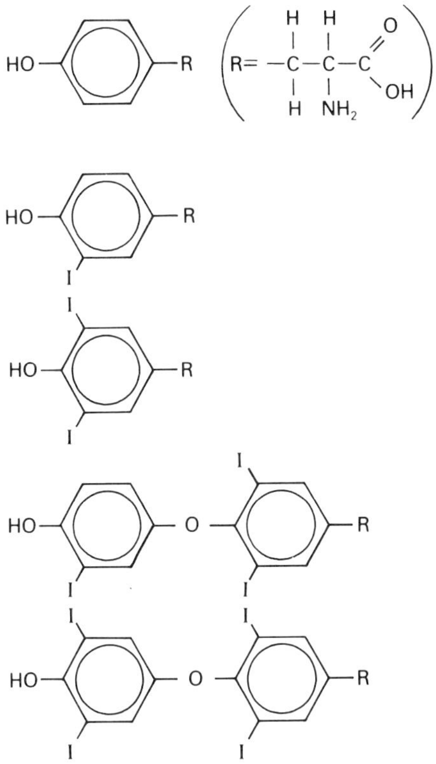

Tyrosine

3-Monoiodotyrosine (MIT)

3,5-Di-iodotyrosine (DIT)

3′,3,5.-Tri-iodothyronine (T_3)

3′,5′,3,5-Tetraiodothyronine (thyroxine, T_4)

Fig. 8.5 Structures of iodotyrosines and iodothyronines.

mins may also be inherited as autosomal dominants and produce familial dysalbuminaemic hyperthyroxinaemia. Such changes in binding proteins may result in misleading elevation or reduction of total T_4 and T_3 levels, but the patients are usually euthyroid because the levels of free unbound hormone which govern the patient's thyroid state are normal.

Anomalous total T_4 and T_3 results can be corrected for abnormal TBG levels either by direct measurement of TBG, to derive a T_4/TBG ratio, or by an indirect measure of the remaining binding sites availabe to bind thyroid hormones. The latter is obtained by mixing the serum with a known quantity of radio-isotope labelled T_3 and a resin able to bind T_3; a proportion of the label will become attached to the serum proteins according to the number of binding sites available. The percentage of radio-isotope bound to the resin can then be used to derive a free thyroxine index (FTI=total $T_4 \times T_3$ resin uptake/100).

Newer techniques for the measurement of free thyroid hormone levels are not usually influenced by the amount of TBG present in the serum, but some methods may be affected by the presence of anomalous albumins.

Thyroxine is produced entirely by the thyroid, but T_3 is also produced by peripheral conversion from T_4 in cells of the liver, kidney, heart, anterior

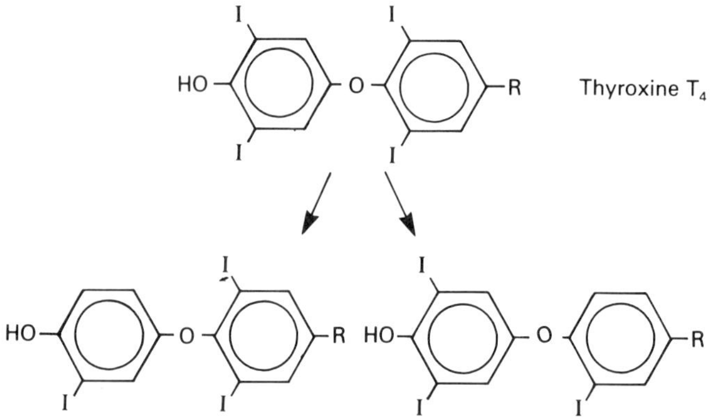

Thyroxine T_4

3'.3.5-Tri-iodothyronine, T_3 (active)

3'5'.3-Tri-iodothyronine, reverse T_3 (inactive)

Fig. 8.6 Deiodination of thyroxine (T4) to tri-iodothyronine (T3) or reverse T3.

pituitary and other tissues. Thyroxine is deiodinated into the active metabolite T_3 or its inactive metabolite reverse T_3 (rT3), a mirror image of the former (Fig. 8.6).

The mechanisms controlling the conversion of T_4 to either T_3 or rT_3 are ill understood but in severely ill patients suffering from a variety of non-thyroid diseases less T_3 and more rT_3 is produced. Such conditions may result in a low T_4 or low T_3 state yet the patient is not hypothyroid as confirmed by a normal serum thyrotrophin (TSH) (see later).

Control of Thyroid Function

The synthesis and release of thyroid hormones is controlled by thyrotrophin (thyroid stimulating hormone, TSH) produced by the anterior pituitary gland which is in turn regulated by thyrotrophin releasing hormone (TRH) from the hypothalamus (Fig. 8.7). Thyroid stimulating hormone is a glycoprotein consisting of alpha and beta subunits linked by non-covalent bonds. The alpha subunit is similar to that of three other glycoprotein hormones (LH, FSH human chorionic gonadotrophin, HCG) but the beta subunits differ. Dissociated alpha and beta subunits are not biologically active but become active when combined.

Thyroid stimulating hormone stimulates the production of T_4 and T_3 by the thyroid, and the circulating levels of these hormones in turn exert a negative feedback effect on TSH and possibly also TRH production. Conversion of T_4 to T_3 within the anterior pituitary suppresses TSH secretion whereas falling serum T_4 levels stimulate TSH release. In normal individuals the levels of the circulating thyroid hormones are maintained within very narrow limits. Thyrotrophin releasing hormone may govern the physiological set-point of the TSH

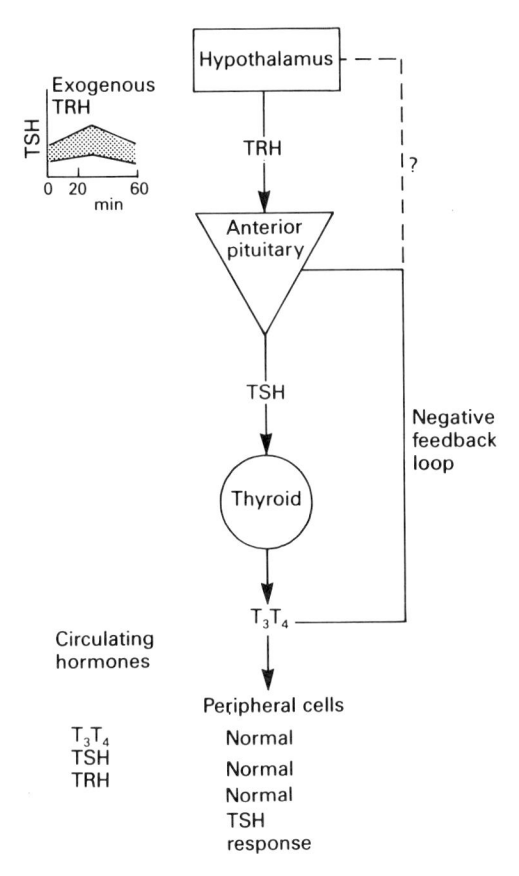

Fig. 8.7 Normal control of thyroid function. TRH, thyrotrophin releasing hormone. TSH, thyroid stimulating hormone. T3, tri-iodothyronine. T4, thyroxine.

response but its exact physiological role is uncertain because serum TRH concentrations are very difficult to measure.

Thyrotrophin releasing hormone is a tripeptide which has been synthesized in the laboratory and is available for diagnostic use. A 200 µg bolus of TRH given intravenously produces a rise in TSH which peaks after about 20 min (at 4–25 mU/l) and falls rapidly but not completely to the baseline by 60 min. The rise in TSH is proportional to the baseline value and the advent of sensitive TSH assays has largely obviated the need for the TRH test (Fig. 8.8).

Peripheral Effects of Thyroid Hormones

Thyroid hormones act on several tissues by a variety of mechanisms. They are concerned in the transport of aminoacids and electrolytes to the interior of cells, the synthesis or activation of specific enzymes within cells and the enhancement of intracellular events which may lead to changes in cell size and

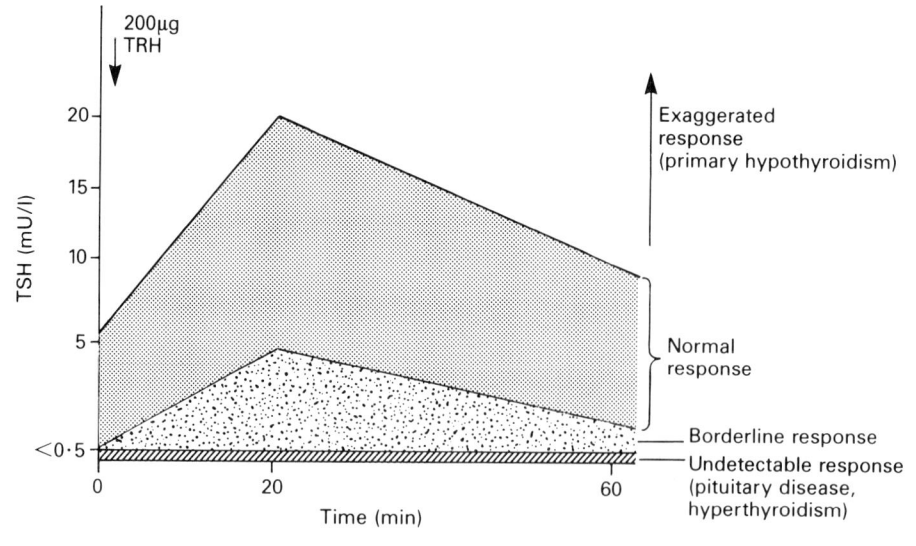

Fig. 8.8 The thyroid stimulating hormone (TSH) response to thyrotrophin releasing hormone (TRH).

activities. They play a major role in growth and the regulation of protein, lipid, carbohydrate and mineral metabolism, and thermogenesis.

Tri-iodo thyronine binds to specific receptor sites in cell nuclei and induces the formation of a variety of species of messenger RNA coding for proteins such as growth factors and enzymes which enhance lipolysis in adipose cells, modulate gonadotrophin secretion in pituitary cells, or maintain cell growth in hair. In liver, kidney and muscle, thyroid hormones regulate the activities of the sodium pump and glycolytic pathways. In these tissues the major cellular effects are mediated via the mitochondria, which regulate energy production by oxidative phosphorylation. The energy produced by the oxidation of substrates is transformed into widely utilizable high-energy phosphate bonds of adenosine triphosphate (ATP). In the brain, thyroid hormones are not concerned in thermogenesis but are important for normal development and regulate the activities of neurotransmitters and their receptors.

The peripheral effects of thyroid hormones in humans are not easily measured. Measurement of basal metabolic rate by indirect calorimetry is a cumbersome procedure which is little used in clinical practice, but does reflect the overall energy production by the body and is increased in hyperthyroidism and decreased in hypothyroidism. Other effects may be observed such as heart rate and the relaxation time of tendon reflexes, but these are crude measures which are obviously abnormal only in fairly extreme disturbances of thyroid function. Sadly, sensitive tests of peripheral thyroid hormone action are lacking in clinical practice, which is why it is so often difficult to judge an individual's true thyroid status.

Effects of Iodine

Daily iodine requirements in a normal adult are approximately 150 μg but iodine intake varies considerably in individuals, even in non-iodine deficient areas from 50 to 500 μg or more. Iodine is mainly found in fish, milk and dairy products, eggs and meat. The iodine content of vegetables, except spinach, is low. Iodine is almost entirely absorbed from the gut with negligible excretion in the faeces but it is excreted in the urine and this can be used as an estimate of iodine intake. Twenty-four hour urine excretion of less than 50 μg is taken to reflect iodine deficiency and if less than 25 μg the deficiency is severe.

Chronic iodine deficiency is endemic in many parts of the world, particularly in mountainous areas such as the Andes and the Himalayas where the iodine is leached out of the soil. In such areas the prevalence of goitre and hypothyroidism is high. There is also a high prevalence of a condition known as endemic cretinism. This is characterized by irreversible intellectual and physical impairment with defects of speech, hearing and gait often, but not invariably, accompanied by hypothyroidism and stunted growth. The incidence of endemic cretinism has been greatly reduced in areas where iodine deficiency has been corrected by the use of prophylactic iodine in the form of iodized oil given by injection to women of reproductive years, or iodized salt and iodized bread. An individual suffering from iodine deficiency will conserve iodine by reducing its excretion and preferentially secreting T_3 rather than T_4. Such individuals have an increased uptake of ^{131}I and low T_4 levels but may have normal T_3 levels even in the face of the raised TSH level found in severe iodine deficiency.

Iodine excess

The acute administration of small amounts of iodine to normal individuals does not alter significantly the uptake of ^{131}I given simultaneously, but in large quantities inhibition of organification occurs. This phenomenon, known as the Wolff–Chaikoff effect after the investigators who first described it, is transient as the thyroid escapes from inhibition after about 48 h due to adaptation of the iodide transport mechanism. Large quantities of iodine, such as may be administered by the use of iodine-containing contrast media in radiological investigations, thus temporarily blunt thyroid function. Therapeutic use of this phenomenon may be made in the preparation of patients with large vascular goitres for surgery by the administration of Lugol's iodine for a few days before operation. Tablets containing a large quantity of iodine could be taken immediately after exposure to ionizing radiation in a nuclear accident in order to prevent the uptake of radio-iodine by the thyroid.

Chronic iodine excess can result in the down regulation of thyroid function by mechanisms which are not fully understood and may lead to hypothyroidism and goitre even in the absence of known underlying thyroid disease. Iodine excess may result from the ingestion of drugs or other agents containing large quantities of iodine such as amiodarone (used for cardiac arrthymias), Felsol (a cough mixture), or Kelp (a seaweed preparation popular as a health food). In some individuals, presumed to have underlying autonomous thyroid nodules or Graves' disease, but protected by relative iodine deficiency from becoming hyperthyroid, the addition of iodine may unmask thyrotoxicosis. The introduction of iodized bread or salt in areas of endemic iodine deficiency has thus frequently led to an increased incidence of thyrotoxicosis as well as a reduction in the incidence of goitre and hypothyroidism. The increased incidence of thyrotoxicosis follows soon after the enhancement of the iodine intake and subsequently declines presumably as the remaining number of susceptible individuals are fewer. This phenomenon named after Jodbasedow may still be observed to occur sporadically even in non-iodine-deficient areas when a susceptible individual may develop thyrotoxicosis following an iodine load.

The effects of amiodarone, mentioned above, are not simply due to its high iodine content (75 mg iodine per 200 mg tablet) as the drug also interferes with the conversion of T_4 to T_3 and its inactive metabolite reverse T_3. This inhibition of T_3 production from T_4 and of the deiodination of reverse T_3 results in high T_4 and reverse T_3 levels but normal or lowish T_3 levels. Therefore, T_3 is a more useful guide to the patient's true thyroid status whilst taking this drug or during the several weeks or months that it takes to clear after withdrawal. Amiodarone may nevertheless occasionally induce either thyrotoxicosis (revealed by a high T_3) or hypothyroidism (revealed by a high TSH) in individuals who are usually thought to have underlying auto-immune thyroid disease.

Radio-isotope studies

Radio-iodine uptake is related to iodine intake in the population and there is evidence that with increasing iodine intake over the years in non-iodine-deficient areas the ^{131}I uptake in normal individuals has gradually decreased. The rate of uptake of ^{131}I is now seldom used in the diagnosis of hyperthyroidism because it is not very precise, is relatively troublesome and costly, and has been superceded by the advent of simpler assays directly measuring the thyroid hormones in the circulation. 131-Iodine or the shorter lasting ^{123}I, or 99-technesium which is trapped but not iodinated, are rapidly taken up by a thyrotoxic gland or nodule. Uptake is very slow in the hypothyroid state, when it is therefore a poor test of thyroid function.

Radio-isotope uptake still has a useful role in the elucidation of certain thyroid conditions such as De Quervain's thyroiditis or the rare iodine trapping or organification defects, but its main use lies in mapping the location of functioning (hot) or non-functioning (cold) thyroid tissue. Thyroid autonomy can be demonstrated by the failure of suppression of ^{131}I uptake to less than 50% of the original uptake after a ten day course of T_3 (20 µg, thrice daily). This T_3 suppression test may involve giving T_3 to someone who is already thyrotoxic, a procedure which is undesirable and seldom necessary. The TRH test has been used instead to clarify borderline thyrotoxic states; a flat TSH response is found in patients with excess thyroid hormone production and a normal response excludes the diagnosis. The response to TRH, however, tests the pituitary response to thyroid hormone feedback and does not always correspond to the results of the T_3 suppression test. A hyperfunctioning autonomous nodule may suppress the function of surrounding normal tissue and if it is necessary to demonstrate the ability of the latter to recover, a radio-isotope uptake test can be repeated after a course of TSH (10 units given IM. for three days) (Fig. 8.9).

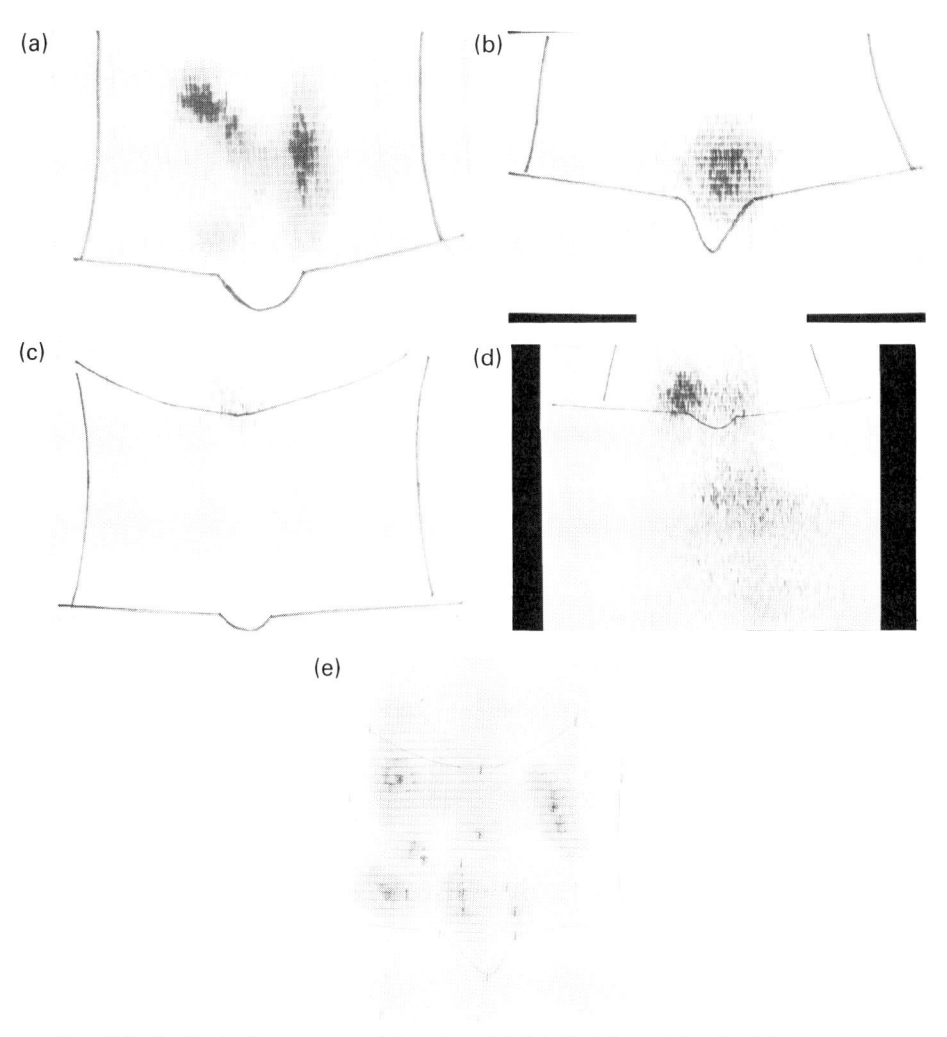

Fig. 8.9 Radio-iodine scans of the thyroid. (a) 'Cold' nodule. (b) 'Hot' nodule. (c) Ectopic thyroid tissue (lingual). (d) Multinodular goitre with retrosternal extension. (e) Metastatic thyroid carcinoma involving local lymph glands. *See also* colour plates between pages 166 and 167.

Thyroid Disease

The major cause of thyroid disease worldwide is iodine deficiency leading to hypothyroidism and goitre. In non-iodine-deficient areas auto-immune thyroid diseases account for most disorders of thyroid function. The term auto-immune thyroid disease embraces a spectrum of disorders ranging from thyrotoxic Graves' disease at one extreme to frank myxoedema at the other, with a range of degree of thyroid dysfunction inbetween. Auto-immunity is indicated by the presence of antibodies directed against various components of the thyroid cell. Thyroid microsomal antibodies and antithyroglobulin antibodies are most commonly measured and these reflect underlying thyroid disease, but do not themselves necessarily cause the damage leading to disordered thyroid function. Other antibodies may stimulate or inhibit thyroid function and growth.

Auto-immune thyroid disease is often associated with other auto-immune diseases such as pernicious anaemia or diabetes mellitus and a miscellany of these conditions are commonly found in families although the mechanism of their inheritance is not fully understood. Thyroid disorders, like other auto-immune diseases, are much more common in women than in men. Auto-immunity does not account for all non-congenital disorders of the thyroid such as thyroid tumours or acute thyroiditis, but these are relatively uncommon.

Hyperthyroidism

Hyperthyroidism or thyrotoxicosis is due to an excess of circulating thyroid hormones, invariably T_3 and usually also T_4 (Table 8.1). The commonest cause is Graves' disease in young and middle-aged women, but in older women it is more commonly associated with a uninodular or multinodular goitre rather than the diffuse goitre characteristically found in Graves' disease. Less commonly hyperthyroidism may result from the administration of excess thyroid hormone by the doctor (iatrogenic hyperthyroidism) or by the patient (thyro-

Table 8.1 Causes of hyperthyroidism

Frequency	Cause
Common	Graves' disease
	Toxic nodular goitre: single
	multiple
Rare	Excess administration of thyroxine: iatrogenic
	factitious
	Excess iodine (Jodbasedow phenomenon)
	Thyroid tumours
	Struma ovarii
	Choriocarcinoma
	Embryonal testicular tumours
	Thyroid stimulating hormone producing pituitary tumour
Transient	Acute/subacute De Quervain's thyroiditis

toxicosis factitia). Other rare causes of hyperthyroidism include excess endogenous thyroid hormone production by thyroid tumours and struma ovarii. Choriocarcinomas, hydatidiform moles and embryonal testicular tumours produce excessive amounts of chorionic gonadotrophins which have a weak affinity for the TSH receptors and can cause hyperthyroidism. Primary TSH producing pituitary tumours are exceedingly rare. Transient hyperthyroidism is a feature of acute or subacute De Quervain's thyroiditis which is presumed to be of viral origin. Hyperthyroidism may be unmasked by the administration of iodine (the Jodbasedow phenomenon) and an exacerbation of thyrotoxicosis can occur acutely after radio-iodine therapy.

The pathogenesis of Graves' disease

Graves' disease is due to circulating thyroid stimulating immunoglobulins (TSI) which bind to the thyroid cell membrane and produce prolonged stimulation of thyroid function. The nomenclature used to describe these immunoglobulins is confusing owing to the variety of techniques used over the years to identify them. Sera from some patients with Graves' disease, when injected into mice or guinea-pigs and pre-labelled with radio-iodine, produce prolonged stimulation of ^{131}I release, hence the earlier used term long-acting thyroid stimulator (LATS). Other sera from such patients fail to demonstrate LATS activity, perhaps because of the species difference or because of the presence of another factor which adsorbs LATS activity. Sera from other patients with Graves' disease may inhibit this adsorption by human thyroid cells permitting LATS activity, hence the term LATS protector (LATS-p). Other techniques measure the ability of sera to displace the binding of labelled TSH to thyroid cell membranes (thyroid binding inhibiting immunoglobulins, TBII) but binding does not invariably mean stimulation of cell function. Stimulation can be demonstrated by the production of cyclic AMP or colloid droplets or release of T_3 from thyroid cells. Thyroid stimulating immunoglobulins can be demonstrated in the sera of most patients with active Graves' disease but are not usually present in the sera of thyrotoxic patients with nodular goitres (Fig. 8.10).

Clinical features of hyperthyroidism (Table 8.2)

The prevalence of hyperthyroidism is about 2% of adult women in the community and it is ten times more common in women than in men. It is most common in the fourth and fifth decades but can occur at any age. The symptoms and signs of florid Graves' disease are usually easily recognized in younger women but the features of hyperthyroidism are often less obvious in the older age group. Typically a patient complains of weight loss despite a good appetite, increased sweating and a preference for a cold rather than a warm environment and increased anxiety. Palpitations, general fatigue, dyspnoea, frequency of bowel action and oligomenorrhoea or amenorrhoea may also occur. There

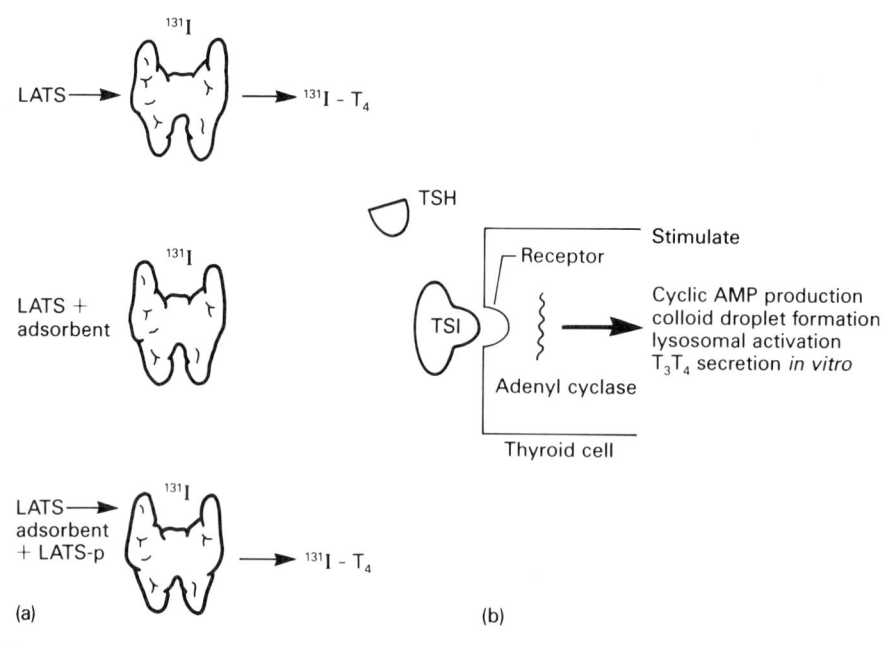

Fig. 8.10 Actions of thyroid stimulating immunoglobulins (TSI). LATS, long-acting thyroid stimulator. LATS-p, LATS protector.

is often a history of thyroid or other auto-immune disease in the family. It is important to ascertain that the patient is not taking any medication that might interfere with thyroid function or thyroid function tests, such as oral contraceptives.

Physical signs include a warm, moist skin and tachycardia or an irregular pulse due to atrial fibrillation. A smooth goitre, often with a bruit, is usually but not invariably palpable in Graves' disease whereas a nodular goitre is more commonly found in older patients. The absence of a goitre does not exclude the diagnosis.

A proximal myopathy may be demonstrated by difficulty in rising unaided from a sitting or squatting position.

Eye signs are not invariably present especially in the older patient, but typically consist of lid retraction giving the eyes a staring appearance and delayed downward movement of the eyelids (lid lag). In the ophthalmopathy of Graves' disease both, but occasionally only one, of the eyes reveal congested conjunctivae and peri-orbital oedema. Swelling of the extraocular muscles pushes the eyes forward resulting in exophthalmos. Failure of closure of the eyelids can lead to keratitis and corneal ulceration. Ophthalmoplegia results from swelling and shortening of the muscle opposing the direction of movement of the eye. Limitation of upward gaze is often one of the early features but any eye muscle can be involved and can lead to distressing diplopia. Rarely the ophthalmopathy causes papilloedema or oedema of the macula with dimi-

Table 8.2 Symptoms and signs of thyrotoxic Graves' disease

	Symptoms	Signs
General	Anxiety, sweating Weight loss Good appetite Heat intolerance	Thin Wasting
Cardiovascular system	Palpitations Breathlessness	Tachycardia Atrial fibrillation High output cardiac failure
Abdomen	Frequent bowel action Diarrhoea	
Urogenital	Frequency of micturition Oligomenorrhoea Amenorrhoea	
Central nervous system	Weakness	Proximal myopathy Periodic paralysis
Skin	Sweating Itching Swelling	Clammy Moist Pretibial myxoedema Acropachy
Thyroid	Swelling	Diffuse goitre ± Bruit
Eyes	Prominent Sore Itchy Double vision Blurring	Lid retraction, lid lag Exophathalmos Conjunctival congestion Ophthalmoplegia Diminished acuity Papilloedema

nished visual activity, when it is termed malignant exophthalmos and can cause blindness. Figure 8.11 shows CT scans of the orbit.

Other extrathyroidal manifestations of Graves' disease include clubbing of the fingers with subperiosteal new bone formation (acropachy), and patches of tender purplish red swellings of the skin usually over the tibia or feet (pretibial myxoedema) (Fig. 8.12). Such features are found in only a small proportion of patients with Graves' disease and do not occur in hyperthyroidism due to nodular goitre. The eye signs and other extrathyroidal features often persist even when the patient is rendered euthyroid.

Hyperthyroidism can occur in pregnancy and may be difficult to distinguish from the features of early pregnancy *per se*. Maternal immunoglobulins cross the placenta and can stimulate the fetal thyroid *in utero* and lead to neonatal Graves' disease. An affected baby has a goitre, exophthalmos, tachycardia, pyrexia and may develop cardiac failure. The condition requires urgent treatment but is self limiting as the maternal immunoglobulins are eliminated over succeeding weeks.

Hyperthyroidism is relatively uncommon in young children but can cause hyperkinetic activity and other behavioural changes and premature growth spurt. In young women the major differential diagnosis is often between

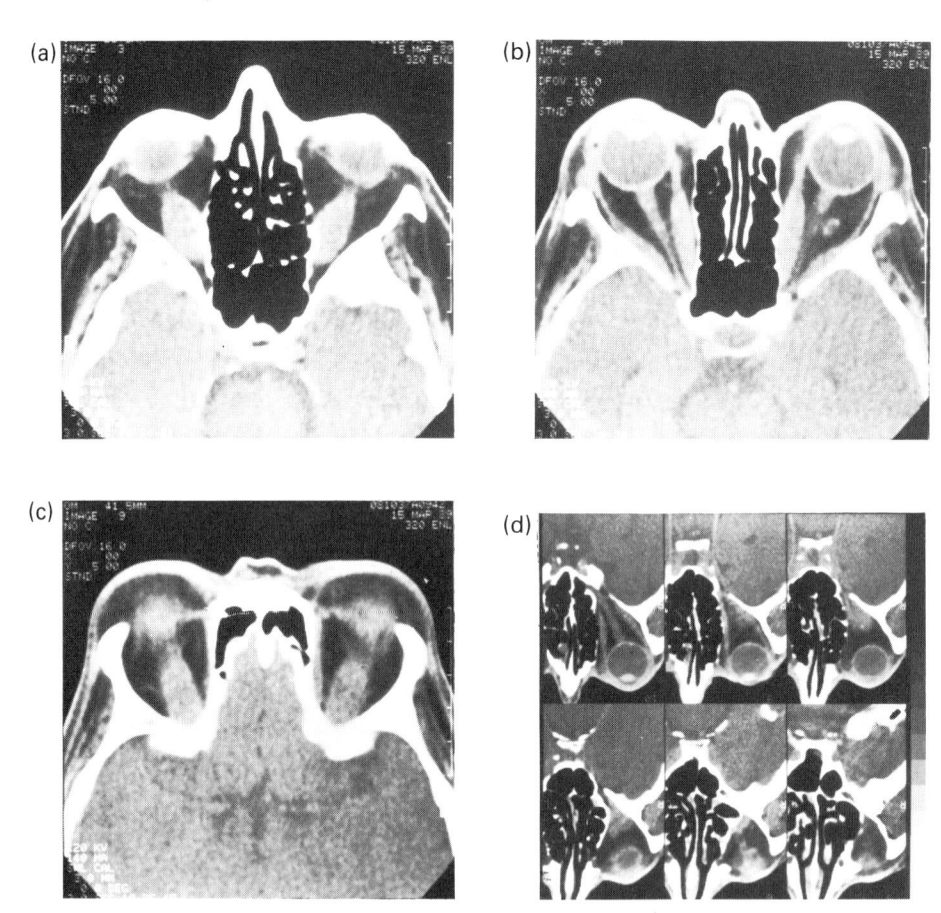

Fig. 8.11 Scans of the orbit showing swelling of extraocular muscles in Graves ophthalmopathy. (a) Inferior rectus muscle involvement. (b) Medial rectus muscle involvement. (c) Superior rectus muscle involvement. In contrast (d) shows sections through the orbit of a patient with unilateral exophthalmos due to a retro-orbital pseudotumour with normal extraocular muscles.

hyperthyroidism and an anxiety state *per se*. Menopausal symptoms may also mimic hyperthyroidism. In older women many of the typical features of hyperthyroidism may be masked and the diagnosis should always be entertained in otherwise unexplained weight loss, atrial fibrillation, heart failure or myopathy.

A thyrotoxic crisis is fortunately uncommon these days but may still occur in patients who are undiagnosed or incompletely treated and subject to major stress or surgery. It is caused by a sudden surge in release of thyroid hormones which can cause arrhythmias, cardiac failure, hyperpyrexia, delirium, and finally coma and death.

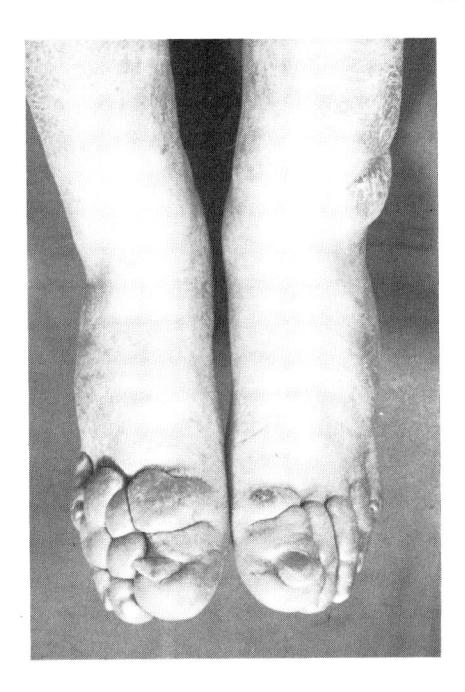

Fig. 8.12 Pretibial myxoedema. *See also* colour plates between pages 166 and 167.

Diagnostic tests (Fig. 8.13)
The clinical diagnosis of hyperthyroidism can usually be readily confirmed by the finding of an elevated free T_4 or a free thyroxine index (see above). If the free T_4 is at a borderline level a serum free T_3 may still be raised, as it is often elevated before T_4 and can be regarded as a more sensitive test of hyperthyroidism (in contrast to hypothyroidism). A diagnosis of T_3 toxicosis should only be made when in addition to the clinical features of hyperthyroidism there is also evidence of thyroid autonomy as evidenced by a flat TRH test or a failure of T_3 suppression. Thyroid stimulating hormone measured in a sensitive assay should be undetectable but if there is doubt a TRH test can be used. A normal rise in TSH after TRH excludes the diagnosis whereas a flat response is consistent with hyperthyroidism but may also be found in euthyroid patients previously treated for Graves' disease and with nodular goitres (Fig. 8.13 and 8.8). Radio-isotope studies help to distinguish a hot nodule from a diffuse goitre.

The Thyroid

Treatment

The choice of treatment lies between drugs, surgery and radio-iodine, or a combination of these. The advantages and disadvantages of each method should be discussed with the patient before reaching a mutual decision as to the most appropriate treatment for that individual.

Medical therapy

The antithyroid drugs most commonly used are carbimazole which is converted to its active metabolite methimazole, and propylthiouracil. Both act by inhibiting the synthesis of thyroid hormones. The starting dose is 30–60 mg of carbimazole or 300–600 mg propylthiouracil daily in divided doses. Treatment is continued until the patient becomes euthyroid which usually takes 6 to 10 weeks. The levels of circulating thyroid hormones are commonly found to return to normal before the patient can be judged to be euthyroid clinically. Excessive treatment is marked by a fall of T_4 below the normal range and a rise

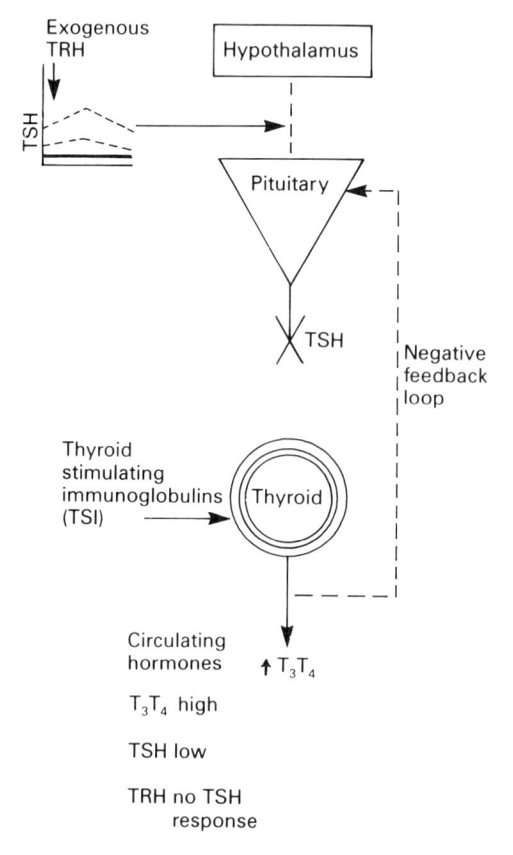

Fig. 8.13 Diagnostic tests of hyperthyroidism. TSH, thyroid stimulating hormone. TRH, thyrotrophin releasing hormone. T_3, tri-iodothyronine. T_4, thyroxine.

in TSH. Treatment can be continued either by reducing the daily dose of antithyroid drug so as to maintain the patient euthyroid clinically and biochemically, or by continuing with a blocking dose of the antithyroid drug but adding a physiological dose of thyroxine (usually about 150 μg daily) to prevent hypothyroidism. Treatment with carbimazole or propylthiuracil alone requires frequent close supervision to prevent overtreatment or escape due to undertreatment. The combination of antithyroid drug and thyroxine has the advantage of preventing such fluctuations in the thyroid status so long as the patient is prepared to take the larger number of tablets required.

It usually takes about six months for the levels of thyroid stimulating immunoglobulins to become undetectable but it is conventional to continue antithyroid drugs for 12 to 18 months to lessen the chance of relapse after stopping treatment. Relapse nevertheless occurs in about 50% of patients within a year of stopping the drugs in which case more definitive treatment is usually advised (see below), or a further course of antithyroid drugs can be given. There is no satisfactory test which can predict at the beginning which patient is likely to relapse after treatment although persistence of thyroid stimulating antibodies or of failure to suppress with T_3 at the end of treatment is associated with early relapse.

A small proportion of patients are allergic to the antithyroid drugs. Reactions such as skin rashes, arthralgia, sore throat and neutropenia develop early in hypersensitive individuals and patients should be advised to stop the drug immediately and seek urgent medical attention. Rarely agranulocytosis can develop. Hypersensitivity to both carbimazole or to propylthiouracil is not usually common so if there is a reaction to one the patient can be treated with the other once the initial reaction has subsided. Nevertheless hypersensitivity to both drugs in the same patient has been reported so careful observation is essential.

Propranolol, a beta-adrenoreceptor blocking drug, controls some of the sympathetic features of hyperthyroidism such as tachycardia, anxiety and sweating, but does not prevent weight loss. It may mask the diagnosis in a patient already on the drug. It interferes with the conversion of T_4 to T_3 but the patient remains biochemically hyperthyroid and T_4 levels are not significantly affected. It is nevertheless a useful adjunct to therapy and can be used to moderate symptoms pending confirmation of the diagnosis or during the initial treatment with antithyroid drugs and radio-iodine therapy, or in preparation for surgery (see below).

Medical treatment is preferred in young children and teenagers and in younger adults and those older patients who do not want surgery or radio-iodine. A patient who is pregnant or who may become pregnant should be treated with the minimum dose of antithyroid drug to maintain her euthyroid status and not with the combination of carbimazole and thyroxine. Carbimazole and propylthiouracil cross the placenta and large doses can render the fetus hypothyroid, but this does not occur with the small doses (carbimazole, 5–10 mg daily) that are all that are usually needed to control the mother.

Failure to control maternal hyperthyroidism with a modest dose of carbimazole may necessitate partial thyroidectomy in mid-pregnancy. Carbimazole is usually stopped two weeks before delivery and the patient is unlikely to relapse then, but may well do so in succeeding months. Carbimazole is excreted in the breast milk in minute quantities and it is conventional to advise against breast feeding. There is however little hazard to the infant and it may be reasonable to breast feed and have the infant's thyroid function checked occasionally.

Neonatal Graves' disease requires treatment with carbimazole in a dose proportional to body weight and can be tailed off after about two months. Potassium iodide drops, propranolol and digoxin in paediatric dosage may also be needed in the initial treatment.

A thyroid crisis requires urgent treatment with carbimazole given intravenously or 100 mg given by nasogastric tube followed by oral iodide. Lugol's solution contains total iodide of 130 mg/ml and up to 0.3 ml, well diluted with milk or water is given three times/day. Propranolol, digoxin and diuretics may also be given to control the cardiac effects. Dexamethasone may also be beneficial as large doses of steroids may interfere with the production of T_3 from T_4.

Surgical treatment
Partial thyroidectomy is followed by a fairly rapid decline in thyroid stimulating immunoglobulin levels and is an effective cure for hyperthyroidism in the majority of cases so treated. Relapse nevertheless occurs in about 5% of patients and the cumulative incidence of hypothyroidism is often underestimated because of lack of long-term follow up, but may reach 25% or more over 10 years. There is also the risk of damage to the parathyroid glands and the recurrent laryngeal nerve and of pre-tracheal bleeding post-operatively. Surgery is certainly indicated if the gland is so large that it can cause tracheal compression although this is not commonly the case in thyrotoxicosis, and is often favoured in patients with largish goitres in the belief (unproven) that they are more likely to relapse after medical treatment. Failure of, or relapse after medical treatment is also a reason for advocating surgery or radio-iodine therapy, depending on the age, condition and choice of the patient. A hot nodule is equally effectively treated by surgery or radio-iodine with little risk of any complications.

Patients who are to undergo elective partial thyroidectomy are best rendered euthyroid by medical treatment first, and the antithyroid drugs discontinued immediately after operation. Lugol's iodine may be given for a few days pre-operatively in patients with very vascular goitres but it is not otherwise necessary although it is still preferred by some surgeons. Surgery can be performed under propranolol cover alone if necessary, but requires very close supervision especially in the immediate post-operative period as escape can occur if doses are inadvertently omitted and can lead to thyroid crisis.

Post-operative hypocalcaemia may occur transiently and require treatment with calcium supplements if mild, or vitamin D if more severe or more permanent. Biochemical hypothyroidism, reflected by a rise in TSH, may be a transient rather than a permanent occurrence a few weeks after surgery, but overt hypothyroidism should not be allowed to occur. The need for permanent thyroxine replacement should nevertheless be reassessed after about six months.

Radioiodine therapy
131-Iodine in large doses destroys thyroid cell activity and prevents their replication. The dose required can vary from 80 to 400 mBq (2 to 10 mCi), the smaller dose being more likely to be associated with a higher relapse rate, and the higher dose with a greater incidence of hypothyroidism which is of the order of 20% in the first year and may reach 50% or more after 10 years. For this reason some physicians advocate the use of a large dose, with the deliberate intention of rendering the patient hypothyroid and starting replacement thyroxine early, rather than using a small dose risking either relapse or the late insidious development of hypothyroidism. Elaborate calculations of dosage based on radio-iodine uptake and estimates of the size of the gland have not been shown to have any better outcome than the use of an empirical dose.

It may take several weeks or a few months for the radio-iodine to take full effect, and thus it may be appropriate to treat the patient medically starting a week or so after giving ^{131}I and stopping after six months to determine the effect of the radio-iodine. Alternatively propranolol can be given to control some of the symptoms whilst the radio-iodine takes effect, which can be monitored by following the free T_4 and TSH levels. It may be wise in any case to cover the initial phase of radio-iodine treatment with propranolol to protect against the possible exacerbation of thyrotoxicosis that can occur due to transient thyroiditis following the radio-iodine.

Radio-iodine therapy is appropriate in older patients or those who are unfit or unwilling to have surgery, and for relapse after surgery. It is effective treatment for hot nodules and the risk of hypothyroidism is very low in this situation. Radio-iodine has been used to treat thyrotoxicosis in all age groups in the USA, but in the UK it has been conventional to avoid giving it to women in their reproductive years. It should not be given to anyone who might possibly become pregnant within a year because of the potential effect on the fetus. There is no evidence that radio-iodine therapy for thyrotoxicosis is liable to increase the risk of thyroid cancer.

Management of ophthalmopathy
The management of the ophthalmopathy of Graves' disease depends on the severity of the condition. It is important to ensure that the patient is maintained in a euthyroid state as the worst examples of ophthalmopathy often seem to occur in patients with a history of relapses or inadequate treatment of thyrotoxicosis, although ophthalmopathy can develop in patients who are not and have never been hyperthyroid. Mild lid lag and protrusion of the eyes insufficient to prevent closure of the eyelids does not warrant treatment with agents

that are seldom effective and carry significant side effects. Irritation and conjunctival congestion may be helped by regular use of methylcellulose eyedrops. Guanethidine eyedrops also help in some patients but others find them more irritating. Exposure of the cornea can result in abrasions and ulceration but the eye can be protected by tarsorrhaphy. Diplopia is troublesome and is most easily relieved by using an eye patch, but many patients are embarrassed by their piratical appearance. Surgical treatment of diplopia may be necessary once any thyroid dysfunction has been corrected and stabilized, but such procedures are usually limited to correcting any diplopia on forward gaze and the patient is likely to continue to have double vision in other directions. Ophthalmoparesis *per se* seldom responds to steroids which are reserved for the sight threatening development of malignant exophthalmos, which requires urgent treatment. Prednisolone in large doses, 60–100 mg daily, can produce a dramatic improvement in visual acuity with reduction of papilloedema, but side effects soon develop and may outweigh the benefits. Other therapies that have been used include cyclosporin and other immunosuppressive drugs such as azathioprine, plasmapheresis, surgical decompression of the orbit, and external radiation. The relative merits of these treatments are not easy to evaluate because published studies usually reflect experience with a combination of therapies in patients with varying severities and duration of ophthalmopathy. Orbital decompression rapidly reduces pressure on the eyeball and protrusion but further surgery may be needed to correct diplopia. Early claims for the efficacy of plasmaphoresis have not been confirmed. External radiation is not immediately effective but has been used to supplement other treatment.

Hypothyroidism

Whilst iodine deficiency is the commonest cause of hypothyroidism worldwide, in non-iodine-deficient areas it is usually due to destructive auto-immune processes which affect older women much more commonly than men (Table 8.3). Additionally a significant proportion of cases of hypothroidism are due to

Table 8.3 Causes of hypothyroidism

Iodine deficiency
Auto-immune thyroiditis
Post-surgery
Post-radio-iodine therapy
Dyshormonogenesis
Acute/subacute thyroiditis
   silent thyroiditis
   post-partum thyroiditis
Drugs
   Overtreatment with carbimazole or propylthiouracil
   Chronic iodine excess
   Lithium
Secondary to pituitary/hypothalamic disease

previous therapy with either surgery or radio-iodine. Hypothyroidism is relatively uncommon in childhood but may then be due to dyshormonogenesis when it is usually associated with a goitre. Hypothyroidism may also occur secondary to pituitary disease or hypothalamic disorders. Transient hypothyroidism may also be a feature of thyroiditis, whether painful or silent, and can result from overtreatment with antithyroid drugs.

Clinical features

Hypothyroidism is insidious in onset and as it most commonly affects middle-aged and older women the symptoms are frequently attributed to the menopause or the ageing process by the patient and even the doctor. The symptoms are non-specific and include general fatigue, a slowing down of physical and mental processes, increased sensitivity to cold, constipation and weight gain. The physical signs of hypothyroidism may not be apparent in the earlier stages of the disease but in the overt stage include cold thickened skin (myxoedema), a puffy facial appearance with peri-orbital oedema, dry coarse hair and a hoarse voice. Delayed relaxation of the tendon reflex may be found in severe myxoedema but is often not present in less florid stages. All the systems of the body may be involved and other features which may be elicited on systematic enquiry or lead to presentation via a specialist include:

Psychiatric:	depression, psychosis and dementia
Neurological:	muscle weakness, cramps, stiffness or myotonia, carpal tunnel syndrome, ataxia, dysarthria, coma, fits
Cardiovascular:	bradycardia, cardiac failure, pericardial effusion, intermittent claudication
Gynaecological:	menorrhagia or oligomenorrhoea
Rheumatological:	joint stiffness and swelling
Haematological:	anaemia, usually normocytic and normochromic but can be macrocytic

The thyroid gland is frequently not palpable.

Mxyoedema coma is fortunately uncommon as it is often fatal, but the diagnosis should be considered in any elderly person found neglected at home and brought into hospital unconscious or stuperose. The patient is often hypothermic and myxoedema may be difficult to distinguish from any other cause of hypothermia.

The above features of primary hypothyroidism are seldom so apparent in hypothyroidism secondary to pituitary or hypothalamic disease where other hormone deficiencies tend to predominate. Minor degrees of hypothyroidism may not be recognized clinically but can be detected biochemically.

Diagnostic tests (Fig. 8.14)

The most sensitive test of primary hypothyroidism is a serum TSH. An elevated TSH level indicates some degree of hypothyroidism whereas a normal TSH

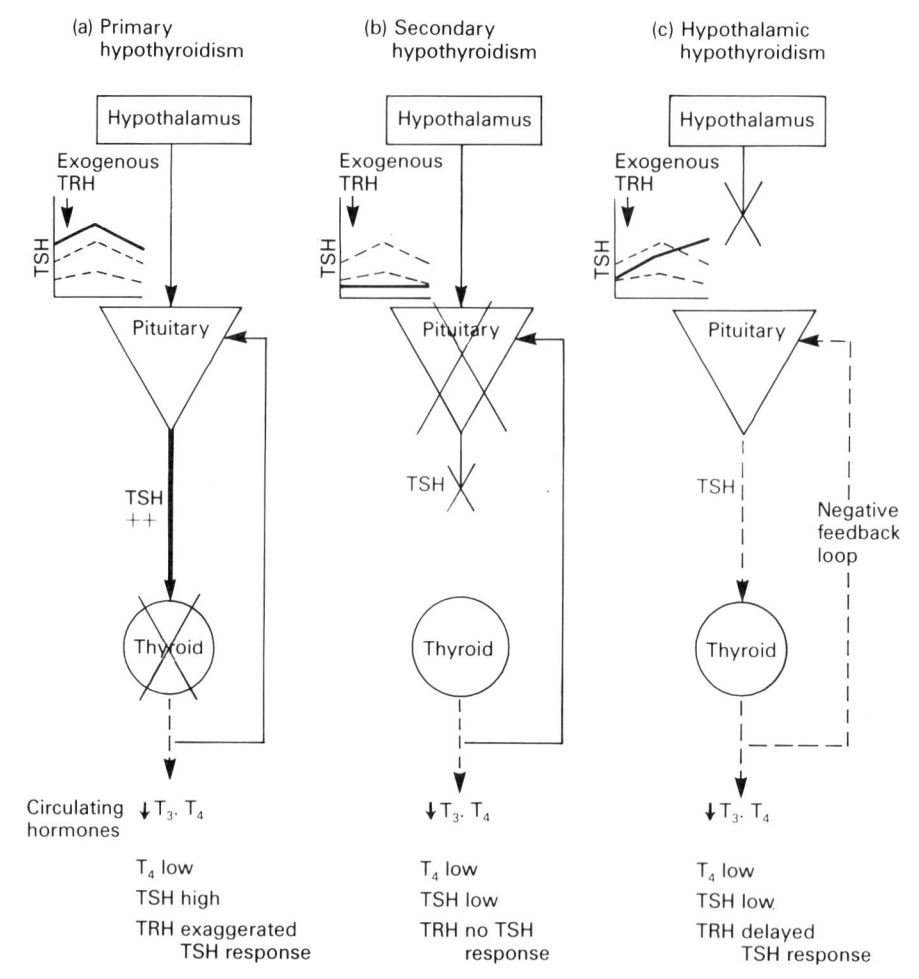

Fig. 8.14 Diagnostic tests for hypothyroidism. (a) Primary hypothyroidism. (b) Secondary hypothyroidism. (c) Hypothalamic hypothyroidism.

excludes the diagnosis. In severe hypothyroidism the serum T_4 will be low but in milder cases the T_4 can be in the low normal range. Tri-iodothyronine is not a useful diagnostic test in hypothyroidism because it is often normal as the thyroid compensates by preferential secretion of T_3 rather than T_4.

Serum total T_4 may be misleadingly low in a number of conditions, such as hypoproteinaemic states including the nephrotic syndrome or liver disease, familial TBG deficiency and altered TBG binding due to competition from drugs such as phenytoin or anabolic steroids. This can be corrected by derivation of a free thyroxine index or direct measurement of free T_4 levels. Both total and free T_4 levels may, however, be reduced in severe acute or chronic non-thyroid illness due to the increased conversion of T_4 to the inactive metabolite reverse T_3, but TSH levels then remain normal (Table 8.4).

In hypothyroidism secondary to pituitary or hypothalamic disease serum TSH measured by sensitive assay should be low or undetectable and the free T_4 will also be low. The TRH test is not as good a discriminator as might be expected: a flat response supports the diagnosis but varying degrees of blunted response are often found. A delayed TSH rise with 60 min values higher than 20 min values is typical of hypothalamic disease. Rarely a patient with long-standing untreated primary hypothyroidism may be found to have an enlarged pituitary fossa due to a feedback tumour, and the high TSH will distinguish this from pituitary tumours of other origin.

The ECG in hypothyroidism typically shows low voltage complexes, minor ST segment depression or T-wave flattening as well as bradycardia, but these changes are non-specific and not invariably present. The serum cholesterol is frequently raised and falls with treatment of the hypothyroidism. There is no simple satisfactory test of the peripheral effects of thyroid hormones in clinical practice at present.

Treatment

Once the diagnosis of hypothyroidism is confirmed thyroxine replacement therapy is commenced with 50 μg daily and increased in 50 μg steps at two weekly intervals to 150 μg daily. This is usually sufficient to render the patient euthyroid clinically and biochemically although it may take longer than six weeks to restore all the tissue effects to normal. Individual thyroxine requirement may vary from 100 to 200 μg/day. The dose of T_4 should be adjusted to ensure that the TSH level returns to normal and on this dose the T_4 level is usually in the high normal range or slightly higher, but the T_3 level is almost invariably normal and may be a better measure of the adequacy of replacement therapy than the T_4 level.

Replacement therapy should be more cautious in the elderly or in anyone with ischaemic heart disease, starting with 25 μg daily and increasing in 25 μg increments at two week intervals. If an exacerbation of angina occurs the dose

Table 8.4 Causes of low T_4 states in clinically euthyroid patients

Low thyroxine binding globulin (TBG)	Hypoproteinaemia
Normal thyroid stimulating hormone (TSH)	Drugs
	Hereditary
Normal TBG	Acute non-thyroid illness
Normal TSH	Chronic non-thyroid illness
Normal TBG	Auto-immune thyroiditis
Positive antibody	Subclinical hypothyroidism
Normal or raised TSH	

of T_4 should be reduced and the angina treated with a beta-blocker such as propanolol before further increments of T_4 are gradually re-introduced.

If the patient is suffering from secondary hypothyroidism it is essential that any cortisol deficiency is corrected before thyroxine replacement therapy is commenced, to avoid the risk of precipitating a hypoadrenal crisis.

The treatment of myxoedema coma is empirical as it is not a situation that is amenable to a controlled trial. The patient should be rewarmed gradually using a space blanket and adequate ventilation maintained if necessary by mechanical means. Tri-iodothyronine can be given intravenously in 20 μg doses repeated every 12 h until the patient is sufficiently awake to commence oral replacement. Alternatively T_3 can be given by nasogastric tube but absorption may be variable and uncertain. Other authors have advocated the use of a single large bolus of T_4 up to 500 μg intravenously, but its subsequent conversion to the active metabolite T_3 may be delayed or uneven. There is always a risk of cardiac arrhythmias developing and it is essential to monitor the patient closely. The cortisol response to stress may also be impaired so it is wise to give intravenous hydrocortisone, 100 μg intravenously six hourly, until the patient is able to take oral therapy then gradually tail down the dosage. Steroids can be discontinued if a plasma cortisol level taken initially before treatment was commenced is subsequently shown to have been appropriately elevated. Once the patient is through the critical early recovery stage, which may take 24 to 48 h or more, then thyroid hormone replacement can be continued using T_4 orally in gradual increments as previously outlined.

Thyroxine replacement therapy for primary or secondary hypothyroidism needs to be continued for life yet a small proportion of patients forget or fail to take their medication which necessitates long-term follow up. A rise in TSH in a patient with primary hypothyroidism previously shown to be euthyroid on T_4 usually indicates non-compliance. A fall in T_4 level would raise the same suspicion in secondary hypothyroidism but the TSH would be of no value in this situation.

Congenital Hypothyroidism

In normal infants there is a rise in TSH within hours of birth followed by a rise in T_3 levels which have been low *in utero*. The elevated TSH levels normally subside within 2–3 days, but persistent elevation of TSH indicates thyroid failure due to either an absent or ectopic thyroid (Fig. 8.15). Routine screening for elevated TSH levels on day five reveals that congenital hypothyroidism occurs in approximately 1:3500 of all births in European countries and in the USA. Prompt treatment with thyroxine should prevent the physical and mental retardation that inevitably otherwise occurs and may not be recognized clinically for many months.

In areas of endemic iodine deficiency low iodine levels in the mother can lead to the development of goitrous hypothyroidism and cretinism in the offspring.

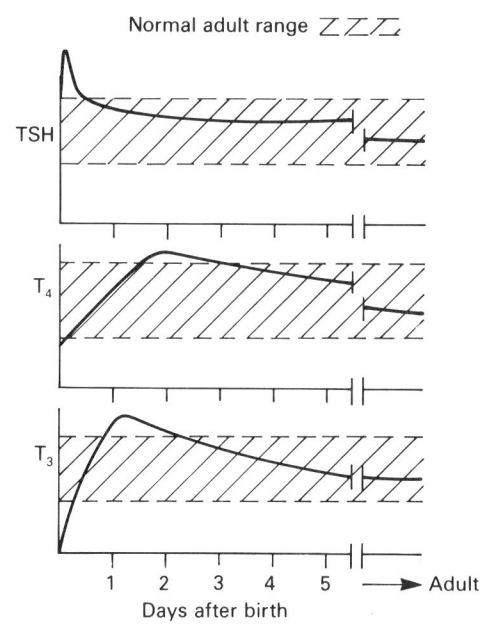

Fig. 8.15 Changes in fetal thyroid hormone levels following birth. TSH, thyroid stimulating hormone. T_3, tri-iodothyronine. T_4, thyroxine. Shading shows normal adult range.

This can be prevented by the prophylactic intramuscular injection of iodized oil to women of reproductive years or very early in pregnancy.

Thyroiditis

The term thyroiditis is used rather too loosely to embrace a variety of conditions of different aetiologies and manifestations. Hashimoto originally described four patients with goitre in whom the histology of the gland was characterized by diffuse lymphocytic infiltration, atrophy of some parenchymal cells with eosinophilic infiltration of other cells and fibrosis. With the advent of methods for detecting circulating antibodies the term Hashimoto's thyroiditis has been used indiscriminately to include anyone with thyroid antibodies, whereas it might be more properly reserved for those with the typical goitre.

Asymptomatic autoimmune thyroiditis

This term describes the condition in which circulating antibodies to thyroglobulin or thyroid microsomes are detectable although the patient has no symptoms and usually does not have a goitre. The presence of such antibodies has nevertheless been shown to correlate with histological evidence of underlying focal lymphocyte infiltration. Thyroid antibodies can be detected in about 10%

of adult women and 1% of men, being more common in older age groups. Many people with antibodies survive a normal life-span without any deterioration in thyroid function, but others insidiously progress to hypothyroidism. The earliest evidence of such a development is a rise in serum TSH. Patients with antibodies and a mildly raised TSH develop overt hypothyroidism at the rate of approximately 5% per annum.

Acute or subacute (De Quervain's) thyroiditis

This condition is characterized by a painful swelling of the thyroid as a result of diffuse inflammation often attributed to but seldom proven to be due to preceding viral infection. There is a rapid discharge of stored thyroid hormones initially with the resultant biochemical picture of hyperthyroidism, but if a radio-iodine uptake test is performed it is very low in contrast to the high uptake in true hyperthyroidism due to Graves' disease. The ESR is markedly raised in the acute stage. The condition is self-limiting but may be very unpleasant whilst it lasts and can relapse. Treatment is symptomatic with simple analgesics but if these do not suffice then steroids in the form of prednisolone, initially 40 mg daily, effectively suppress the inflammation and relieve the pain. The initial discharge of thyroid hormones is typically followed by a phase of low thyroid activity which may last several weeks and require thyroxine replacement whilst the thyroid recovers, but permanent hypothyroidism is rarely a sequel.

Silent or painless thyroiditis

A biochemical picture of hyperthyroidism associated with a low radio-iodine uptake may sometimes be found in the absence of any history of pain or other feature to suggest acute or subacute thyroiditis. The patient usually presents with mild features of hyperthyroidism but none of the extrathyroidal features of Graves' disease. The condition may not be diagnosed if a radio-iodine uptake test is not performed. It is relatively uncommon in Europe, whereas it is said to account for about 10% of cases of hyperthyroidism in the USA. This condition is also self-limiting and usually runs its course over a few weeks rather than the few months more typical of painful thyroiditis. Its aetiology is unknown, but is thought by some to be a variant of subacute thyroiditis rather than an auto-immune process.

Post-partum thyroiditis

Pregnancy influences the course of auto-immune processes and modifies thyroid disease. It is thus common to find that pre-existing thyrotoxicosis is easily controlled with minimal doses of antithyroid drugs during pregnancy and may remit on withdrawal of the drug only to relapse a few weeks or 2–3 months post-partum. Similarly in patients with thyroid antibodies who are asymptomatic, the titre of the antibodies declines during pregnancy and they may disappear entirely only to rebound post-partum. This rebound may be accompanied by transient hyperthyroidism, with low radio-iodine uptake, in some patients and may be followed by a period of hypothyroidism as in silent thyroiditis. In other patients the rise in antibody titres is associated with a rise in TSH and the development of hypothyroidism 3 to 6 months post-partum, but not necessarily permanently. The phenomenon of post-partum thyroiditis is thus very varied in its form but would appear to be due to the effects of pregnancy on underlying auto-immune processes rather than an inflammatory response. The condition is likely to remain silent clinically but should not be forgotten as a possible cause of post-partum depression.

Reidel's thyroiditis

This is a very uncommon condition of unknown aetiology in which the thyroid is almost entirely replaced by fibrous tissue which extends beyond the gland and encases surrounding tissues. The condition may be difficult to distinguish clinically from anaplastic carcinoma. It may also be associated with fibrosis elsewhere such as retroperitoneal fibrosis. Hypothyroidism usually develops and requires replacement therapy. Surgical treatment is confined to the relief of pressure effects.

Goitre

Goitre is endemic in iodine-deficient countries where more than 20% of the population may have visible thyroid enlargement which is usually nodular. In non-iodine-deficient areas goitre is sporadic and is most commonly associated with auto-immune disease, but it is not always possible to establish the cause (Table 8.5).

Goitre is found at least four times more commonly in women than in men. Diffuse goitre is much commoner in young women whereas the prevalence of nodular goitre increases with age in women but not in men.

Physiological enlargement of the thyroid occurs during puberty and in pregnancy. Diffuse goitre is characteristically found in Graves' disease. Hyperthyroidism in old people is more commonly associated with nodular goitre. Goitrogens include antithyroid drugs and other agents which may interfere with thyroid hormone synthesis and release such as lithium, iodine-containing drugs and foodstuffs devised from seaweed, soyabean and cassava.

Goitre in childhood is uncommon and may be associated with hypothyroidism due to familial or congenital dyshormonogenesis in which there is a defect in one of the enzymes governing the steps of thyroid hormone synthesis or release. Pendred's syndrome is the name given to the combination of congenital deafness with goitre due to an organification defect.

Goitre in adults is most commonly benign due to colloid nodules of varying sizes which may degenerate and become cystic or fibrosed. The aetiology is

Table 8.5 Causes of goitre

Endemic		Iodine deficiency	
Sporadic	Diffuse	Physiological	Puberty
			Pregnancy
		Pathological	Graves' disease
			Dyshormonogenesis
			Thyroiditis
		Drugs	Antithyroid: carbimazole propylthiouracil
			Lithium
			Iodine-containing, e.g. cough mixtures
		Foodstuffs	Cassava
			Seaweed
			Soya bean
	Nodular (single or multiple)	Benign	Colloid cysts
			Adenoma
		Malignant	Papillary carcinoma
			Follicular carcinoma
			Medullary carcinoma
			Anaplastic carcinoma
		Granuloma	Sarcoid
			Tuberculosis
		Lymphoma	
		Reidel's thyroiditis	

unknown but may be due to factors which stimulate growth rather than function of the gland.

Solitary nodules in the thyroid may be due to cysts, degenerative colloid nodules which may be haemorrhagic, benign adenoma or malignant papillary, follicular or medullary (C-cell) carcinoma. Other rare causes of nodules in the thyroid include lymphoma and granuloma of sarcoidosis, tuberculosis or syphilis. Benign adenomas are common and are well encapsulated. Papillary carcinoma is the commonest form of thyroid malignancy. The capsule is frequently incomplete and metastases to local lymph glands are common. Follicular carcinomas vary in size and degree of differentiation and metastases may be widespread. Anaplastic carcinomas grow rapidly and invade the whole gland and surrounding tissues.

Clinical features

The patient usually presents with a lump in the neck, noticed by herself or a relative or found incidentally as part of a medical examination. Systematic enquiry should be made to assess possible thyroid overactivity or underactivity. Particular enquiry should be made about medication to exclude goitrogens such as proprietary cough mixtures, which may contain iodine. A past history of external radiation to the neck area particularly in childhood enhances the likelihood of malignancy. A painful goitre is uncommon and is usually due to subacute (De Quervain's) thyroiditis but may follow a therapeutic dose of ^{131}I and very rarely can be due to acute suppuration.

A large gland may extend retrosternally and can cause tracheal compression leading to stridor, or involve the recurrent laryngeal nerve presenting with a hoarse voice.

A solitary nodule or history of a rapidly enlarging gland or a finding of enlarged cervical glands always raises the possibility of malignancy. It is often difficult on clinical examination alone to determine whether or not a nodule is truly solitary and whether it is solid or cystic. A solitary midline swelling may be due to a thyroglossal cyst. Medullary carcinoma may be associated with multiple neuromas in the eyelids, lips and tongue, and evidence should be sought for associated hyperparathyroidism and phaeochromocytoma. Anaplastic carcinomas are usually hard and irregular, and fixed to surrounding structures. A wooden hard gland is also found in the rare Reidel's thyroiditis.

Investigations

Investigations are directed towards finding the cause and effects of the goitre. Thyroid function should be assessed to confirm whether the patient is euthyroid, hyperthyroid or hypothyroid. Patients with a goitre who are apparently clinically euthyroid may nevertheless be subclinically hypothyroid reflected by a normal T_4 but slightly raised TSH, or subclinically hyperthyroid with a normal T_4 but mildly elevated T_3. A suppressed sensitive TSH or a flat TSH response to TRH may be found in patients with multinodular goitre who are otherwise biochemically euthyroid. The presence of circulating thyroid antibodies indicates an underlying auto-immune process but these are common and seldom discriminatory in determining the cause of the goitre.

An ultrasound scan will help to reveal whether the goitre is diffuse or nodular, and whether a nodule is cystic or solid, but it does not give information on the function of the tissue. An isotope uptake test will help to localize areas of functioning and non-functioning tissue and define the position and size of a goitre (Fig. 8.9). Radio-iodine studies may also be helpful in determining the cause of dyshormonogenic goitre (see page 214). Whilst a cystic lesion on ultrasonic scan and an active nodule on radio-iodine scan are more likely to be benign than malignant neither investigation can provide a definitive diagnosis which must ultimately depend on the histological findings.

Fine needle aspiration of a nodule by skilled hands together with cytological expertise can provide a direct answer as to whether the lesion is benign, malignant or equivocal without the need for expensive and time consuming scans. Expert cytology can also save a number of operations by confining exploration to those with malignant changes or equivocal neoplasia. Where, however, cytological expertise is not available surgical exploration is advised for cold solid nodules.

Management

Benign goitre

Most goitres are ultimately shown to be benign and not associated with any thyroid dysfunction. The patient needs reassurance that there is no evidence of malignancy and the gland can be left alone. If the goitre is large a trial of thyroxine therapy may be justified even in the absence of a raised TSH because a proportion of such glands may shrink, although the majority do not respond.

Surgery is indicated if the goitre is causing pressure effects and may be warranted for cosmetic reasons, although the latter must take into consideration the inevitable scar and possible morbidity associated with partial thyroidectomy.

Hyperthyroidism or hypothyroidism require appropriate treatment. A patient with an autonomous nodule who is clinically and biochemically euthyroid may be kept under observation until hyperthyroidism develops, often first revealed by a rise in T_3, when treatment either with radio-iodine or surgery is equally effective.

Management of painful subacute thyroiditis is discussed on page 238.

Thyroid malignancy

Fine needle aspiration cytology cannot readily distinguish follicular adenoma from follicular carcinoma and is usually reported as follicular neoplasia which requires surgical exploration. Benign adenomas are completely encapsulated and hemithyroidectomy is sufficient. Follicular carcinomas and papillary carcinomas vary in size and degree of differentiation, the capsule is incomplete and metastases are common. Total thyroidectomy and removal of affected local lymph glands as far as possible by a skilled surgeon is advisable. If such expertise is not readily available then partial thyroidectomy is advised followed by total thyroid ablation with a large dose of radio-iodine. The patient then requires maintenance therapy with T_4 or T_3 to prevent hypothyroidism and suppress any TSH drive to regenerate thyroid tissue. If the thyroid has been effectively ablated then serum thyroglobulin should become undetectable and its reappearance would suggest recurrence of the tumour. The maintenance T_3 is then discontinued for 10 days or T_4 for a month and a thyroid scan using a high dose of radio-iodine is repeated to localize any recurrent tissue which will require further ablative treatment. Measurement of thyroglobulin as a tumour marker in this context may save the patient unnecessary prolonged periods off thyroid hormone replacement whilst repeat scans are performed, which otherwise used to be performed at annual intervals.

The prognosis of well-differentiated thyroid carcinomas depends on the size and stage of the tumour at diagnosis. A younger patient with a solitary small tumour removed surgically and treated with thyroid ablation has an excellent prognosis with a likelihood of 20 or more years disease free. On the other hand an older patient presenting with metastatic spread, particularly if it involves bone as well as lungs and local invasion, has a markedly reduced life-expectancy, even when treated on the same principles.

The patient with medullary carcinoma should be investigated to exclude phaeochromocytoma and parathyroid adenoma prior to thyroid surgery. Medullary carcinoma is treated by thyroidectomy and excision of lymph node metastases where possible, but is not particularly sensitive to radiation. Plasma calcitonin levels can be measured to determine the response to treatment and recurrence of metastases. First degree relatives should also be screened for medullary carcinoma and associated endocrine tumours.

Anaplastic and other poorly differentiated tumours have a very poor prognosis. Treatment is with palliative external radiation and surgery is usually avoided although it may occasionally be necessary to relieve pressure symptoms.

Further Reading

Delange, F. (1988). Neonatal hypothyroidism: recent developments. *Ballière's Clinics in Endocrinology and Metabolism* **2**, 637–652.

Franklyn, J.A. and Sheppard, M.C. (1988). Thyroid nodules and thyroid cancer–diagnostic aspects. *Ballière's Clinics in Endocrinology and Metabolism* **2**, 761–775.

Ingbar, S.H. and Braverman, L.E. (eds) (1986). *Werner's The Thyroid: A Fundamental and Clinical Text*, 5th edition. J.B. Lippincott Co., Philadelphia.

Jansson, R., Dahlberg, P.A. and Karlsson, F.A. (1988). Postpartum thyroiditis. *Ballière's Clinics in Endocrinology and Metabolism* **2**, 619–635.

Toft, A.D. (ed.) (1985). Hyperthyroidism. *Clinics in Endocrinology and Metabolism* **14**, No. 2.

9

THE ADRENAL GLANDS

Development and Anatomy

Each adrenal gland consists of a cortex and medulla which are of separate embryological origin. The cortex is derived from mesoderm and the medulla originates from ectodermal cells of the neural crest. The adrenal glands develop between the fourth and eighth weeks of fetal life. The medullary glands migrate to invade the developing cortex and occupy a central position within the gland. Residual accessory tissue of cortical or medullary cells or both may occasionally be found along the lines of their original migration.

In the adult the adrenal glands are located at the upper pole of each kidney and are roughly triangular in shape with the base invaginated. They have a rich blood supply from the aorta, inferior phrenic and renal arteries. Arterioles form a plexus in the capsule from which capillaries run centrally through the cortex to form sinusoids which interconnect and drain through the medulla to form a central vein. The left adrenal vein drains into the left renal vein whereas the right adrenal vein drains directly into the inferior vena cava (Fig. 9.1).

The cortex consists of three zones. The outer layer, the zona glomerulosa, lies just beneath the capsule and consists of clusters of compact cells. The middle layer, the zona fasciculata, consists of bundles of larger cells and the inner layer, the zona reticularis, is composed of smaller cells loosely arranged in the sinusoids.

The medulla consists of a complex network of preganglionic sympathetic nerve fibres from the coeliac ganglia and large foamy secretory cells containing granules. These cells stain brown with silver stains, hence the term chromaffin tissue.

Physiology of the Adrenal Cortex

The adrenal cortex is the source of most of the steroid hormones produced in the body other than those derived from the gonads and placenta. The adrenocorticosteroids are essential for life and may be grouped into three types according to their principal metabolic activities:

Glucorticoids: Mainly cortisol produced in the zona fasciculata and zona reticularis

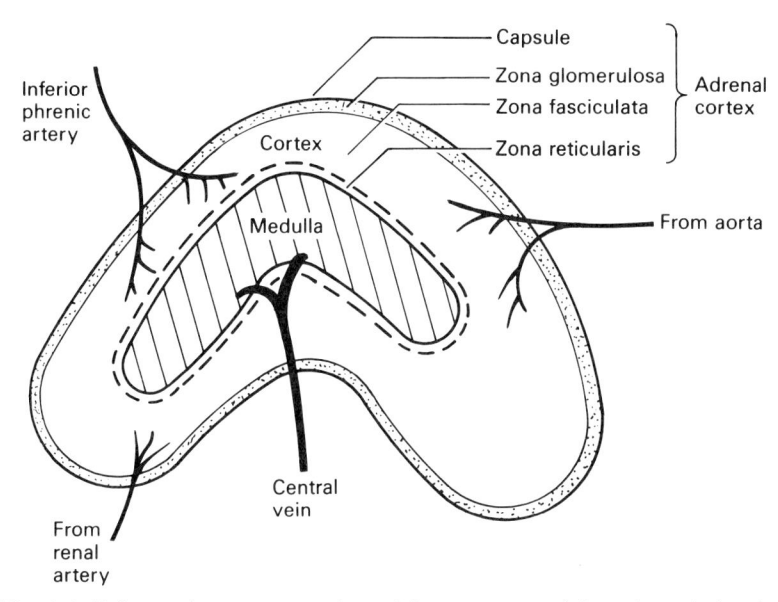

Fig. 9.1 Schematic representation of the anatomy of the adrenal gland.

Mineralocorticoids: Mainly aldosterone produced only in the outer zona glomerulosa
Sex steroids: Mainly androgens produced in the zona reticularis

The basic structure of the steroid ring is shown in Fig. 9.2 and the position of the carbon atoms in the ring are numbered 1 to 17. All those adrenocorticosteroids which have biological activity have a ketone group in position 3 and a two carbon side chain on position 17 with a ketone group on position 20 and a hydroxyl group on position 21. The adrenocorticosteroids thus have 21 carbon atoms whereas androgens have 19 because they have no carbon atoms on positions 20 and 21, and oestrogens 18 because they also lack a carbon atom on position 19. All the steroids are synthesized from cholesterol in a series of steps each of which is controlled by an enzyme (Fig. 9.6). Lack of one of the enzymes will result in an accumulation of the steroid prior to the blocked step and a deficiency of the steroids usually produced in subsequent steps (see congenital adrenal hyperplasia).

Glucocorticoids affect carbohydrate metabolism by enhancing gluconeogenesis, i.e. promoting glucose formation, but also by inhibiting its utilization by antagonizing the action of insulin. Excess glucocorticoids are thus diabetogenic and a deficiency can lead to hypoglycaemia. Glucocorticoids also increase protein breakdown and excess leads to negative nitrogen balance.

Another important physiological role of glucocorticoids is their anti-inflammatory activity. Increased glucocorticoid activity leads to a fall in eosinophils and lymphocytes, but to an increase of the neutrophil count. Large amounts of glucocorticoids suppress the inflammatory response and antibody

246 The Adrenal Glands

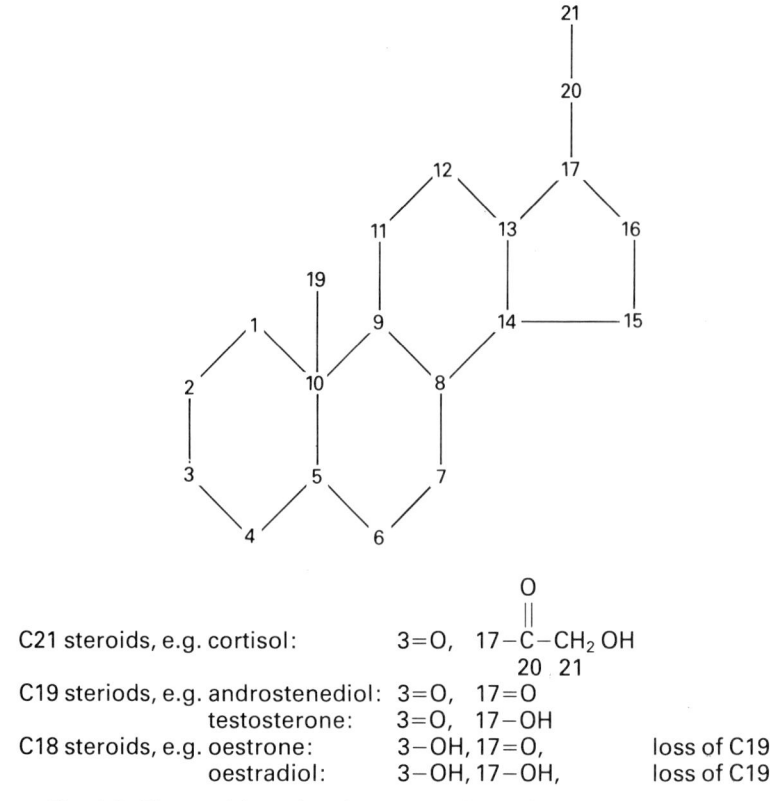

```
                                    21
                                    |
                                    20
                                    |
                        12         17
                     11/   \13   /
                              \16
                19    |    |    |
                 \1   9    14——15
                 /  \  /  \  /
                2   10    8
                |    |    |
                3    5    7
                 \  / \  /
                  4    6
```

C21 steroids, e.g. cortisol:	3=O, 17−C̈−CH₂OH
	20 21
C19 steriods, e.g. androstenediol:	3=O, 17=O
testosterone:	3=O, 17−OH
C18 steroids, e.g. oestrone:	3−OH, 17=O, loss of C19
oestradiol:	3−OH, 17−OH, loss of C19

Fig. 9.2 The position of carbon atoms in the basic steroid ring.

formation. Cortisol levels increase markedly in response to physical and psychological stress. Glucocorticoids have weak effects on sodium retention and potassium excretion but such effects may become more important with high dosage of such steroids.

Glucocorticoid synthesis and release is under the control of adrenocorticotrophin hormone (ACTH) from the pituitary, which is in turn regulated by corticotrophin releasing hormone (CRH) from the hypothalamus. There is circadian activity with peak levels around 0900 h and low levels at midnight. Cortisol exerts a negative feedback effect on ACTH secretion (Fig. 7.8). Cortisol circulates in the blood largely bound to an alpha-globulin, cortisol binding globulin.

Mineralocorticoids act predominantly to promote sodium influx and potassium efflux from cells. This is most evident in the renal tubule where the effects can be measured in terms of sodium and potassium output, but there are several other factors governing the regulation of sodium, potassium, water and hydrogen ion balance by the kidney which may predominate.

Aldosterone secretion is controlled predominantly via the renin–aldosterone

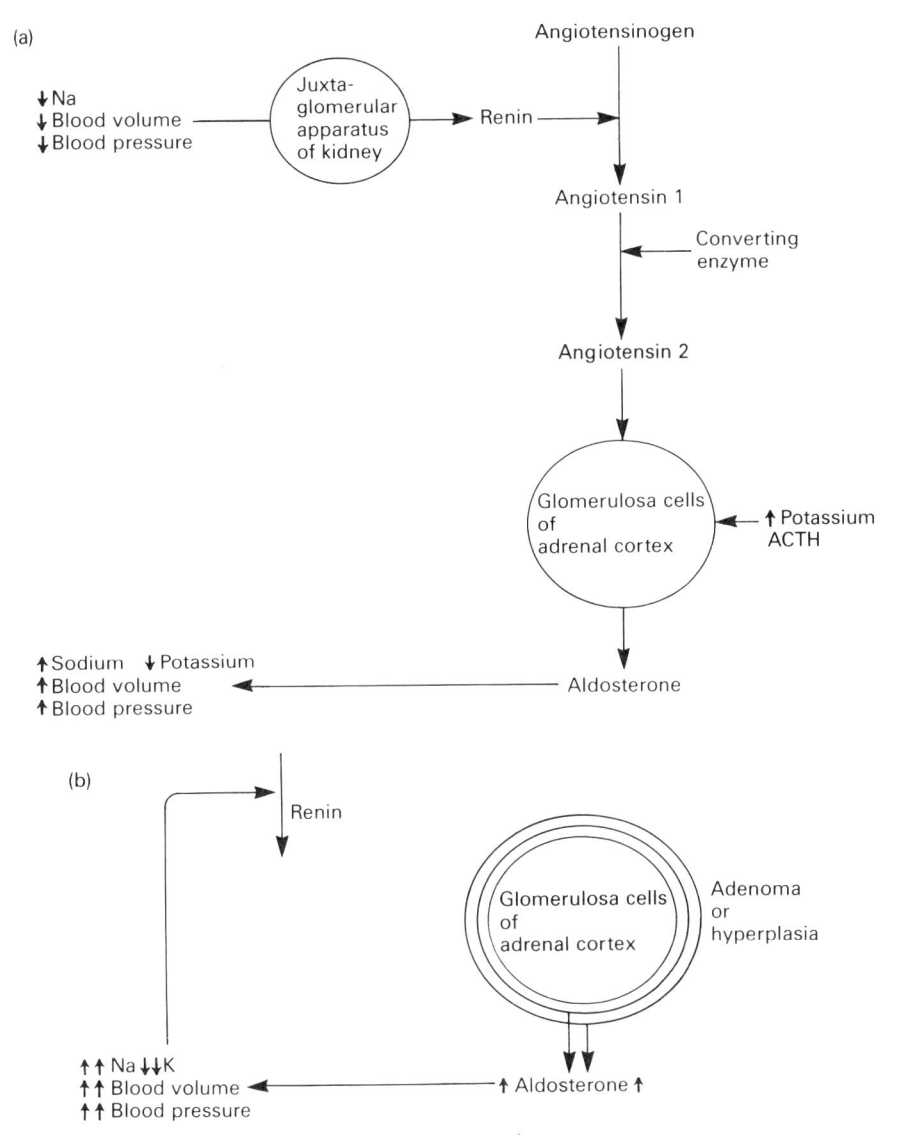

Fig. 9.3 (a) Control of aldosterone secretion. (b) Conn's syndrome. ACTH, adrenocorticotrophic hormone.

axis (Fig. 9.3a). A reduced blood volume or low sodium state stimulates renin secretion from the juxtaglomerular apparatus and renin catalyses the conversion of circulating angiotensinogen to angiotensin 1. Angiotensin converting enzyme, present in the lungs and vascular tissue, in turn converts angiotensin 1 to angiotensin 2 which acts on the zona glomerulosa to release aldosterone. Aldosterone may be released directly in response to hyperkalaemia and is also influenced by ACTH, but the latter is not a dominant effect as mineralocorticoid activity is maintained by the zona glomerulosa after hypophysectomy, whereas the zona fasciculata and reticularis atrophy and their functions are lost.

Androgen secretion from the adrenal cortex is relatively minor compared with gonadal production and is not sufficient to maintain secondary sexual characteristics in the castrated male, nor to counter the effects of the loss of ovarian function in the post-menopausal female. Overproduction of androgens from the adrenal in pathological states, such as congenital adrenal hyperplasia, may nevertheless lead to important pathophysiological effects.

Metabolism of Adrenocorticosteroids

About 90% of cortisol is bound to an alpha-globulin but the latter has a very low affinity for aldosterone. The biological half-life for cortisol is about 90 min whereas it is only approximately 20 min for aldosterone. The adrenocorticosteroids are degraded in the liver into biologically inactive metabolites which are conjugated with glucuronic acid or sulphate, making them more water soluble. The metabolites excreted via the kidneys can be measured in 24-h urine collections as:

(a) free cortisol—which measures unbound cortisol
(b) 11-OH corticosteroids—which measure all steroids including cortisol with an OH group on C11 (Fig. 9.2)
(c) 17-OH corticosteroids—which measure cortisol and all its precursors with an OH group on C17
(d) 17-oxysteroids (also called 17-ketosteroids)—which measure the adrenal androgens dehydroepiandosterone (DHEA) and androstenedione. A proportion of testosterone from the testis is also converted to androstenedione.

Clearly alterations in liver and kidney function and in protein binding (such as during pregnancy) will affect considerably the urinary output of these steroids.

Diseases of the Adrenal Cortex

Diseases of the adrenal are relatively uncommon compared with the prevalence of diabetes or thyroid disease but they are important because they can be life-threatening and are treatable.

Hypofunction

Addison's disease

When Thomas Addison first described the eponymous condition which he recognized as being due to destruction of the adrenal glands, the commonest

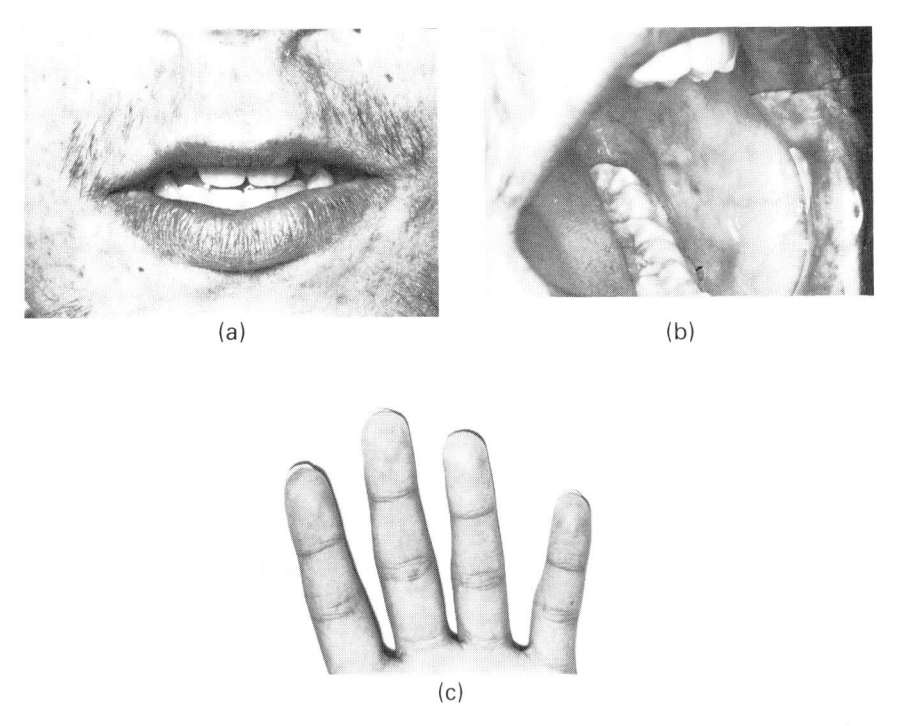

Fig. 9.4 Clinical features of Addison's disease. (a) Lips and face. (b) Buccal mucosa. (c) Palmar creases. *See also* colour plates between pages 102 and 103.

cause was tuberculosis and this remained the case until the advent of successful antituberculous therapy. Spontaneous primary adrenal failure is now most likely to be due to auto-immune destruction of the gland, but adrenal failure may also become manifest following long-term treatment with suppressive doses of steriods when the drug is withdrawn. It may also result from metastatic carcinoma or from haemorrhage into the adrenals such as may occur in meningococcal septicaemia or rarely after severe trauma.

Clinical features
Addison's disease may present acutely, or it may develop insidiously only to be revealed when the patient is unable to respond to intercurrent illness or stress.

Acute adrenal insufficiency presents with profound shock. The patient is hypotensive and dehydrated due to the loss of both mineralocorticoid and glucocorticoid function. The classical bronzed pigmentation of the skin and mucous membranes described in Addison's disease will not be evident if the acute failure is the result of a sudden insult such as haemorrhage, but is more likely to be found in the patient who has been developing the condition gradually (Fig. 9.4). Chronic adrenal insufficiency is characterized by non-specific symptoms of general lassitude, malaise, progressive weakness, diarrhoea and vomiting, weight loss, thirst and polyuria. There may be a history of other auto-immune diseases such as thyroid failure, premature ovarian failure or pernicious anaemia in the family or even in the patient. A history of previous long-term steroid therapy must be excluded. Evidence of increased pigmentation should be sought particularly over pressure points, in the palmar creases and the buccal mucosa (Fig. 9.4). Postural hypotension is a common feature. Muscle weakness can be so profound as to lead to paresis.

Investigations

In suspected acute adrenal failure blood should be taken for plasma cortisol, urea, electrolytes and glucose, but treatment should be initiated without waiting for the results. Typically the serum K^+ is elevated, the Na^+ reduced and urea moderately raised, but these findings are not invariably present depending on the severity of the condition at the time of diagnosis. The blood glucose may be low, the plasma cortisol inappropriately low for the degree of stress and endogenous ACTH levels are high. The proof of the diagnosis ultimately rests on the demonstration that the adrenal is incapable of producing an adequate cortisol response to an ACTH load. The latter test is carried out when the patient is on replacement therapy with a steroid such as dexamethasone which does not interfere with the cortisol assay. A dose of 0.25 mg of synthetic ACTH (Synacthen) is given intramuscularly and the cortisol level measured basally and at 30 and 60 min. An increment of more than 200 nmol/l to a level of over 500 nmol/l is usually deemed to be an adequate response which excludes the diagnosis (Fig. 9.5).

A plain abdominal X-ray or ultrasonic scan of the adrenals is seldom likely to show calcification these days and is probably not justified unless there is a strong suspicion of tuberculosis. Adrenal antibodies are likely to be positive but cannot always be demonstrated.

Treatment

Acute adrenal failure is a medical emergency. The patient requires intravenous saline to rehydrate and to correct the hypovolaemia, as well as intravenous hydrocortisone initially in large doses such as 100 mg every six hours. The steroid dosage can then be gradually reduced stepwise and eventually given orally. The usual maintenance dose of hydrocortisone is 20 mg in the morning and 10 mg in the evening. The patient will also need mineralocorticoid replacement therapy in the form of fludrocortisone, 0.05–0.1 mg daily. The optimum replacement dose should be judged by the patient's clinical response in terms of their sense of well-being, reduction of pigmentation, maintenance of normal blood pressure and normal electrolytes.

The patient should be supplied with a steroid card to carry at all times and advised of the need to double the dose of hydrocortisone in response to the stress of any intercurrent illness without waiting to see a doctor. Should the patient become severely ill or be unable to maintain oral therapy because of vomiting they should be advised to seek medical attention immediately.

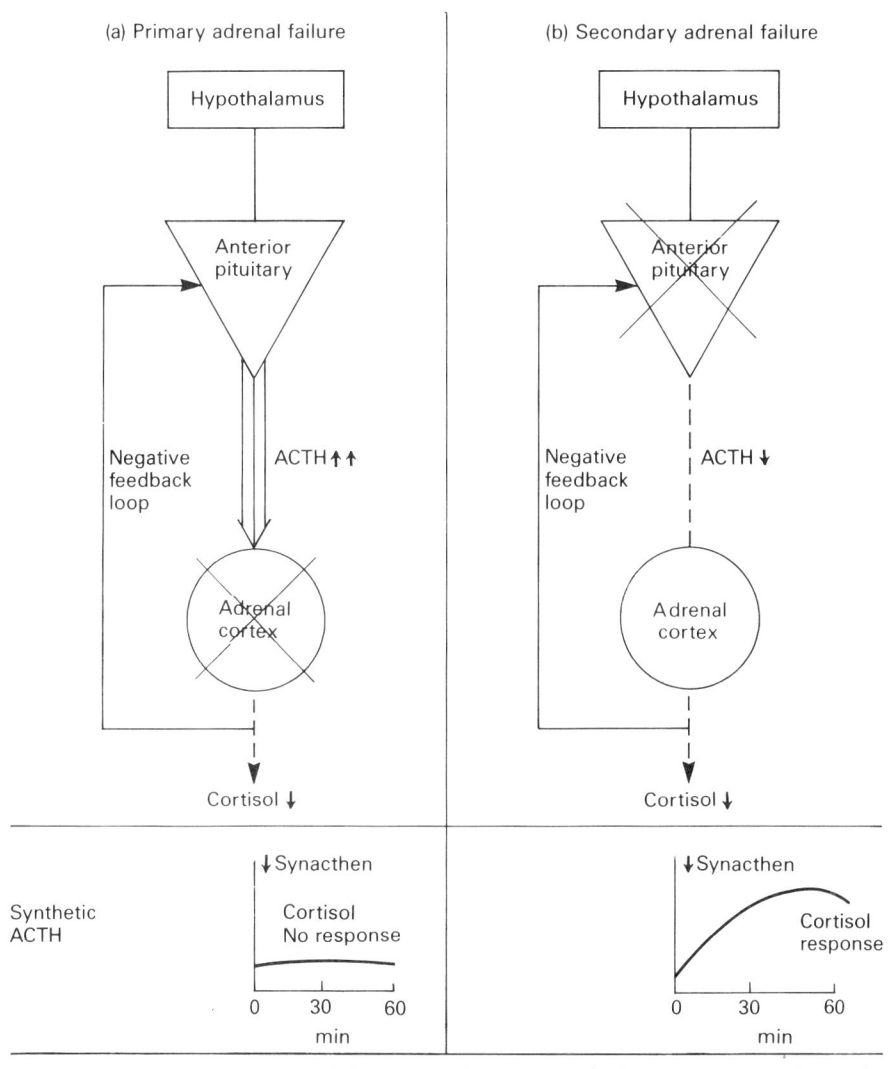

Fig. 9.5 Diagnostic tests of (a) Addison's disease (primary adrenal failure), (b) adrenal failure secondary to pituitary failure. ACTH, adrenocorticotrophin hormone.

Secondary hypoadrenalism
Adrenal failure secondary to pituitary or hypothalamic disease results from lack of ACTH drive affecting the zona fasciculata and reticularis but not the zone glomerulosa. The result is lack of cortisol production but maintenance of aldosterone activity.

The commonest cause is a pituitary tumour in adults, but a craniopharyngioma is more likely in childhood. Pituitary infarction following massive post-partum haemorrhage (Sheehan's syndrome) is now fortunately relatively uncommon. Long-term steroid therapy can also permanently suppress the pituitary part of the pituitary–adrenal axis as well as the adrenal itself.

Clinical features   Secondary hypoadrenalism presents in a similar way to primary hypoadrenalism with respect to the symptoms of cortisol deficiency, namely anorexia, nausea, lassitude and general weakness, but there is lack of pigmentation (due to the lack of ACTH). The preservation of aldosterone activity also means that although the blood presure may be lowish there is often an absence of postural hypotension and hypovolaemia. Other features of pituitary failure are commonly present such as loss of libido, amenorrhoea and secondary sexual characteristics (Chapter 7).

Investigations   Basal plasma cortisol is low in secondary hypoadrenalism but the adrenal is still capable of responding to synthetic ACTH. The pituitary lesion is demonstrated by the lack of cortisol response to an insulin-induced hypoglycaemic stress test (Fig. 9.5b) (Chapter 7).

Treatment   Secondary hypoadrenalism requires replacement glucocorticoid in the form of hydrocortisone (20 mg a.m. and 10 mg p.m.) or prednisolone (5 mg a.m. and 2.5 mg p.m.) but there is usually no need for mineralocorticoid replacement.

Congenital adrenal hyperplasia

Enzyme defects in the synthesis of the adrenal steroids can lead to deficiency of cortisol, aldosterone or androgens. A defect in the pathway of cortisol formation results in increased ACTH output which in turn increases the amount of precursors up to the level of the block. The increased precursors may be diverted along other pathways, depending on the level of the block, and lead to hyperplasia and increased production of aldosterone or androgens.

A defect in the cortisol pathway will result in the clinical features of hypoadrenalism.

A defect in the aldosterone pathway will result in a salt-losing state. Conversely a defect which leads to enhanced aldosterone production will lead to sodium retention and hypertension.

Lack of androgens in the developing fetus will result in a female phenotype regardless of the genetic sex (Chapter 10). Conversely excessive production of adrenal androgens will lead to virilization of the fetus. The result of such abnormalities of hormone production, which are often partial rather than complete, may be the development of ambiguous external genitalia or external appearances which are inappropriate to the internal anatomy of the sexual organs and chromosomal sex (Chapter 10).

Defects of adrenal steroid synthesis are rare with the exception of the 21-hydroxylase defect. The major defects and their consequences are sum-

Congenital Adrenal Hyperplasia 253

```
                        Cholesterol
                            ↓
                       Pregnenolone  — — — — — →  DHEA
                            ↓                      ↓
Deoxycorticosterone ←— Progesterone  ————————→ Androstenedione
        ↓                   ↓                      ↓
  Corticosterone      17-OH Progesterone        Testosterone
        ↓                   ↓
   Aldosterone        11 Deoxycortisol
                            ↓
                         Cortisol
```

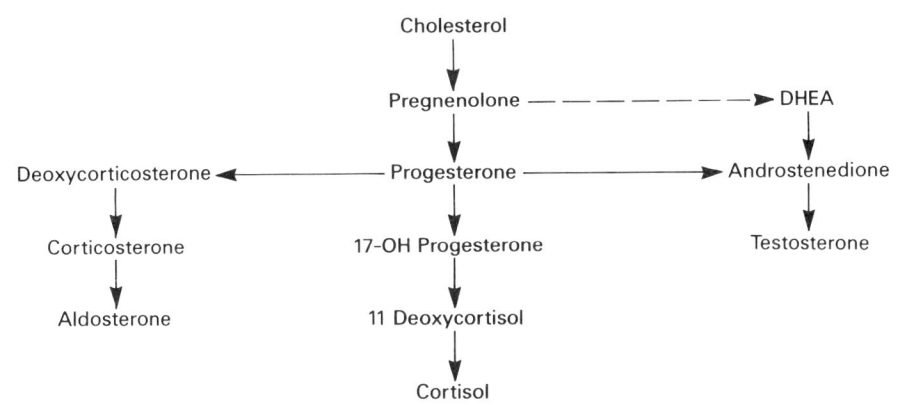

Fig. 9.6 Steps in steroid synthesis from cholesterol. DHEA, dehydroepiandosterone.

marized below and can best be understood by reference to Figs 9.6 and 9.7 which identify the level of each block.

(a) 20–22-Desmolase deficiency blocks the conversion of cholestrol to pregnenolone, an essential early step in the formation of all the steroid hormones, with resultant lack of cortisol, aldosterone and testosterone. The effects are severe and the infant (of female phenotype) rarely survives despite treatment with cortisol, saline and mineralocorticoid (Fig. 9.7a).

(b) 3-β-Hydroxysteroid dehydrogenase deficiency results in lack of cortisol and aldosterone. The production of DHEA, a weak androgen, is increased but its conversion to androstenedione and testosterone is impaired. Infants present with hypoadrenalism and a salt-losing syndrome, ambiguous genitalia in the male and mild virilization in the female. Treatment is required with cortisol, mineralocorticoid and salt supplements. Later surgical correction of abnormal genitalia and androgen supplements of boys at puberty will be necessary (Fig. 9.7b).

(c) 17-Hydroxylase deficiency results in impaired cortisol and androgen production but enhanced mineralocorticoid formation with resultant salt retention and hypertension. The defect in sex hormone formation also affects the testis and ovary so males may present with pseudohermaphroditism and females with lack of secondary sexual development. Sex hormone replacement therapy is necessary as well as cortisol to suppress the ACTH drive (Fig. 9.7c).

(d) 21-Hydroxylase deficiency results in impairment of cortisol and of aldosterone production but enhanced androgen formation. In its severe form the major presenting feature is a salt-losing state but in milder forms it may present because of virilization of the female or precocious pseudopuberty in the male. Large quantities of pregnanetriol, which derives from 17-OH progesterone the precursor to the block, are excreted in the urine. Treatment

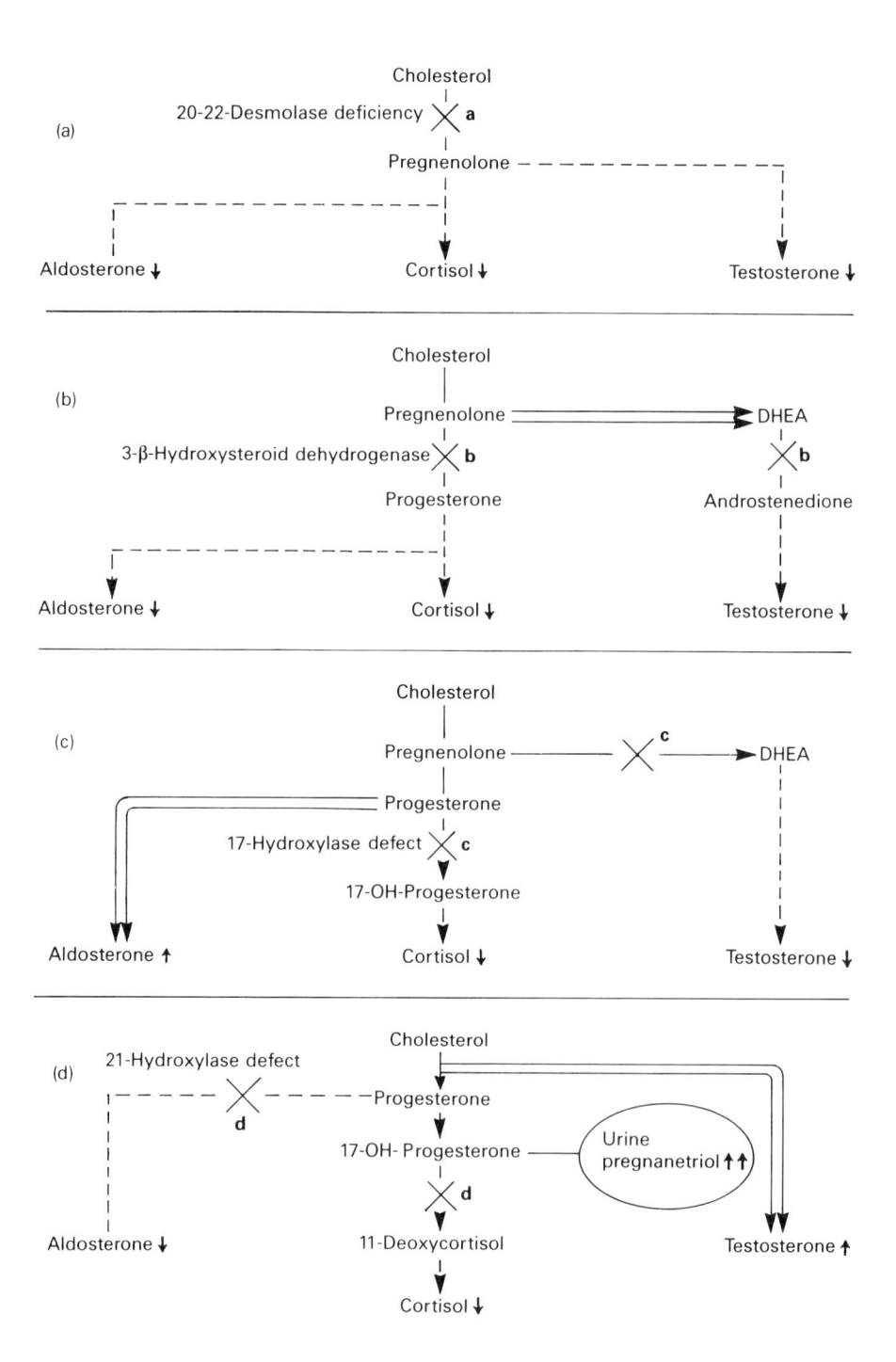

Congenital Adrenal Hyperplasia

(e)

```
                    Cholesterol
                        |
    ↑Deoxycorticosterone←──────────────┐
            |                          |
            ✗ e                        |
            ↓                          |
    Corticosterone          11 Deoxycortisol ─── (Urine tetrahydro S ↑↑)
        |                        |
        |              11-β-Hydroxylase ✗ e
        |              defect
        ↓                        ↓
    ↓Aldosterone            ↓Cortisol                    Testosterone ↑
```

(f, g)

```
                            Cholesterol
                                |
    ↑Deoxycorticosterone ───────┤
            |                   |
    ↑Corticosterone             |
            |                   |
18-Hydroxylase defect ✗ f       |
            |                   ↓              ↓
18-Hydrogenase defect ✗ g     Cortisol     Testosterone
            ↓
    Aldosterone ↓↓
```

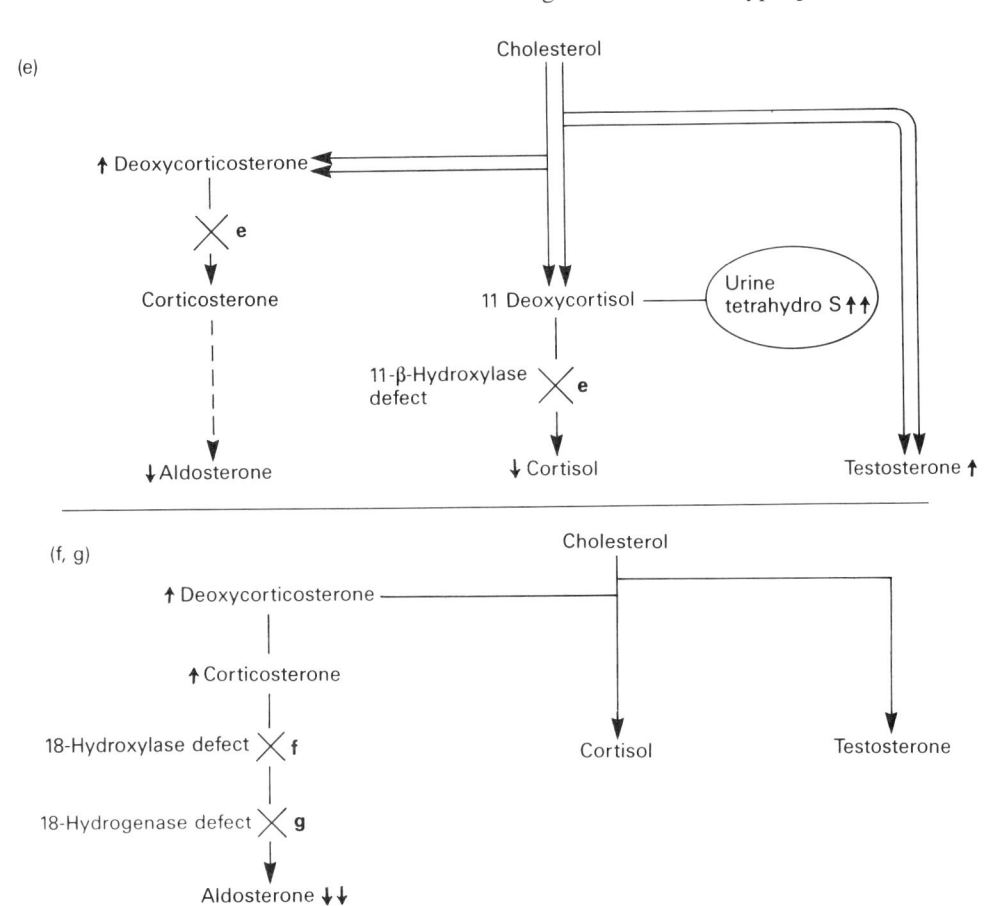

Fig. 9.7 (a–g) Defects in steroid synthesis. (a) 20-22-Desmolase deficiency. (b) 3-β-Hydroxysteroid dehydrogenase deficiency. (c) 17-Hydroxylase defect. (d) 21-Hydroxylase defect. (e) 11-β-Hydroxylase defect. (f) 18-Hydroxylase defect. (g) 18-Hydrogenase defect.

is with cortisol and mineralocorticoid depending on the degree of aldosterone deficiency (Fig. 9.7d).

(e) 11-β-Hydroxylase defect blocks the penultimate step in the synthesis of cortisol and the conversion of deoxycorticosterone to corticosterone and hence aldosterone. The precursor 11-deoxycortisol accumulates and has salt-retaining properties which more than compensate for the decreased aldosterone production and leads to hypertension. The tetrahydro-S derivative of the precursor is excreted in large quantities in the urine. Androgen production is increased leading to virilization. Treatment is with cortisol. Metyrapone is a drug which acts by inhibiting 11-β hydroxylation and may be used diagnostically and therapeutically in Cushing's syndrome (Fig. 9.7e).

(f) 18-hydroxylase and (g) 18-dehydrogenase defects affect the penultimate and ultimate steps, respectively, of aldosterone synthesis with a resultant salt-losing syndrome. Cortisol and androgen production are normal (Fig. 9.7f, g).

Adrenal Hyperfunction

Cushing's syndrome

Harvey Cushing first described his eponymous syndrome in 1912. The term Cushing's disease is conventionally reserved for the syndrome when it is due to pituitary production of excess ACTH leading to bilateral adrenal hyperplasia, as originally recognized by Cushing. The majority of spontaneous cases are indeed of pituitary origin but the syndrome may also be due to an adrenal adenoma or carcinoma, or an ectopic source of ACTH usually from a bronchial neoplasm. The use of large doses of steroids for any length of time will produce a similar clinical picture and the description of the clinical features which follows should serve as a reminder of the complications of steroid therapy.

Clinical features (Table 9.1)
The patient usually complains of obesity but the distribution of fat is mainly on the face and trunk rather than the limbs. The round face is commonly described as moon-faced, and the exaggerated fat pad above the shoulders gives rise to the description of buffalo hump but this feature can be found in simple obesity. The limbs are thin and weak due to proximal myopathy. The skin is thin and

Table 9.1 Clinical features of Cushing's syndrome

Appearance	Round, reddened 'moon' face
	Mild hirsutism
	Acne
	Increased pigmentation (Cushing's disease)
	Obesity of trunk
Cardiovascular system	Hypertension
	Fluid retention
Abdomen	Dyspeptic symptoms
	Obese
	Purple striae
Spine	Back pain
	Osteoporosis
	Vertebral collapse
Central nervous system	Depression, psychoses
	Wasting
	Proximal myopathy
Skin	Thin, easy bruising
	Poor wound healing
Metabolic	Diabetes mellitus
	Hypokalaemia

bruises easily and stretch marks, usually found on the abdomen, thighs or buttocks, have a purple discolouration. Abrasions or ulcers of the skin are slow to heal. The female patient particularly may complain of acne and hirsutism of the face and present with oligomenorrhoea or secondary amenorrhoea. Pigmentation is increased in Cushing's disease but not in Cushing's syndrome due to other causes, but this can be difficult to judge because of the high colour of the cheeks and the individual's varying complexion.

The patient may also complain of backache due to osteoporosis and vertebral collapse or of indigestion due to peptic ulceration. Hypertension and diabetes are commonly but not invariably found. The patient's mental state may be disturbed and depression or other psychoses can be the presenting feature of the condition or cause the underlying diagnosis to be overlooked.

Patients with an ectopic ACTH syndrome are more likely to present with the clinical features of the underlying tumour, usually weight loss and wasting, rather than the typical features of Cushing's syndrome outlined above unless due to a very slow growing tumour such as carcinoid. The diagnosis may be suspected clinically from the markedly increased pigmentation usually associated with excessive ACTH production, or from the hypokalaemia noted on the electrolyte screen which is usually much more profound than in Cushing's disease.

Differential diagnosis
The differential diagnosis usually lies between Cushing's syndrome and so-called simple obesity, particularly if the obese patient is also hypertensive and diabetic. The distribution of the body fat is the main distinguishing feature and the skin is usually thickened in simple obesity and striae are pale rather than purplish. It should also be remembered that whilst obesity is common, Cushing's syndrome is rare.

The polycystic ovary syndrome may also cause diagnostic difficulty because of the associated obesity, hirsutism and oligomenorrhoea.

Patients with alcoholism may also develop a pseudo-Cushingoid appearance.

Diagnostic tests
The most useful screening test to exclude a diagnosis of Cushing's syndrome is measurement of 24 h urinary free cortisol excretion. The normal range is 35 to 255 nmol/24-h. Values comfortably within the normal range make the diagnosis highly unlikley (but Cushing's disease can rarely be cyclical). Stress can cause elevated levels and to establish a diagnosis of Cushing's syndrome it is necessary to demonstrate evidence of hypercortisolism under resting conditions and also loss of the normal diurnal cortisol rhythm. The 0900 h plasma cortisol is often within the normal range but the midnight cortisol is elevated (normal less than 170 nmol/l).

In normal individuals cortisol production is suppressed by a low dose of 0.5 mg of dexamethasone six hourly, whereas in Cushing's syndrome there is impairment of the normal feedback mechanisms with failure of suppression by

258 The Adrenal Glands

low dose dexamethasone and also lack of stimulation by insulin-induced hypoglycaemia.

Once the diagnosis of Cushing's syndrome is established it is necessary to differentiate between pituitary, adrenal and another source (Fig. 9.8).

Adrenal adenoma or carcinoma
Excess cortisol from an adrenal tumour leads to suppression of ACTH which should therefore be undetectable. Previously the unreliability of assays for ACTH made it necessary to seek evidence for the adrenal origin of the syndrome by indirect tests of dexamethasone suppression and metyrapone

(a) Cushing's disease	(b) Cushing's syndrome	(c) Ectopic ACTH
ACTH Raised	ACTH Undetectable	ACTH High
Dexamethasone: (8mg daily) - Suppresses 24 h urinary 17-OH cortisteroid output	Dexamethasone: (8mg daily) Fails to suppress 17-OH corticosteroid output	Dexamethasone: (8mg daily) Fails to suppress 17-OH corticosteroid output
Metyrapone: Further increases 24 h urinary 11-OH corticosteroid output	Metyrapone: No effect on 11-OH corticosteroid output	Metyrapone: No effect on 11-OH corticosteroid output

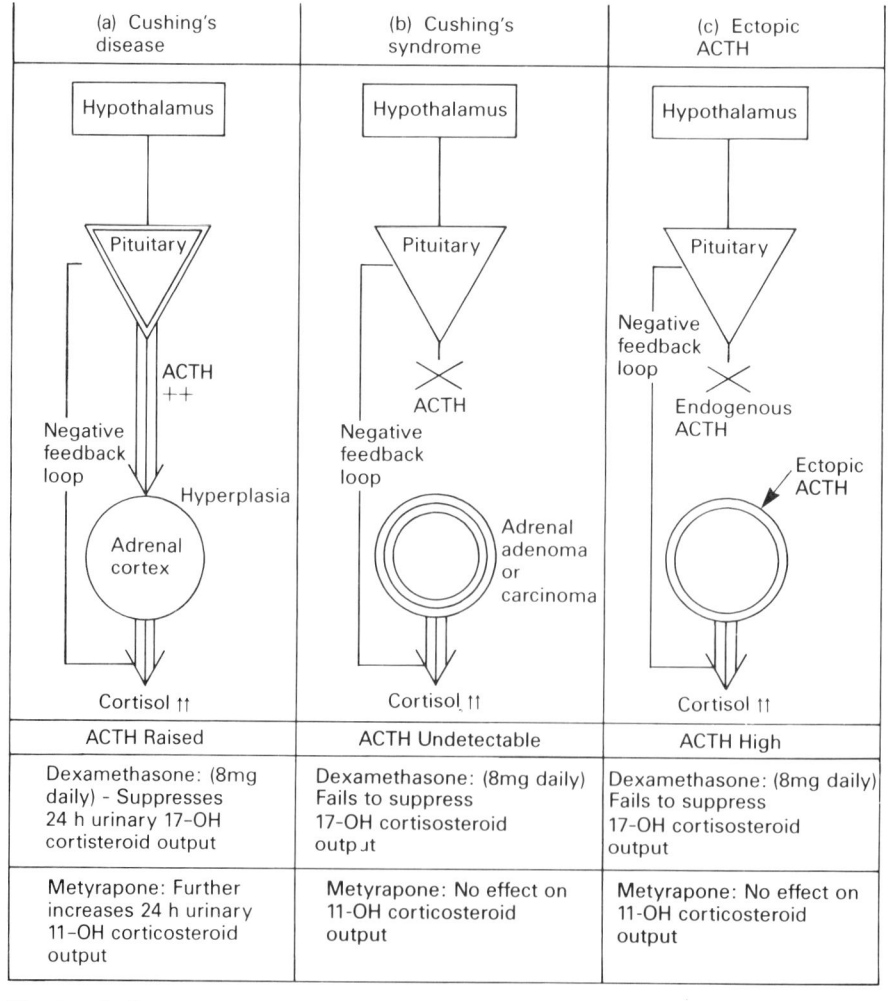

Fig. 9.8 Differential diagnosis of Cushing's syndrome. ACTH, adrenocorticotrophic hormone. (a) Cushing's disease. (b) Cushing's syndrome. (c) Ectopic ACTH.

stimulation. Large doses of dexamethasone (2 mg six hourly) usually fail to suppress cortisol production by an adrenal tumour. Metyrapone in a dose of 250 mg every four hours, if tolerated by the patient, whilst blocking the synthesis of cortisol at the penultimate step thus sending a signal to increase ACTH output, fails to increase the production of the 11-deoxycortisol precursor, measured in the urine as 17-hydroxycorticosteroid (17-OHCS), in patients with adrenal tumours.

A CT scan of the adrenals will help to localize the tumour prior to surgery. Adrenal adenomas are usually unilateral but carcinomas are said to account for about 10% of adrenal tumours and may be bilateral, locally invasive and metastasize.

Pituitary adenoma
Excess ACTH from the pituitary leading to bilateral adrenal hyperplasia is the commonest cause of Cushing's syndrome. Plasma ACTH is raised or within the normal range but inappropriately so for the raised levels of plasma cortisol. Pituitary-dependent Cushing's disease is not totally autonomous thus suppression of cortisol production may occur with large (2 mg) but not small (0.5 mg) doses of dexamethasone. Similarly metyrapone, blocking cortisol synthesis, enhances further ACTH output and increases the production of the 11-deoxycortisol precursor measured in the urine as 17-OHCS.

The skull X-ray seldom shows any enlargement of the pituitary fossa in Cushing's disease although the boundaries may not be easily defined because of osteoporosis. A CT scan may or may not reveal a microadenoma as the ACTH-producing cells are often quite dispersed. Proof that the ACTH is coming from the pituitary and not an ectopic source may sometimes be difficult to establish even with selective venous catheterization.

Ectopic ACTH syndrome
The clinical situation in which this syndrome is suspected is usually distinct from that of typical Cushing's disease but not invariably so. Levels of ACTH are often markedly higher but may overlap with those found in Cushing's disease. Tumours producing ectopic ACTH do not respond to metyrapone. The primary tumour is usually an oat-cell bronchial neoplasm but it may not be obvious on a plain chest X-ray. Causes of ectopic ACTH syndrome are shown in Table 9.2.

Table 9.2 Causes of ectopic ACTH syndrome

Oat cell carcinoma of bronchus	+++
Carcinoid tumours	++
Pancreatic tumours	++
Phaeochromocytoma	+
Medullary carcinoma of thyroid	+
Gastrointestinal tumours	+
Prostatic carcinoma	+
Renal carcinoma	+

Treatment

Medical treatment is seldom fully effective in blocking the excessive cortisol production, whatever the origin of the Cushing's syndrome, for any length of time. Metyrapone in large doses often causes unacceptable gastrointestinal side effects and may not be sufficient by itself to block cortisol synthesis. If effective then the patient will need additional supplementary replacement steroids to remain euadrenal and not hypoadrenal. Aminoglutethamide, which is cytotoxic to both adrenal and thyroid cells, may be used in addition to metyrapone to control cortisol production, but it frequently causes an erythematous rash and other toxic effects.

Surgical removal of a benign adrenal adenoma is the treatment of choice and should effect a cure. The patient is best rendered as near euadrenal as possible by medical treatment prior to operation and will need supplementary steroid therapy to cover the stress of surgery. Post-operatively the patient may need replacement steroids for several months until the contralateral adrenal recovers from the suppression caused by the original adenoma.

It may not be possible to remove an adrenal carcinoma if extensive local invasion or metastases have occurred. Local radiation and medical treatment with cytotoxic agents such as opDDD may offer some palliation but the prognosis is poor.

Pituitary-driven Cushing's disease is most logically treated by removing the pituitary lesion where possible. Trans-sphenoidal hypophysectomy in skilled hands is usually the treatment of choice but is not always effective and some degree of hypopituitarism may be the price to be expected, particularly if clearance of the fossa is necessary at operation because no discrete microadenoma is visible. Similar results are claimed for trans-sphenoidal implantation of radioactive seeds of gold or yttrium. If direct treatment of the pituitary is not effective or not practicable for whatever reason then it may be necessary to advise total bilateral adrenalectomy in order to remove the source of cortisol production. Maintenance glucocorticoid and mineralocorticoid therapy will then become essential to prevent adrenal insufficiency. External radiation is then given to the pituitary to try to prevent the continuing activity of the ACTH cells which can lead to excessive pigmentation and expansion of the pituitary fossa known as Nelson's syndrome. The results of external radiation alone in the treatment of Cushing's disease have been disappointing. Cushing's disease remains one of the more difficult endocrinopathies to cure completely.

Conn's syndrome

Primary hyperaldosteronism is due to an adenoma or hyperplasia of the glomerulosa cells of the adrenal cortex. Carcinoma is extremely rare. The excessive production of aldosterone leads to sodium retention with increase in blood volume and rise in blood pressure which in turn suppress renin levels (Fig. 9.3b).

Primary hyperaldosteronism needs to be distinguished from secondary

Table 9.3 Causes of hyperaldosteronism

Primary	Adrenal adenoma or carcinoma	Aldosterone ↑
	Adrenal hyperplasia	Renin ↓
Secondary	to excessive stimulation of normal adrenals	Aldosterone ↑
	↓ Blood volume, e.g. nephrotic syndrome, cirrhosis	Renin ↑
	↓ Sodium, e.g. salt-losing nephritis	
	Renal ischaemia, e.g. renal artery stenosis	
	Malignant hypertension	
	Reninoma (very rare)	

hyperaldosteronism which is due to excessive stimulation of normal adrenals as a result of reduction of blood volume (for example, in the nephrotic syndrome or cirrhosis), loss of sodium (for example, in salt-losing nephritis) or renal ischaemia (for example, in malignant hypertension or renal artery stenosis), which all lead to high renin levels. A primary reninoma is very rare (Table 9.3).

Clinical features
The condition is relatively rare but is said to be slightly more common in females than in males. It nevertheless probably accounts for less than 1% of all cases of hypertension. The diagnosis is usually suspected in a patient who is found to be hypokalaemic as well as hypertensive. It is important to exclude diuretics as a cause of the hypokalaemia. Less commonly the patient may present with the clinical features of hypokalaemia such as weakness, flaccid paralysis, tetany or paraesthesiae. Polydipsia, polyuria and oedema if present are all mild.

Investigations
Plasma electrolytes usually reveal low potassium and mildly raised sodium levels but they can be within the normal range, particularly if the patient has a relatively low salt intake. Urinary potassium excretion is increased. It is necessary to establish the presence of raised aldosterone levels and suppressed renin levels under controlled conditions. The blood samples need to be carefully prepared according to laboratory instructions. The patient is tested in the recumbent and in the elevated posture before and after a week of sodium restriction (10 mmol/day) and of sodium loading (150 mmol/day). In the patient with Conn's syndrome renin levels should remain suppressed and the aldosterone levels elevated despite assumption of upright posture and after sodium loading. Hyperplasia is demonstrated biochemically by suppression of the hyperaldosteronism after a course of dexamethasone.

An adenoma is more common than hyperplasia as a cause of Conn's syndrome but the adenoma may be small and not easy to demonstrate even with a CT scan of the adrenals. An iodocholesterol scan or sampling via an adrenal vein catheter may help to localize a small tumour.

Table 9.4 Effects of stimulation of alpha- and beta- adreno receptors

	Alpha-receptor	Beta-receptor
Cardiovascular system	↑ Systolic blood pressure ↑ Diastolic blood pressure ↑ Contractility	↑ Systolic blood pressure ↑ Heart rate ↑ Contractility ↑ Cardiac output
Peripheral blood flow		
Coronary	Constriction	Dilatation
Skin		
Striated muscle		
kidney		
Smooth muscle		
Bronchial	—	Relaxation
Gut	Contraction	Relaxation
Bladder	Contraction	Relaxation
Pancreatic secretion	Decreased	Increased
Lipolysis	—	Increased
Glycogenolysis	±	Increased
Sweating	Increased	
Central nervous system	Pupil dilatation Anxiety Alertness	

Treatment
Surgery is usually the treatment of choice for a proven adenoma and should cure the hyperaldosteronism and the hypertension. Some patients, however, are not fit for or do not want surgery and the condition can be treated medically even when due to an adenoma as well as for hyperplasia. Spironolactone is an aldosterone antagonist and is quite well tolerated in modest dosages of 200 mg daily, but above 400 mg daily it often causes unacceptable side effects, particularly gynaecomastia in males. Amiloride may be used as an alternative.

Physiology of the Adrenal Medulla

The adrenal medulla secretes the catecholamines adrenaline (epinephrine) and nonadrenaline (norepinephrine) into the circulation in response to stimulation via preganglionic (cholinergic) sympathetic nerves. Noradrenaline is also a neurotransmitter secreted by sympathetic post-ganglionic nerve endings. Both adrenaline and noradrenaline are released together by the medulla and have multiple effects on many target organs. In general noradrenaline predominantly affects alpha-receptors whereas adrenaline affects both alpha- and beta-receptors (Table 9.4). Whilst it is generally assumed that the adrenal medulla plays a major role in the sudden release of catecholamines in preparation for 'fight or flight' no major harm seems to follow its removal unlike the adrenal cortex, loss of which is fatal without replacement therapy.

Various other substances such as met-encephalin and somatostatin are produced by the medulla but their physiological roles are uncertain.

Synthesis and Release of Catecholamines

Adrenaline and noradrenaline are derived from phenylalanine in a series of steps represented in Fig. 9.9. The enzymes responsible for each step in the sequence are found in the brain as well as the adrenal medulla, and are also present in sympathetic nerve endings (except for the enzyme converting noradrenaline to adrenaline). The chromaffin granules in the medulla store both noradrenaline and adrenaline and the conversion of the former to the latter may be modulated by glucocorticoids from the cortex. The catecholamines released into the circulation in response to neurological stimulus are either taken up by tissues where they are stored or degraded or are excreted in the urine. Enzymes in the liver and kidneys convert most of the catecholamines to normetadrenaline or metadrenaline which may be further converted to HMMA (4-hydroxy 3-methoxy mandelic acid, also known as VMA—vanillyl mandelic acid) and can be measured in the urine.

Measurement of Catecholamines

Direct measurement of plasma adrenaline and noradrenaline is now possible in some laboratories but for screening purposes 24-h urine collections for the

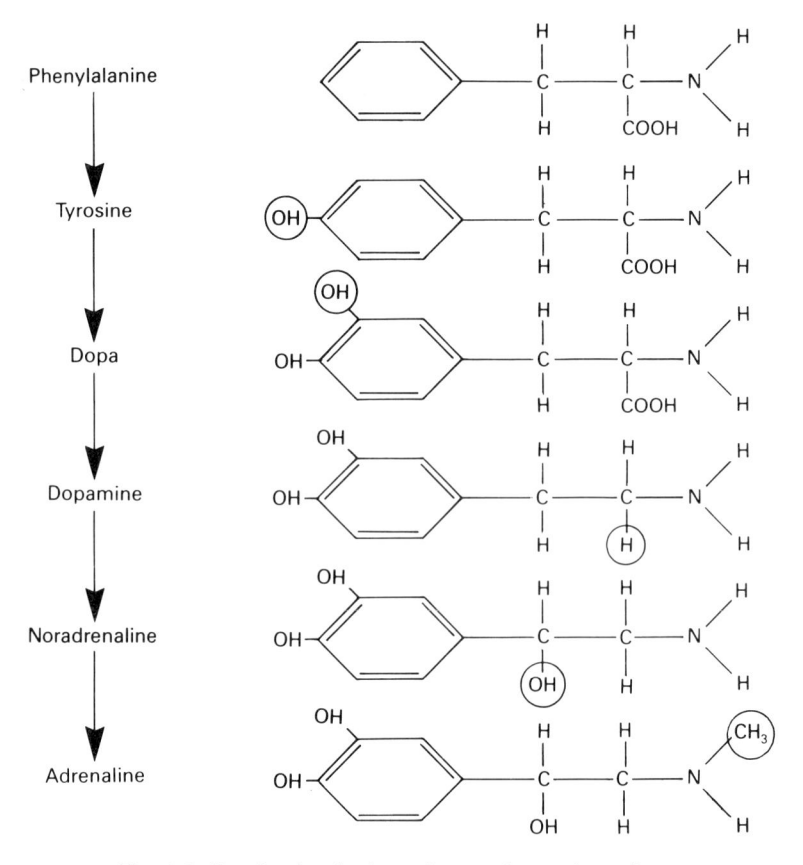

Fig. 9.9 Synthesis of adrenaline and noradrenaline.

measurement of metanephrines or normetanephrines or HMMA are still usually required. Many factors may interfere with the measurement of these substances and include:

(i) Physiological effects, e.g. stress, exertion or illness
(ii) Dietary effects, e.g. coffee, bananas in large quantities
(iii) Drug effects (a) those which affect the patient, e.g. monoamine oxidase (MAO) inhibitors, beta-blocking agents, (b) those which interfere with the assay method being used.

Close collaboration with the laboratory before undertaking the sampling is advisable.

Pathology of the Adrenal Medulla

Tumours of the adrenal medulla include neuroblastomas which are relatively common amongst the malignant tumours of childhood, ganglioneuromas which are more benign and affect older children and young adults, and phaeochromocytomas which occur mostly in adults.

Phaeochromocytoma

Phaeochromocytomas are uncommon but may be familial. They may be associated with familial neurofibromatosis (von Recklinghausen's disease) or with multiple endocrinopathy neoplasia (MEN) (Chapter 6) syndrome type 2a, both of which usually exhibit autosomal dominant inheritance. Patients with medullary carcinoma of the thyroid (Chapter 8) should be screened for phaeochromocytoma and vice versa. Phaeochromocytoma may also be associated with MEN 2b which can occur sporadically and is characterized by a Marfanoid habitus, thickened lips and mucosal neuromas.

Clinical features

Phaeochromocytoma can mimic numerous other conditions and the diagnosis is easily overlooked. It may present as panic attacks excessive sweating, cardiac arrhythmias, paroxysmal or sustained hypertension, headaches, abdominal crisis (due to haemorrhage into the tumour) or with diabetes mellitus. It may thus mimic an anxiety state, hyperthyroidism, subarachnoid haemorrhage or hypertension from any cause. It is uncommon for the tumour to be large enough to present as an abdominal mass but care must be taken on palpation of the abdomen and during investigation not to compress the lesion and provoke a surge of adrenaline or noradrenaline release.

Investigations

Where possible direct measurement of plasma total catecholamines (normal <1 µg/l) can be used to confirm the diagnosis. Alternatively 24-h urinary metadrenaline (normal <20 µg) and normetadrenaline (normal <70 µg) or HMMA (VMA) may be measured. It is important that the estimations are undertaken when the patient is not under stressed conditions, yet at a time when the paroxysmal nature of the problem may be caught. It is therefore wise to arrange for two or three consecutive 24-h urine collections to be made before excluding the diagnosis.

Once the biochemical evidence for the diagnosis has been established it is necessary to locate the tumour. Ninety per cent of phaeochromocytomas are to be found in the adrenal medulla but they can occur anywhere along the sympathetic chain from the neck to the pelvis. A CT scan of the adrenals will locate most tumours but selective catheterization and venous sampling may be necessary before others can be localized.

Management

Surgical removal of the adrenal tumour is the treatment of choice but it is advisable to block the effects of secreted catecholamines medically before surgery or any other procedure such as catheterization or intravenous pyelography. Medical treatment may also be needed urgently to control a hypertensive crisis. Initial treatment should aim to block alpha-receptor activities. Phenoxybenzamine can be given by intravenous infusion 0.5 mg/kg body weight in 250 ml of 5% dextrose over 2 h and then orally in a dose to 10 to 20 mg every 6 or 8 h. Further treatment to block beta-receptor activities can then be added, such as propranolol 40 mg thrice daily. It is better to avoid treatment with beta-blockade alone as this may lead to an exacerbation of the alpha-adrenergic effects and precipitate a hypertensive crisis.

Further Reading

Burke, C.W. (1985). Adrenocortical insufficiency. *Clinics in Endocrinology and Metabolism* **14**, 947–976.

Cryer, P.E. (1985). Phaeochromocytoma. *Clinics in Endocrinology and Metabolism* **14**, 203–220.

Hall, R. and Besser, M. (eds) (1989). *Fundamentals of Clinical Endocrinology*, 4th edition. Churchill Livingstone, Edinburgh.

Howlett, T.A., Rees, L.H. and Besser, G.M. (1985). Cushing's syndrome. *Clinics in Endocrinology and Metabolism* **14**, 911–946.

New, M.I., White, P.C., Speiser, P.W., Crawford, C. and Dupont, B. (1989). Congenital adrenal hyperplasia. In *Recent Advances in Endocrinology and Metabolism*, No. 3, pp. 29–76. Edited by Edwards, C.R.W. & Lincoln, D.W. Churchill Livingstone, Edinburgh.

10

THE GONADS

Development

Control of gonadal development and hence of sex differentiation lies in the sex chromosomes which are designated X and Y. In the normal human female the chromosome pattern or genotype is XX whereas in the male it is XY. Much of the material required for sexual development is carried on the X chromosome and is required by both sexes. In order to prevent a double dose of this material developing in all but the germ cells in females one of the X chromosomes is inactivated in somatic cells and forms the so called Barr body seen in the nucleus of female cells. The number of Barr bodies is thus one less than the number of X chromosomes.

The genotype governs the physical development of the individual or phenotype although this may be modified by hormonal and other factors during development. The basic phenotype is female thus in the absence of a Y chromosome the internal and external genitalia will be of female type. The presence of a Y chromosome leads to the expression of a male factor which determines the differentiation of the primordial gonad towards a testis rather than an ovary, and the production of testosterone and other factors which in turn lead to the suppression of the female (Mullerian) ducts and development of the male (Wolffian) ducts (Fig. 10.1).

The Internal Genitalia

The primordial germ cells in the wall of the yolk sac migrate to the primitive gonad developing in the urogenital ridge. During the second month of fetal life two pairs of ducts, the Mullerian and the Wolffian ducts, develop and connect the gonads to the urogenital sinus (Fig. 10.1a). In the female the Mullerian system develops to form the Fallopian tubes and the uterus and the upper third of the vagina, and the Wolffian system regresses (Fig. 10.1b). In the male the developing testis produces both a factor which suppresses the Mullerian ducts and testosterone which is required to promote and maintain the development of the Wolffian system to form the epididymis and vas deferens and later the seminal vesicles (Fig. 10.1c).

Lack of both primitive gonads will result in persistence of the Mullerian ducts

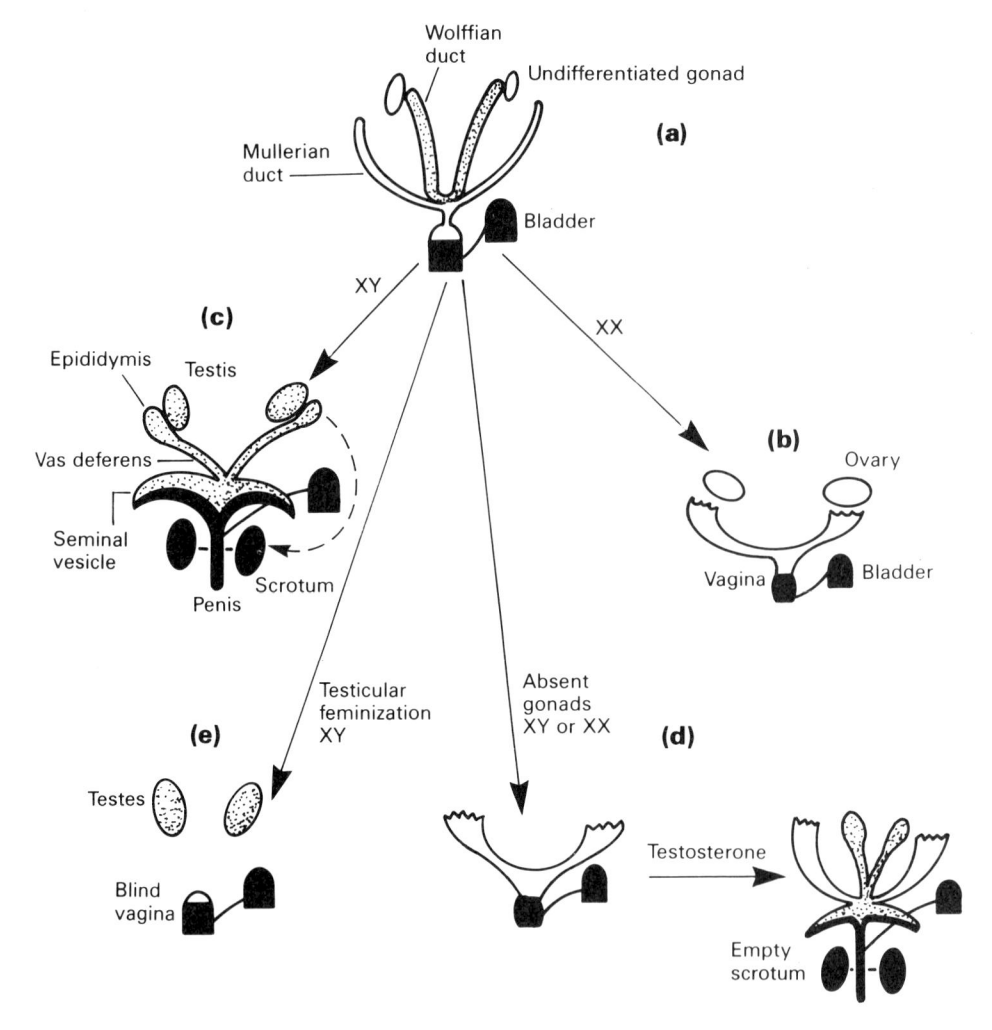

Fig. 10.1 Development of internal genitalia. (a) Undifferentiated gonad. (b) Normal female. (c) Normal male. (d) Lack of primitive gonads. (e) Testicular feminization syndrome.

so the internal genital system will be female (Fig. 10.1d). Lack of testes or lack of the factor which suppresses the Mullerian ducts, or lack of effective testosterone will result in failure of development of the Wolffian ducts and will also result in persistence of female internal genitalia.

The External Genitalia

The external genitalia develop from the same primitive tissues in both sexes. In the female the genital tubercle forms the clitoris and the labioscrotal folds become the labia major and minora. The lower two-thirds of the vagina develop as a pouch from the urethral fold which joins up with the lower end of the fused Mullerian ducts. In the male the testis produces testosterone which is converted by an enzyme 5-α-reductase to dihydrotestosterone (DHT) in the tissues which form the external genitalia. This promotes the formation of the penis and scrotum.

Exposure to excessive androgens early in fetal life may lead to masculinization of external genitalia in the female, or later in fetal development will result in clitoromegaly. Lack of testosterone or of the enzyme 5-α-reductase, or of the receptors responsive to DHT will result in feminization of external genitalia in the genotypic male.

The Testis

By the end of the second month of fetal life the developing gonads are recognizably either testes or ovaries. The testis consists of epithelial cords which later become seminiferous tubules, and interstitial (Leydig) cells which secrete testosterone. The Leydig cells respond to stimulation by placental human chorionic gonadotrophin (HCG) which peaks at about 12 weeks gestation and subsequently subsides. The Leydig cells subsequently decrease in size and activity and do not become prominent again until puberty. The testes gradually descend from their position on the posterior abdominal wall to enter the scrotum only shortly before birth. The mechanisms governing their descent are not known.

The testes remain very small during the first eight or nine years of life and then they begin to enlarge as the seminiferous tubules increase in size and activity. The stimulus for this increase is the development of pulsatile secretion of the gonadotrophins luteinizing hormone (LH) and follicle stimulating hormone (FSH) in response to pulses of gonadotrophin releasing hormone from the hypothalamus. These pulsations begin at night but increase in amplitude and frequency and eventually occur throughout the day before puberty can be completed. Luteinizing hormone stimulates the activities of the Leydig cells and FSH stimulates the development of spermatogenesis for which androgens are also necessary. Testosterone exerts a negative feedback effect on LH secretion and FSH may be controlled by inhibin which is probably produced within the Sertoli cells which exist within the tubules and sustain the germ cells (see Fig. 7.10).

Spermatogenesis occurs in the seminiferous tubules. Initially the stem cells or spermatogonia divide by mitosis maintaining the diploid number of chromosomes. Subsequent meiotic divisions ensure that each cell contains only the haploid number of chromosomes with either an X or Y sex chromsome. The whole process of development of the mature sperm from the early stem cell takes approximately 70 to 90 days.

The sperm are stored in the epididymis and subsequently pass down the vas deferens to be mixed with fluid from the seminal vesicles and prostate to form the semen. The normal ejaculate is between 2 and 6 ml in volume and contains over 20 million sperm/ml, of which more than 60% show normal morphology and motility.

Normal Puberty in Males

The first clinical sign of puberty is an increase in testicular volume and wrinkling of the scrotal skin. The average age of onset of these change is about 11 years in boys in the UK. Later, pubic hair appears scantily at first around 12 years of age and thickens increasingly over a year or two. The penis enlarges at about 13 years of age and spontaneous erections and emissions occur. Deepening of the voice, coarsening of the skin and acne are all features of increasing testosterone secretion and affect individuals to varying degrees. The pubertal growth spurt reaches its peak velocity in boys at about 14 years of age, i.e. after the sexual developments. There is a wide variation of two or three years from the average in the age of onset of puberty.

The Ovary

In the fetus between the 8th and 20th week the oogonia divide repeatedly, initially by mitosis but subsequently by meiosis to form oocytes. Each oocyte is surrounded by granulosa cells and forms a primordial follicle which remains dormant until puberty and subsequent events. The ovary at birth contains more than enough primordial follicles for a lifetime's reproductive cycles and many atrophy.

The ovaries remain quiescent for several years until events in the hypothalamus or in higher centres initiate pulsatile secretions of gonadotrophin releasing hormone (GnRH) and thus of the gonadotrophins LH and FSH. Pulsations of LH and FSH initially occur at night but subsequently occur throughout the day before puberty is completed. Follicle stimulating hormone as its name implies stimulates the maturation of the follicles and early in puberty several follicles enlarge as can be demonstrated by ultrasound. Subsequently as puberty advances and the menstrual cycle begins only one follicle develops fully with each cycle but the mechanisms by which this dominant follicle is selected remain unclear. Other follicles which may enlarge early in the cycle atrophy.

The Normal Menstrual Cycle (Fig. 10.2)

The first half of the cycle is known as the follicular phase during which time the follicle is maturing and meiosis is completed within the ovum. An increase in oestrogen levels in the blood occurs before ovulation and once the follicle has matured oestrogen levels begin to fall and progesterone levels begin to rise. These changes modulate the hypothalamic/pituitary control of gonadotrophin

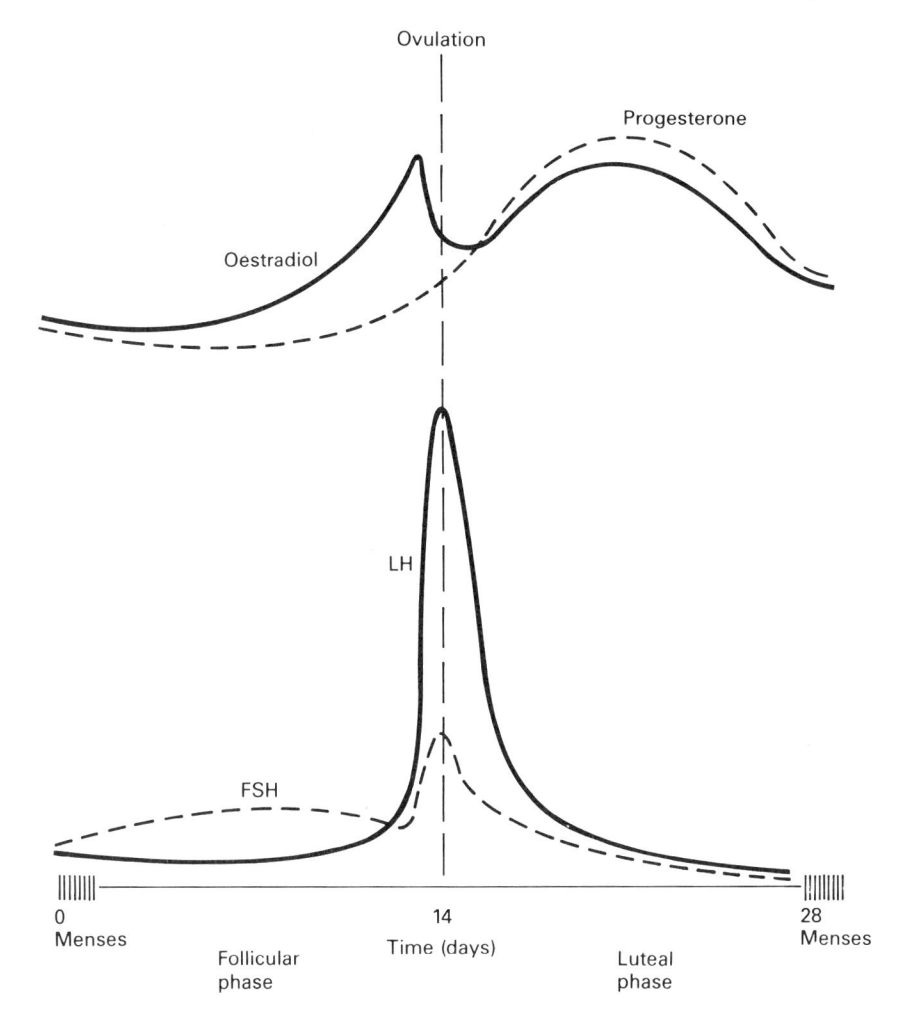

Fig. 10.2 Changes in luteinizing hormone (LH), follicle stimulating hormone (FSH), oestradiol and progesterone during the normal menstrual cycle.

release with a resultant surge of LH over 24 to 48 h which causes rupture of the follicle and release of the ovum. The residual granulosa cells of the follicle are transformed into the corpus luteum, which continues to produce progesterone, and the second half of the cycle is known as the luteal phase.

During the follicular phase of the cycle the increasing oestrogen levels cause the endometrium lining the uterus to proliferate. Subsequently in response to progesterone during the luteal phase it becomes secretory in preparation for implantation by a fertilized ovum. Should that occur the implanted trophoblast generates HCG which sustains the activities of the corpus luteum. In the event of fertilization not occurring the corpus luteum fails and the progesterone levels fall with resultant shedding of the endometrium at menstruation.

Normal Puberty in Females

The first feature of puberty in the female is the development of the breast buds and areola enlargement which occurs on average at about the age of 10 years in girls in the UK. The breasts continue to enlarge and pubic hair appears. Vaginal and uterine secretions increase. Pigmentation of the nipples also develops. Menstruation begins at about 13 years of age but this menarche can occur normally within the range 10 to 16 years. Growth is stimulated by both oestrogens and androgens, the latter mainly from the adrenals, and the peak growth spurt occurs earlier in pubertal development in girls than in boys, usually before the onset of menstruation.

The first few menstrual cycles are often anovulatory and irregular but subsequently with adequate gonadotrophin stimulation ovulation occurs and menstruation follows 14 days later. The average cycle is of approximately four weeks duration and menses last 3 to 5 days.

Pathological Sexual Disorders

The approach to this section is best understood in terms of disturbances of the normal processes of sexual development outlined in the previous sections.

Chromosomal Abnormalities (Table 10.1)

Male phenotype

Klinefelter's syndrome due to an XXY constitution is said to occur in 1 in 700 males. Primary sex differentiation is normal initially but the germ cells de-

Table 10.1 Chromosomal abnormalities

Male phenotype	
47 XXY	Klinefelter's syndrome, infertile
47 XXY/46 XY	Klinefelter's mosaic, may be fertile
48 XXXY	
49 XXXXY	Very rare, mentally retarded
Male Turner's syndrome	Somatic changes, but XY
Female phenotype	
45 XO	Turner's syndrome
47 XXX	Normal ovaries, tall, impaired IQ
47 XXX/45 XO	Mosaic
Pure gonadal dysgenesis	
46 XX	Failure of puberty
46 XY	Uterus present
	Variable gonadal remnant
	Potential gonadal malignancy
Testicular feminization	
46 XY	No uterus or tubes

generate leaving only Sertoli cells and Leydig cells. The testes remain pea-sized even in adulthood but variable amounts of androgens are produced and partial puberty occurs. The degree of androgenization may be such that the patient does not present until later in adulthood because of infertility. Others present with pubertal failure or gynaecomastia but the latter is not invariably present, nor are such patients inevitably tall. Plasma testosterone levels may be normal or low and FSH levels are invariably raised. Levels of LH are usually also raised but less markedly than FSH depending on the testosterone levels. True Klinefelter's syndrome patients are of course azoospermic but the rarer mosaic 47XXY/46XY can be fertile. Patients need counselling about the cause of their infertility. Some patients may benefit in terms of development and sexual performance from testosterone supplements.

The karyotypes 48XXXY and 49XXXXY are very rare and are also associated with sterile testes and with mental deficiency.

Female phenotype

Turner's syndrome due to an X0 constitution is said to occur in approximately 1:2500 females. The patient has streak ovaries which consist of stroma but no follicles (although the latter may be found in patients with a mosaic karyotype XX/X0).

Turner's syndrome is associated with other somatic features which may lead to its recognition at an earlier age, but many patients do not present until failure of puberty with primary amenorrhoea. They are usually of short stature, much less than the third centile for height, and have cubitus valgus (an increased carrying angle) and often a shortened fourth or other metacarpal bone. Webbing of the neck is usually but not invariably present and the chest is flat with widely spaced nipples but undeveloped breasts. There is also an association with congenital heart disease, particularly coarctation of the aorta but also atrial and ventricular septal defects, which are said to be found in approximately 20% of patients.

The gonadotrophin levels are invariably raised and oestrogen levels are low leading to late fusion of the epiphyses, i.e. a delayed bone age. The patient will benefit from cyclical oestrogen replacement therapy to foster the development of secondary sex characters, correct the amenorrhoea and prevent premature osteoporosis. Growth hormone treatment should be considered before sex hormone replacement causes fusion of the epiphyses. The patient will remain infertile and will need counselling at the appropriate age. *In vitro* fertilization of a donated ovum and implantation into the hormonally treated and prepared uterus remains a possibility.

Pure gonadal dysgenesis

If the gonads fail to develop from the earliest stages of fetal development then the phenotype will be female in appearance regardless of the underlying genotype. The problem is not likely to present until the patient fails to undergo puberty. At that point plasma oestrogens will be low and gonadotrophins high. The lack of gonads may be demonstrated by ultrasound or CT scan and confirmed at laparoscopy if necessary. A uterus will be present even if the underlying genotype is XY and not XX. If the genotype is XY then careful search will be necessary to exclude or remove any internal gonadal remnant because of the increased risk of malignancy in such tissue.

Testicular feminization

This rare condition is due to a gene defect coding for the androgen receptor and is probably an X-linked disorder. The patient has an external female phenotype but an XY genotype. The testes are present so that the factor which leads to suppression of the Mullerian ducts is produced and there is no uterus or tubes. The testes produce testosterone but the lack of receptors means that it is ineffective so the Wolffian ducts disappear and the external genitalia remain female in appearance. The vagina ends as a blind sac (Fig. 10.1e). The unopposed action of oestrogens results in normal breast development and patients usually present because of primary amenorrhoea. The testes may be palpable in the groin or be intra-abdominal and show no evidence of spermatogenesis although there may be hyperplasia of the Leydig cells. There is an increased risk of malignancy in the ectopic gonads. Plasma testosterone levels are in the same range as for normal adult males.

The patient will have been raised as female and this self perception should not be disturbed although it will be necessary to explain that the amenorrhoea and infertility cannot be corrected because of the absent uterus. It will also be advisable at some point to remove the gonads because of the risk of malignancy although replacement hormone therapy will be necessary subsequently. The vagina may need enlargement by gradual stretching with dilators, or even surgery to allow satisfactory intercourse.

5-alpha-Reductase deficiency

In this rare autosomal recessive condition the patient is unable to convert testosterone to the dihydrotestosterone necessary for development of normal male external genitalia. The internal genitalia are male because the testes produce the Mullerian suppression factor and the testosterone necessary to develop the Wolffian ducts. The female appearance of the external genitalia means that the patient will have been reared as a female but at the time of puberty signs of virilization occur with enlargement of the phallus, deepening of the voice and male behaviour. Removal of the gonads, hormone replacement therapy and adjustive surgery may all be needed.

True hermaphroditism

This condition in which there are both XX and XY chromosomes and both testis and ovary or ovotestes is extremely rare. The patient is likely to be noted to have ambiguous genitalia at birth. The exact anatomical defects will depend on whether male or female factors predominate; a testis on one side and an ovary on the other can lead to male internal genitalia and female internal genitalia on the respective sides.

Abnormal genitalia

Cryptorchidism

It can be difficult to be sure of the presence of the testes in the scrotum at birth or in early childhood because they are retractile, but it should be possible to establish that they can be brought into the sac. Unilateral cryptorchidism is commoner than bilateral failure of descent. Examination of the child in a warm bath may help. Careful palpation of the inguinal canal and groin may localize the retractile gonad but failure to find a gonad necessitates further investigation The incidence of testicular failure and of malignancy is much greater in ectopic and intra-abdominal testes. If the testes do not descend normally within the first year of life then treatment with a short course of HCG (1500 IU twice weekly for six weeks) can be tried and if this fails surgical orchidopexy is indicated. If undescended testes are left untreated beyond two years they are likely to remain undescended until puberty and fertility will be impaired.

Ambiguous genitalia

At birth if the external genitalia are not clearly either normal male or normal female urgent investigation is necessary to determine the cause and appropriate treatment.

The abnormality may simply be a minor deformity of development such as a urethral orifice which opens before the tip of the penis and does not necessarily signify any underlying chromosomal or hormonal disturbance. On the other hand it may be difficult to determine whether the organ is a small penis in a genotypic male, or a large clitoris in a genotypic female exposed to androgens as a result of congenital adrenal hyperplasia (Chapter 9).

Urgent analyses of the buccal smear and chromosomal pattern should enable the genotype to be established (Table 10.1). Hormonal investigations will be helpful in XY patients who have ambiguous genitalia and XX patients who are masculinized to determine the type of enzyme deficiency responsible for the adrenal hyperplasia.

The management of the patient will depend on the cause but in principle the child will be reared according to its genotype with correction of the genitalia by surgery at appropriate stages. There may however be considerable difficulty in gender assignment and sensitive management is required from people with expertise in the subject.

If the defect is only partial or is not recognized at birth and presents much later then it is likely that the patient will continue to be managed according to the sex which has already been assigned to them as they will be psychologically so adjusted.

Pubertal Abnormalities

Precocious puberty

Puberty may be said to be precocious when it occurs before the age of 8 years in girls or 10 years in boys. It is necessary to establish whether the early development is due to the early maturation of the normal hypothalamic–pituitary–gonadal axis (true precocious puberty) or due to early development of secondary sexual characteristics in the absence of gonadal maturation (pseudo-precocious puberty) (Table 10.2).

True precocious puberty may be constitutional in that there is a family history of early development in one or other parent, or it may be due to a pathological cause such as a pineal tumour, post-encephalitis or meningitis.

Pseudo-precocious puberty will result from exposure to androgens or oestrogens at an inappropriate stage of development. Causes include adrenal, testicular and ovarian tumours, congenital adrenal hyperplasia (Chapter 9) and even more rarely, teratomas.

Clinical investigations include a careful family history, symptomatic enquiry for any evidence to suggest intracranial pathology and, in particular, examination for any signs of raised intracranial pressure or an abdominal or testicular mass. Laboratory investigations include the chromosome pattern, plasma androgens or oestrogens in conjunction with gonadotrophins (the levels of the latter will be low in pseudo-precocious states), and urinary steroid estimations (see congenital adrenal hyperplasia). Management will depend on the cause: true constitutional early development may simply require reassurance and sympathetic support. Organic causes of true sexual precocity are often less amenable to therapy although the use of long-acting analogues of gonado-

Table 10.2 Causes of precocious puberty

True precocious puberty
(Early development of hypothalamic–pituitary–gonadal maturation)
Constitutional
Pathological   Pineal tumours – Pineocytoma
                                    Pineoblastoma
                                    Teratomas
                    Post-encephalitis
                    Post-meningitis
                    Toxoplasmosis
                    Polyostotic fibrous dysplasia

Pseudo-precocious puberty
(Early secondary sexual development in the absence of gonadal maturation)
Pathological   Adrenal tumours
                    Ovarian tumours
                    Testicular tumours
                    Congenital adrenal hyperplasia
                    Intracranial tumours
                    Teratomas

Table 10.3 Causes of delayed puberty

	Cause
Constitutional	Often familial
Primary gonadal failure	See Tables 10.4 and 10.6
Secondary gonadal failure	Pituitary disease
	Hypothalamic disorders
	See Tables 10.4 and 10.6
Non-endocrine disease	Chronic debilitation
	Malnutrition
	Malabsorption
	Emotional deprivation

trophin releasing hormone leading to down regulation of the receptors should be effective. The causes of pseudo-precocity may be more treatable but will not be responsive to GnRH analogues. The anti-androgen cyproterone acetate may be used to arrest precocious sexual development.

Delayed puberty

Delayed puberty is a common cause of referral for a specialist opinion. It is difficult to give a precise time when puberty can be said to be delayed but most girls will have gone through puberty by 14 and boys by 16 years of age although it can be normal up to 18 years. Children will often be brought along earlier by anxious parents, depending on their expectations or the pressures on the child as a result of being amongst the last in the class who has yet to develop secondary sexual characteristics (Table 10.3).

The causes of delayed puberty may be constitutional, when there is often a family history of late onset of puberty in one or other parent, or due to primary gonadal failure or gonadal failure secondary to hypothalamic/pituitary disease (see Tables 10.4 and 10.6). Initial assessment should include details of the family history of parental and sibling development, the patient's own developmental milestones, any evidence of systemic disease, eating habits and weight change, and physical and scholastic attainments. The examination should also include weight and height measured accurately and recorded on centile growth charts, and particular evidence sought for any signs of an intracranial lesion (visual field defects, etc.), pubertal development such as a few wisps of pubic hair, enlargement of the testes or the development of the breast buds in the female. In the absence of any signs of pubertal development initial laboratory screening tests might reasonably include basal gonadotrophin levels, thyroid function tests, skull X-ray, radiological bone age and chromosomal analysis. Raised LH and FSH, (hypergonadotrophic hypogonadism) will indicate primary gonadal failure of whatever cause, whereas low or normal LH and FSH (hypogonadotrophic hypogonadism) will not distinguish between the prepubertal state and hypogonadism secondary to hypothalamic or pituitary disease.

Further investigations may establish such causes of secondary hypogonadism as craniopharyngioma or pituitary tumour but it is at present impossible to separate with certainty simple constitutionally delayed puberty from isolated gonadotrophin releasing hormone deficiency. The latter condition may be associated with anosmia or other congenital midline defects such as cleft palate when it is known as Kallman's syndrome. The presence of multiple cysts in the ovaries on pelvic ultrasound will favour normal prepubertal ovaries whereas the lack of such cysts is more consistent with GnRH deficiency.

Management
If there are early signs of puberty then it may suffice to reassure the patient and parents that all will be well and to document further growth and development as it occurs over succeeding months. If, however, there are no signs of puberty and no obvious cause has been found or the problem is thought to lie at the hypothalamic level then pubertal changes can be provoked by administration of pulsatile GnRH therapy. This requires pulses of GnRH to be given every 90 min initially at night and subsequently throughout 24 h to mimic the normal progression of GnRH pulsatility at puberty. GnRH therapy cannot be given continuously or down regulation of the receptors will occur and pubertal development will be suppressed. It should be remembered that normal pubertal changes take place over many months and time should be allowed for the necessary psychological adjustments to occur as well as the physical changes. Once puberty has been passed therapy can be discontinued to observe whether sexual function is maintained spontaneously, which should be the case in constitutionally delayed puberty but will not occur in isolated GnRH deficiency where further hormone replacement therapy will be needed.

Gonadotrophin releasing hormone therapy will not be effective in patients with a pituitary lesion but they should respond to HCG therapy, which should again be given in modest dosage initially, say 1500 IU twice or three times a week intramuscularly over several months to induce pubertal changes. Maintenance therapy will be necessary with cyclical oestrogens and progesterone in the female and testosterone in the male.

Human chorionic gonadotrophin therapy will be ineffective in patients with primary gonadal failure who can only be treated with hormone replacement therapy to develop their secondary sexual characteristics and who will remain infertile.

Hypogonadism in females

Hypogonadism in females may present with delayed puberty or primary amenorrhoea, or be acquired later in life and present with secondary amenorrhoea and loss of libido. It may also become apparent during the course of investigating other conditions such as hirsutism or galactorrhoea.

The causes of hypogonadism (Table 10.4) can be grouped according to whether there is primarily failure of the ovaries (associated with raised LH and

Table 10.4 Causes of female hypogonadism/Amenorrhoea

	Cause
Primary ovarian failure	Chromosomal abnormalities – Primary amenorrhoea
	Congenital hypoplasia – Primary amenorrhoea
	Auto-immune
	Ovariectomy
	Menopause
	Radiation
	Cytotoxic chemotherapy
Excess androgens	Congenital adrenal hyperplasia
	Masculinizing tumours
	Polycystic ovaries
	Androgenic steroids
Pituitary–hypothalamic disorders	Pituitary tumours
	Craniopharyngioma
	Hyperprolactinaemia
	Isolated gonadotrophin or gonadotrophin releasing hormone deficiency – Primary amenorrhoea
	Trauma
	Infection
	Granuloma, e.g. sarcoidosis
	Functional – Depression
	Anorexia nervosa
	Psychogenic
	Post-oral contraception
Associated with other non-endocrine disease	Malnutrition
	Obesity
	Malabsorption
	Anorexia

FSH, hence the term hypergonadotrophic hypogonadism) or the ovaries fail secondary to pituitary or hypothalamic disease (associated with low LH and FSH levels, and termed hypogonadotrophic hypogonadism). Amenorrhoea may also result from excessive androgenization and can also be functional, that is to say not directly attributable to disease of the pituitary or ovaries *per se* but a central effect mediated via the hypothalamic pathways. The commonest cause of amenorrhoea in women of reproductive years is pregnancy which must be excluded before any other investigations of secondary amenorrhoea are undertaken.

Primary ovarian failure
A chromosomal abnormality such as Turner's syndrome, or congenital gonadal hypoplasia is likely to present with primary amenorrhoea or delayed puberty. Later in life secondary amenorrhoea due to premature primary ovarian failure is likely to be due to auto-immune disease and may be associated with other auto-immune disorders such as vitiligo, premature greying of the hair, Addison's disease (Chapter 9) or primary hypothyroidism (Chapter 8). There is often a family history of one or other of these disorders. It will of course also

occur following surgical removal or irradiation of the ovaries. Normal spontaneous cessation of ovarian function, the menopause, occurs at about the age of 50 years in women in the UK.

Ovarian failure secondary to pituitary–hypothalamic disease
A pituitary tumour is the commonest cause of secondary ovarian failure, although in the younger age group a craniopharyngioma is more likely. Either may present as primary amenorrhoea or failure of pubertal development in childhood or with secondary amenorrhoea in the older age group, or hypogonadism found secondarily to other features of pituitary tumours such as a visual field defect (Chapter 7). A prolactinoma is the likeliest pituitary tumour and the patient may present with galactorrhoea as well as amenorrhoea (Chapter 7). Hypogonadism may also be a feature of other pituitary tumours including chromophobe adenomas, and tumours causing acromegaly (Chapter 7) or Cushing's disease (Chapter 9).

Isolated gonadotrophin deficiency will present as primary amenorrhoea and failure to undergo puberty, with or without anosmia or other congenital defects of Kallman's syndrome.

Trauma causing section of the pituitary stalk will also cause amenorrhoea and galactorrhoea. Rarely basal infection such as meningitis or a granuloma such as tuberculosis or sarcoidosis can also cause amenorrhoea.

Functional causes of amenorrhoea mediated via the hypothalamus but not usually due to primary hypothalamic disease include depression, anxiety and other psychogenic disturbances. Post-contraceptive pill amenorrhoea for up to three months is common but requires investigation if it persists for longer than six months. It may be due to any of the causes listed above which therefore need to be excluded, but is often then attributable to a disturbance of the hypothalamic rhythm of gonadotrophin releasing hormone activity.

Amenorrhoea is also associated with severe disturbances of weight either due to malnutrition, malabsorption or anorexia on the one hand or obesity on the other. Amenorrhoea may also occur during any serious illness whatever the cause. Regaining normal weight after severe weight loss such as may occur in anorexia nervosa is not necessarily followed by immediate recovery of menstrual function. If amenorrhoea persists for more than six months after regaining weight then therapeutic intervention with an agent such as clomiphene may be necessary to trigger the cycle.

Virilization (Table 10.5)
Hypogonadism associated with increased androgens may be due to congenital adrenal hyperplasia (Chapter 9) which usually presents at birth or later with ambiguous genitalia or abnormalities of pubertal development. The commonest defect of steroid hormone synthesis, 21-hydroxylase deficiency, may be partial and present with amenorrhoea and clitoromegaly at a later age. Virilization developing in an older age group should, however, raise the possibility of an androgen-producing tumour of the ovary or adrenal.

Table 10.5 Causes of virilization

Congenital adrenal hyperplasia
Polycystic ovaries
Ovarian tumours – Arrhenoblastoma
Hilus cell tumour
Adrenal tumours – Adenoma
Carcinoma
Hyperplasia (Cushing's disease) secondary to pituitary

Hirsutism is difficult to define objectively because the perception by the patient of what is normal secondary body hair and what is pathological will depend on ethnic background, complexion and social attitudes. Excessive hair developing on the face, breasts or in a masculine distribution on the body is likely to be associated with an increased plasma free testosterone level. It can be difficult to establish whether the increased androgens are of adrenal or ovarian origin. Normal 24-h urinary free cortisol levels to exclude Cushing's syndrome, normal 17-α-hydroxyprogesterone to exclude late onset 21-hydroxylase deficiency, and normal DHEA sulphate will exclude most adrenal causes (Chapter 9).

Polycystic ovaries are commonly but not invariably associated with obesity, oligomenorrhoea or amenorrhoea and mild hirsutim. Levels of LH are typically mildly elevated, although FSH levels are usually normal, and testosterone levels are either at the upper limit of normal for women (<2–3 nmol/l) or slightly raised. Ultrasound or a CT scan will usually reveal the multicystic ovaries with thickened capsules without the need for laparoscopy. The exact cause of polycystic ovaries remains unknown.

Investigation of hypogonadism
A careful history and examination will be likely to point to the correct diagnosis in most instances and laboratory investigations selected accordingly for confirmation. The diagnosis is not, however, always apparent clinically and screening tests are needed of which the most informative are basal LH and FSH to distinguish hyper- from hypogonadotrophic causes, serum prolactin (Chapter 7), testosterone, free thyroxine (T_4) and thyroid stimulating hormone (TSH), and skull X-ray. Further provocative tests of pituitary/hypothalamic function may be necessary in pituitary disease although the gonadotrophin releasing hormone test has proved disappointing in practice and seldom adds more information to that gained from measuring basal gonadotrophins alone. Chromosome analysis will also be helpful in selected cases.

Management of hypogonadism
Treatment of specific conditions such as congenital adrenal hyperplasia with appropriate glucocorticoid and mineralocorticoid replacement therapy (Chapter 9) and the management of delayed puberty have already been outlined. The management of other causes of hypogonadism will depend not only on the

underlying condition but also on the age, expectations and wishes of the patient. Thus in premature primary ovarian failure it is advisable to restore adequate oestrogen levels with cyclical therapy, not only to maintain libido and normal secondary sexual development but also the suppleness of connective tissues and to prevent osteoporosis. Other younger women with primary ovarian failure will need counselling concerning the disappointment of their own infertility but also of the possibilities and limitations of the options now available to overcome this problem, such as *in vitro* fertilization of a donated ovum, which is beyond the scope of this text and requires specialist expertise.

Successful treatment of the cause of secondary hypogonadism such as removal of a pituitary tumour, or suppression of hyperprolactinaemia with bromocriptine may not only correct the hypogonadism but also restore fertility and patients need counselling accordingly. However, removal of a pituitary tumour may also lead to permanent gonadotrophin deficiency and the patient may then need cyclical replacement therapy. If fertility is still required treatment with HCG and Pergonal under controlled conditions with specialist supervision will be needed.

Patients with functional causes for their amenorrhoea may simply need reassurance that their periods are likely to return spontaneously in due course when the emotional or other contributory factors have resolved. It is, however, difficult to predict when this may happen and in the meantime contraceptive precautions (using non-hormonal methods) may still be advisable. If the patient is anxious that the cycle be restored or no spontaneous period has occurred within six months after correction of the original upset then a trial of clomiphene may be appropriate.

The management of the polycystic ovary syndrome will depend partly on its severity and whether the patient is complaining primarily of hirsutism or amenorrhoea or infertility. It can be difficult for the patient to determine her priorities and for the doctor to treat all aspects satisfactorily. Thus a patient may complain of hirsutism for which the most effective treatment might be cyclical oestrogen with cyproterone acetate. Some patients want to become pregnant. Stimulation with clomiphene, an anti-oestrogen, may provoke a rise in gonadotrophins and successfully induce rupture of a follicle although it may fail or cause painful ovarian swelling. In other patients an explanation of the nature of the cause of the irregular periods may suffice, with advice about alternative methods of contraception because spontaneous ovulatory cycles may still occur. Reassurance should also be given that in the later event of fertility being required and not achieved spontaneously further hormonal stimulation with clomiphene or gonadotrophin therapy may be effective. A wedge resection of the ovaries is seldom performed nowadays but was used to restore ovulation, albeit temporarily.

Hormone replacement therapy (HRT) and the natural menopause
It is widely agreed that cyclical hormone therapy should be given for premature gonadal failure and that oestrogens protect against osteoporosis. Oestrogens

are also commonly given to alleviate troublesome menopausal symptoms such as hot flushes and loss of libido, although many of the symptoms are self-limiting but may recur when therapy is withdrawn. It has therefore been advocated that HRT should be recommended to women approaching the menopause not only to prevent these problems from occurring but also to maintain tissue suppleness and a generally more youthful appearance and sense of well-being. The disadvantages of such therapy include continuation of periods, possible irregular bleeding which would necessitate endometrial curettage to ensure that endometrial hyperplasia had not developed, as this may predispose to malignant changes. There is also an increased risk of venous thrombosis and possibly of cardiovascular disease although hard data on these aspects are difficult to find. These risks are minimized by the use of low doses of naturally occurring conjugated equine oestrogens for 21 days together with a progestogen for the last 12 days of the cycle. In women without a uterus there is no need for progesterone and continuous low dose oestrogen can be given.

Attitudes to the issues involved vary widely amongst women and their doctors and are changing. It is important that the advantages and disadvantages are discussed with the patient and if HRT is chosen by the patient that careful follow up is maintained by the doctor.

Hypogonadism in males

Hypogonadism in males may present because the testes are not found in their correct position early in life (cryptorchidism), or with delayed puberty, or later in life because of loss of libido, impotence or infertility.

Table 10.6 Causes of male hypogonadism. (a) Tubule failure → infertility, (b) Leydig cell failure → testosterone ↓

Primary testicular failure (a and b)	Testicular agenesis
	Bilateral torsion
	Bilateral orchitis
	Bilateral cryptorchidism
	Klinefelter's syndrome (a>b)
	(a) Tubular failure only
	Sertoli cell only syndrome
	Radiation
	Cytotoxic drugs
	Tubular sclerosis (dystrophia myotonica)
	(b) Interstitial cell only
	Disorders of testosterone synthesis
Secondary testicular failure	Isolated gonadotrophin deficiency (LH and FSH) or gonadotrophin releasing hormone
	Pituitary tumours, granulomas
	Hypothalamic disease, craniopharyngioma
	Hyperprolactinaemia
	Functional – depression/anxiety, anorexia
Associated with other non-endocrine disease	Malnutrition
	Malabsorption

LH, luteinizing hormone. FSH, follicle stimulating hormone.

284 The Gonads

The causes (Table 10.6) can be considered in the same manner as previously outlined for women, namely, primary gonadal failure (or hypergonadotrophic hypogonadism), gonadal failure secondary to pituitary or hypothalamic disease (hypogonadotrophic hypogonadism) or functional disturbances mediated via the hypothalamus (Fig. 10.3).

Primary testicular failure
This may predominantly affect the tubules, in which case the problem is likely to present as one of infertility, or the Leydig cells, leading to diminished testosterone production and lack or loss of androgenization, or more commonly both types of cell function may be lost.

Congenital causes of primary testicular failure affecting both tubular and Leydig cell function include testicular dysgenesis (total agenesis will present with a female phenotype), and Klinefelter's syndrome, although in the latter

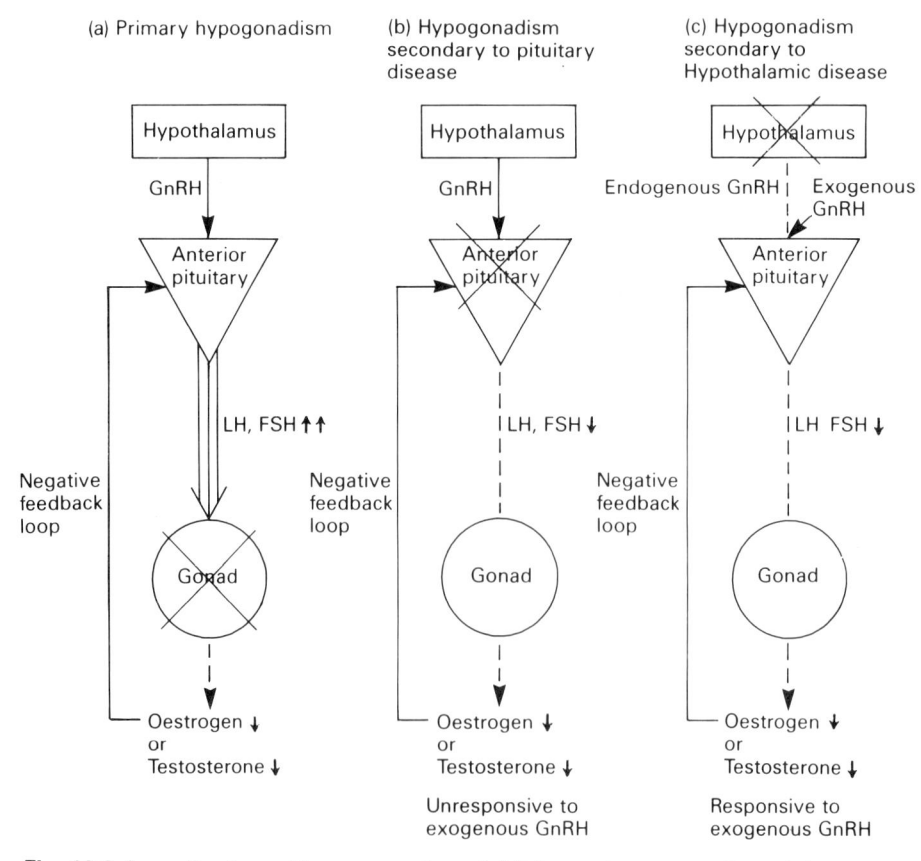

Fig. 10.3 Investigation of hypogonadism. (a) Primary hypogonadism. (b) Hypogonadism secondary to pituitary disease. (c) Hypogonadism secondary to hypothalamic disease. LH, luteinizing hormone. FSH, follicle stimulating hormone. GnRH, gonadotrophin releasing hormone.

tubular function is lost and varying degrees of Leydig cell function are maintained.

Disorders of testosterone production as a result of one or other of the adrenal enzyme deficiencies (Chapter 9) in a genotypic male may result in a pseudohermaphrodite state with varying combinations of internal and external genitalia and unpredictable degrees of Leydig cell function.

The testes in the testicular feminization syndrome produce testosterone from the Leydig cells but it is ineffective due to a receptor disorder in other tissues. The testes in 5-α-reductase deficiency produce testosterone which has some effects but failure of conversion to dihydrotestosterone results in ambiguous external genitalia.

Acquired primary testicular failure may follow bilateral torsion of the testes, or bilateral orchitis, of which the best known cause in adults is mumps, but it may also follow other viral infections. Bilateral cryptorchidism which has not been corrected early in life is also likely to lead to delayed puberty or varying degrees of lack of androgenization and to infertility.

The tubular cells are more susceptible to damage by radiation or cytotoxic drugs than the Leydig cells although both may be affected. Rarely a patient presenting with infertility and azoospermia but normal secondary sexual characteristics may be found to have Sertoli cells but no germ cells when the testis is biopsied.

Secondary testicular failure
Testicular failure secondary to pituitary/hypothalamic disease may also be congenital or acquired. Congenital causes are uncommon but include isolated gonadotrophin releasing hormone deficiency which as in women may be associated with anosmia or other congenital defects (Kallman's syndrome) but is otherwise difficult to distinguish from constitutionally delayed puberty. Even rarer is the condition of isolated LH deficiency which results in a eunuchoid appearance, but the normal FSH activity means that such patients are potentially fertile if given the testosterone needed for normal spermatogenesis.

Craniopharyngioma in younger patients and pituitary tumours in older patients are more common causes of hypogonadotrophic hypogonadism. Prolactinoma or hyperprolactinaemia without an identifiable adenoma are relatively frequent, but galactorrhoea is extremely uncommon in males even in the face of astronomical prolactin levels. Hypogonadism may be a presenting or an incidental feature of other pituitary tumours including non-functioning chromophobe adenomas and acromegaly.

Functional hypogonadism may occur in men as in women. Impairment of sexual function may be due to loss of libido, impotence or failure of gonadal function with softening of the testes and thinning of body hair and can occur with malnutrition due to a variety of diseases. Anorexia nervosa does occur in men but is ten times more common in women. Increased oestrogen production as in cirrhosis, or the administration of oestrogen preparations will diminish male sexual function.

Impotence, that is failure to have or maintain an erection sufficient to achieve satisfactory sexual intercourse, whilst a feature of organic primary or secondary gonadal failure is more likely to be of psychological origin in the absence of any other evidence of endocrine dysfunction, autonomic neuropathy or peripheral vascular disease. The incidence of impotence increases with age and the longer the duration the less likely there is to be a satisfactory resolution of the problem, but temporary impotence associated with emotional distress is common at any age.

Laboratory investigation of hypogonadism in males
The history and examination will point to whether the cause is likely to be either primary or secondary gonadal failure in most instances, with the exception of the difficulties already outlined in distinguishing isolated gonadotrophin releasing hormone deficiency from simple delayed puberty. Baseline investigations should include plasma testosterone, basal LH and FSH to distinguish hyper- from hypogonadotrophic hypogonadism, prolactin, free T_4 and TSH and a skull X-ray. In adults the ability to produce semen which on analysis shows a normal sperm count and motility will exclude most organic causes of hypogonadism. Chromosome analysis should be undertaken in cases of primary gonadal failure, ambiguous genitalia or absent pubertal development. In cases of secondary gonadal failure further investigations of pituitary function may be indicated.

Management of hypogonadism in males
The treatment of particular conditions such as congenital adrenal hyperplasia has been outlined in Chapter 9, and the management of delayed puberty discussed above. Primary gonadal failure presenting in adulthood, whether congenital (e.g. Klinefelter's syndrome) or acquired, is relatively uncommon. It is invariably associated with infertility for which there is no treatment and patients need counselling accordingly. Such patients will, however, benefit from testosterone supplements not only to foster secondary sexual features but also to prevent premature osteoporosis.

The management of secondary gonadal failure will depend on the cause and whether or not fertility as well as restoration of sexual function is required. If the family has been completed treatment will be made relatively simple by maintenance of adequate androgen levels with oral testosterone derivatives such as Restandol (testosterone undecanoate in oleic acid), 40–120 mg daily in divided doses. Alternatively a mixture of testosterone proprionate and other esters can be given by intramuscular injections in the form of Sustanon 100 or 250 mg every two or three weeks. If, however, fertility is to be achieved the problems are more complex. Firstly, it must be remembered that infertility is a problem of a couple and not just one partner so both partners need thorough investigation before embarking on what may be expensive and demanding treatment. Let us assume for the purposes of discussion here that the female partner has been shown to have a normal ovulatory menstrual cycle and patent tubes and the male has been shown to have a pituitary cause for his infertility. Fertility may be restored by the correction of hyperprolactinaemia either with bromocriptine or by removal of an adenoma, (Chapter 7) or by the removal of other pituitary tumours causing Cushing's disease or acromegaly or a chromophobe adenoma. Surgical excision of such tumours may, however, leave the patient hypogonadal. Spermatogenesis can nervertheless be restored by treatment with intramuscular injections of HCG and Pergonal. The response can be monitored by measuring the plasma testosterone levels and the sperm count and therapy adjusted until both are in the normal range. Neither clomiphene nor pulsatile GnRH therapy will be of any value in the treatment of infertility due to pituitary disease, although GnRH therapy would be appropriate in isolated GnRH deficiency.

Further Reading

Brook, C. G. D., Jacobs, H. S., Stanhope, R. *et al.* (1987). Pulsatility of reproductive hormones: applications to the understanding of puberty and to the treatment of infertility. *Ballière's Clinics in Endocrinology and Metabolism* **1**, 23–41.

Clayton, R. N. (1987). Gonadotrophin releasing hormone: from physiology to pharmacology. *Clinical Endocrinology* **26**, 361.

Franks, S. (1989). Polycystic ovary syndrome: a changing perspective. *Clinical Endocrinology* **31**, 87.

Hall, R. and Besser, M. (eds) (1989). *Fundamentals of Clinical Endocrinology*, 4th edition. Churchill Livingstone Edinburgh.

Judd, H. L. (1987). Oestrogen replacement therapy: physiological considerations and new applications. *Ballière's Clinics in Endocrinology and Metabolism* **1**, 177–206.

McLachlan, R. I., Robertson, D. M., De Kretser, D. and Burger, H. G. (1987). Inhibin—a non-steroidal regulator of pituitary follicle stimulating hormone. *Ballière's Clinics in Endocrinology and Metabolism* **1**, 89–112.

11

CALCIUM METABOLISM, PARATHYROID HORMONE AND VITAMIN D

The main store of calcium in the body lies in bone which is continually remodelled by the action of osteoclasts and osteoblasts. Osteoclasts, rich in acid phosphatase, actively resorb bone, whereas osteoblasts, rich in alkaline phosphatase, are concerned in bone formation. In normal individuals the activities of bone resorption and bone formation are closely balanced and are regulated by the actions of parathyroid hormone (PTH) and vitamin D.

Parathyroid Hormone

Parathyroid hormone is produced by the parathyroid glands, of which there are normally four, situated behind the upper and lower poles of the lateral lobes of the thyroid gland. They are small brown bodies normally about 5 mm by 4 mm wide and 1–2 mm thick and are not always easy to find at surgery (see Fig. 8.2). Parathyroid hormone is a polypeptide containing 84 aminoacids of which the first 32 are essential for biological activity. The hormone is derived from larger precursor molecules, pre-pro-PTH and pro-PTH, which are broken down into the active hormone and other fragments. Parathyroid hormone is measured by radio-immunoassay and many of the fragments may interfere with the assay which is not particularly sensitive and it may be difficult to detect low normal concentrations.

Parathyroid hormone acts on the kidney to increase calcium resorption and diminish phosphate reabsorption and on bone to increase calcium resorption, and hence increase serum calcium. Secretion of PTH is inversely related to serum calcium so that a fall in serum calcium leads to increased PTH secretion, and a rise in serum calcium supresses PTH release. The action of PTH is mediated by cyclic AMP so measurement of the latter in plasma or urine can be used as a measure of PTH activity.

The biochemical changes that result from an excess of PTH production include hypercalcaemia, hypercalciuria, hypophosphataemia, hyperphosphaturia and increased urinary hydroxyproline excretion.

Vitamin D

Ninety per cent of vitamin D, in the form of cholecalciferol (D_3), is produced in the skin by the action of sunlight on the precursor 7-dehydrocholesterol (Fig. 11.1). The remainder of vitamin D is ingested in the diet mostly as cholecalciferol (D_3) or ergocalciferol (D_2). Both forms of vitamin D are initially converted in the liver to 25-hydroxy vitamin D and subsequently in the kidney to the active metabolite 1,25-dihydroxy vitamin D or the inactive metabolite 24,25-dihydroxy vitamin D. The active 1,25 dihydroxy vitamin D acts on the small intestine to increase calcium absorption, and also acts on bone to release

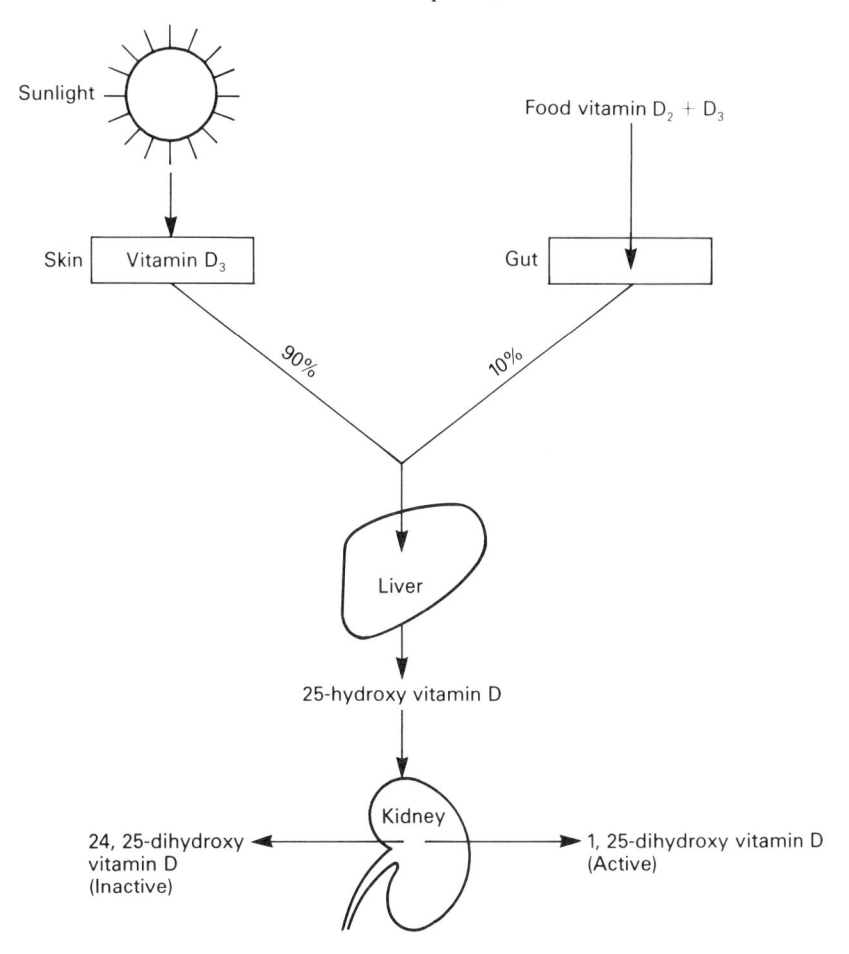

Fig. 11.1 Vitamin D metabolism.

calcium. In situations of calcium deficiency there is preferential secretion of the active metabolite 1,25-dihydroxy vitamin D over the inactive 24,25-dihydroxy vitamin D. Parathyroid hormone also stimulates the production of 1,25-dihydroxy vitamin D. Lack of vitamin D leads to softening of the bone and produces rickets or osteomalacia. Excess vitamin D and excessive PTH cause hypercalcaemia.

Calcitonin is a hormone produced by the parafollicular (C-cells) in the thyroid and has a hypocalcaemic action but its role in the control of human calcium haemostasis does not appear to be a major one under normal physiological conditions. It may be more important in pathological states with increased bone turnover such as Paget's disease, and medullary carcinoma of the thyroid.

Calcium Balance

Although 99% of the calcium in the body is contained within bone only a small amount (approximatley 10 mmol) is exchanged daily, whereas the kidney filters about 200 mmol of calcium per day, most of which is reabsorbed. Intestinal absorption of calcium from the diet is approximately 5 mmol per day (Fig. 11.2). The kidney is thus the major regulator of calcium balance on a daily basis in normal healthy individuals although chronic loss of calcium will result in greater resorption of calcium from bone, with resulting demineralization, in order to maintain calcium haemostasis. Serum calcium is maintained within

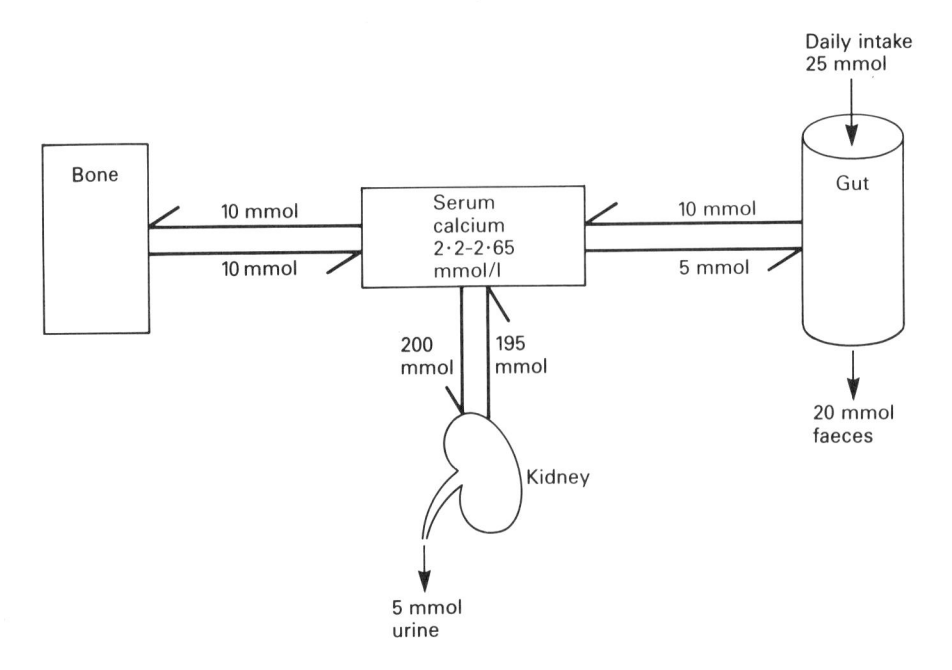

Fig. 11.2 Calcium balance.

narrow limits of 2.20–2.65 mmol/l. Calcium is bound to serum proteins, particularly albumin, so total calcium estimations are significantly affected by changes in serum proteins. In low protein states such as nephrotic syndrome, liver disease or malnutrition with a low serum albumin the serum total calcium will also be low but the ionized calcium, which is the physiologically active form that accounts for about half the total calcium, is normal. Serum globulins also bind calcium, but with a lower affinity than albumin, so in conditions of marked increase in globulins such as myeloma the total serum calcium is increased.

Ionized calcium is more difficult to measure than total calcium and the two correlate well in the presence of normal serum proteins so total calcium estimation is usually performed in a routine laboratory. The result of total calcium estimation must, however, always be interpreted with a knowledge of the serum proteins. Various formulae have been devised to adjust the serum total calcium to an arbitrary standard serum albumin of 42 g/l, but they are seldom necessary. Where an abnormality of calcium metabolism is suspected, but results of serum total calcium are borderline or equivocal, then by arrangement with the laboratory it may be appropriate to measure the ionized calcium.

Hypercalcaemia

Causes of hypercalcaemia are shown in Table 11.1. By far the commonest causes are hypercalcaemia associated with malignancy and primary hyperparathyroidism. Malignant diseases in which hypercalcaemia is relatively common include myeloma and squamous cell carcinoma of the bronchus. Hypercalcaemia may also occur with carcinoma of the breast, larynx and pharynx, oesophagus and tumours of the lower gastrointestinal tract, ovaries and kidneys. In many cases the hypercalcaemia is found in association with secondary bony metastases in advanced carcinoma, but in others the hypercalcaemia is found in the absence of clinical or radiological evidence of spread of the carcinoma to bone. Parathyroid hormone-like substances may be produced

Table 11.1 Causes of hypercalcaemia

Malignancy
  With metastases in bone
  Without metastases in bone
Hyperparathyroidism
  Primary
  Tertiary
Sarcoidosis
Thyrotoxicosis
Vitamin D toxicity
Milk alkali syndrome
Thiazide diuretics

by carcinomas but they are not detectable by PTH assays, and may result in hypercalcaemia without metastases.

Primary hyperparathyroidism is the second commonest cause of hypercalcaemia after malignancy and is said, as a result of biochemical screening, to affect up to 400 per million of the population. It is more common in elderly females. It is usually due to a discrete adenoma of one of the parathyroid glands but may be due to hyperplasia of all the glands, particularly if it is associated with rare inherited conditions. These include familial hyperparathyroidism where no other endocrine disorder is found, multiple endocrine neoplasia type 1 (MEN 1) where hyperparathyroidism is associated with pancreatic islet cell tumours and occasionally pituitary tumours, and multiple endocrine neoplasia type 2 (MEN 2) where it is associated with phaeochromocytoma and medullary carcinoma of the thyroid (Chapter 6).

Secondary hyperparathyroidism may result from any prolonged hypocalcaemic state with resultant stimulus to increased PTH secretion and hyperplasia of the parathyroid glands (see causes of hypocalcaemia below). In chronic renal failure the kidney fails to produce the active 1,25-dihydroxy vitamin D and this can lead to severe hypocalcaemia and bone disease known as renal osteodystrophy. Some patients with renal osteodystrophy subsequently develop hypercalcaemia and it is assumed that the hyperplastic parathyroids have become autonomous, a condition known as tertiary hyperparathyroidism.

Other causes of hypercalcaemia are relatively rare. Sarcoidosis is sometimes associated with hypercalcaemia which is thought to be due to overproduction of 1,25-dihydroxy vitamin D and is responsive to steroids. Thyrotoxicosis is associated with increased bone turnover, and occasionally in severely hyperthyroid patients the serum calcium is raised but is usually corrected by treatment of the thyrotoxicosis. Vitamin D poisoning may occur in patients who are given inappropriate therapy with large doses of calciferol or excessive replacement doses of the more active metabolites such as 1-α-cholecalciferol for hypoparathyroidism after thyroid surgery. Patients on replacement therapy require careful regular monitoring of their serum calcium level to ensure that it remains in the normal range.

Clinical Features

Mild hypercalcaemia is frequently picked up by biochemical screening, particularly in hospitals using multichannel analysers, and is usually asymptomatic. The symptoms and signs of hypercalcaemia are non-specific and often absent unless the hypercalcaemia is severe. Clinical features of more severe hypercalcaemia include general tiredness and lethargy, muscle weakness, polyuria and thirst, constipation, nausea, vomiting, and rarely disturbed behaviour and even impaired consciousness. Physical signs are few apart from evidence of dehydration and proximal muscle weakness. Band keratopathy at the margin of the iris is very rare even in quite prolonged hypercalcaemia. In primary hyperparathyroidism the association with renal stones and peptic ulcer symptoms is relatively uncommon, although it is clearly appropriate to check the serum calcium in patients presenting with renal calculi. Bone pain is uncommon except in rare patients with long-standing untreated primary hyperparathyroidism who have developed bone deformities, pathological fractures and osteoclastomas. Evidence for multiple endocrine neoplasia or a positive family history should be sought.

Patients with hypercalcaemia due to malignant disease usually have evidence of the underlying carcinoma at the time of recognition of the hypercalcaemia. When underlying malignancy is suspected, but not obvious, investigations should be directed at more occult sites such as lung, ovary and kidney.

Sarcoidosis may cause difficulties with the differential diagnosis but it is unusual for hypercalcaemia to be the presenting feature and usually there will be evidence of hilar lymphadenopathy or pulmonary infiltration and uveitis and other organ involvement. Patients with hypercalcaemia due to thyrotoxicosis are usually floridly hyperthyroid. Chronic renal failure must usually be severe and long-standing before hypercalcaemia develops. Patients with chronic renal failure who develop tertiary hyperparathyroidism deposit calcium in the kidneys and in arterial walls which may make the vascular anastomosis necessary for renal transplantation more difficult.

Laboratory Investigation

Repeatedly raised serum calcium with low serum phosphate, with or without raised alkaline phosphatase, in the presence of normal serum proteins is the typical disturbance found in primary hyperparathyroidism. This pattern, however, may be indistinguishable from that found in hypercalcaemia due to malignancy. The serum PTH is raised, or at least measurable and inappropriate for the hypercalcaemia, due to primary hyperparathyroidism, whereas it is undetectable in hypercalcaemia due to malignant disease. Other pointers from the history and examination will indicate the need to screen for suspected malignant disease and findings such as anaemia, high ESR, low albumin, raised globulin and abnormal liver function tests are more likely to be associated with malignancy as they are not features of primary hyperparathyroidism. Renal function tests and thyroid function tests will be obviously abnormal in hypercalcaemia due to renal failure or thyrotoxicosis, respectively. X-rays of the hands will reveal subperiosteal erosions of the phalangeal bones in only about 10% of patients with primary hypoparathyroidism and is thus not very helpful in diagnosis (Fig. 11.3). Other radiological investigations which may be helpful in suspected malignancy which is not overt include chest X-ray, ultrasonic scan of the kidneys and ovaries, mammography and isotope bone scans. Where there is still uncertainty about the diagnosis a trial of steroid therapy which suppresses hypercalcaemia into the normal range favours diagnosis of sarcoidosis, although some malignancies may also respond, and make a diagnosis of primary hyperparathyroidism highly unlikely.

In patients suspected of familial hyperparathyroidism it will be necessary to

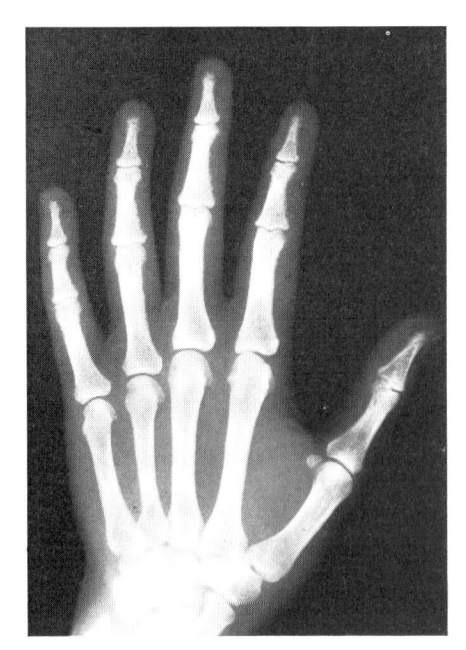

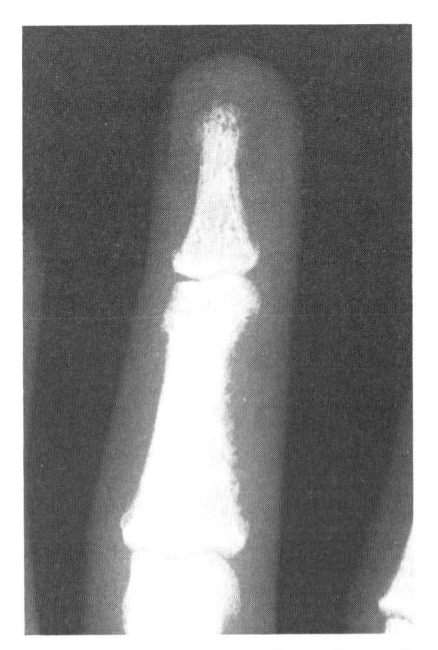

Fig. 11.3 (a) A hand in hyperparathyroidism showing subperiosteal erosions of the phalanges, (b) the same hand in close up.

screen other first degree relatives for hypercalcaemia. If multiple endocrine adenopathy is suspected then it will also be necessary to screen other members of the family as well as the patient for evidence of hyperparathyroidism, phaeochromocytoma and other endocrine tumours as in MEN 1 and MEN 2.

Management of Primary Hyperparathyroidism

Many patients identified by biochemical screening and subsequently shown to have primary hyperparathyroidism have probably had mild asymptomatic hypercalcaemia for a long time before the diagnosis was made.

The only definitive treatment for primary hyperparathyroidism is surgical removal of the abnormal parathyroid(s), but surgery is not necessary in all cases. Clearly if a patient is symptomatic or suffering from any of the complications of the disease then surgery is indicated and most physicians would also advise surgery for the younger patient who may not be symptomatic but is likely otherwise to suffer the consequences of long-term hypercalcaemia such as renal damage, hypertension or bone disease. The only alternative to surgery is conservative management with no active intervention unless hypercalcaemia becomes more severe and symptomatic. Such a conservative approach may be reasonable in an elderly patient in whom hypercalcaemia is almost an incidental finding, although it is important to have established that the underlying diagnosis is indeed primary hyperparathyroidism and the options for treatment must be explained to the patient. Surgery should be performed by an experienced parathyroid surgeon. In the vast majority of cases of primary hyperparathyroidism a simple adenoma will be found and removed, but it is important to identify at least one and preferably all the other normal parathyroid glands. When hyperplasia of all four glands is found as in tertiary hyperparathyroidism then all four glands are removed. However, fragments of one gland can be transplanted, usually to the forearm for easy access without recourse to further neck surgery if the remnant becomes hyperplastic in the future. Post-operatively the serum calcium needs daily monitoring as it may fall below the normal range temporarily and mild hypocalcaemia may persist for several days. This is usually asymptomatic but if more severe then calcium supplements and vitamin D in the form of 1-α-cholecalciferol may be needed.

Management of Hypercalcaemia of Malignancy

The management of hypercalcaemia depends on the severity of the hypercalcaemia and the underlying diagnosis. Mild hypercalcaemia is often asymptomatic and no specific treatment is needed to lower the serum calcium pending investigations to achieve a definitive diagnosis. On the other hand severe hypercalcaemia which is usually due to malignancy may present as a medical emergency and require urgent treatment even though the underlying diagnosis has not yet been established. In a patient with severe hypercalcaemia who is dehydrated and often nauseated or vomiting the first priority is rehydration with intravenous normal saline of at least 3 l/day. Potassium supplements are usually needed to correct or prevent hypokalaemia which is frequently present. Diuretics may be needed if any evidence of fluid overload develops. Other agents which may be used to lower the serum calcium include calcitonin, steroids in large doses, disodium etidronate, phosphates and mithramycin. Calcitonin can be given as 200–400 units of Calcitone intramuscularly every eight hours. Steroids if they can be taken orally, are given as prednisolone, 20 mg every six hours, otherwise intravenous hydrocortisone may be needed initially until oral therapy can be tolerated.

Disodium etidronate, given intravenously in a dose of 7.5 mg/kg/day for three successive days, in 250 ml of normal saline over two hours is effective therapy for hypercalcaemia of malignancy, but great care must be taken if renal function is impaired. Oral phosphates can be given as phosphate effervescent tablets up to 4 g daily in divided doses, but they often cause unacceptable gastrointestinal side effects, particularly diarrhoea. Slow intravenous phosphate infusions can be used with caution in patients in whom the hypercalcaemia is life-threatening. A phosphate solution consisting of 500 ml of 0.1 mol/l phosphate buffer made up of disodium phosphate and monopotassium phosphate gives 50 mmol of phosphorus. The phosphate solution will precipitate calcium in the form of $CaHPO_4$ in extraskeletal tissues and may cause calcification of vessels and other tissues which can lead to later problems. The solution is also very damaging to the skin and underlying tissues if extravasation occurs. Mithramycin given in a dose of 20 µg/kg body weight intravenously as a single bolus injection may also be effective in lowering serum calcium in malignant states.

Once the severe hypercalcaemia has been controlled by the emergency measures outlined above then investigation of the underlying cause can be undertaken. In the meantime the serum calcium should be maintained at tolerable levels by adequate oral fluid intake and oral steroid therapy if responsive. Disodium etidronate can be given orally. The recommended dose is 20 mg/kg/day for up to 30 days as a single dose two hours before a meal. It is essential to monitor the responses by frequent measurement of serum calcium and phosphate. Once the underlying malignancy has been identified it may still be possible to remove the primary tumour and alleviate the cause of the hypercalcaemia, for example, removal of a hypernephroma. Sadly, however, most patients are in an advanced stage of malignancy and treatment can only be palliative. Measures aimed at reducing the hypercalcaemia as outlined above can nevertheless lead to symptomatic relief and help to make the patient less distressed and more comfortable, but are not to be expected to alter the ultimately poor prognosis.

Management of Hypercalcaemia due to Other Causes

Vitamin D toxicity

Immediate cessation of vitamin D therapy is clearly indicated and replacement therapy reintroduced if indicated in a lower dose at a later stage when the serum calcium is normal. If severe hypercalcaemia has developed then intravenous fluids should be given and prednisolone, 20 mg, six hourly given orally until the calcium returns to normal as this suppresses hypercalcaemia in this condition.

Sarcoidosis

The hypercalcaemia is steroid responsive and prednisolone should be given and maintained in the lowest dose necessary to maintain a normal serum calcium. Once the underlying condition is suppressed steroids should be gradually withdrawn as the hypercalcaemia may remit, but further courses of prednisolone will be necessary if hypercalcaemia recurs.

Thyrotoxicosis

The hypercalcaemia should resolve within the four to eight weeks that it usually takes for the hyperthyroidism to respond to antithyroid drugs. If hypercalcaemia persists once the patient is euthyroid then underlying concomitant primary hyperparathyroidism should be suspected.

Hypocalcaemia

Clinical Features

Some symptoms of hypocalcaemia are more likely to be found in acute situations, such as hypoparathyroidism following surgery, rather than chronic mild hypocalcaemia which predominantly effects bone. More acute symptoms include paraesthesiae around the mouth and in the hands, carpopedal spasm, and in severe hypocalcaemia fits may occur. Increased excitability of muscle may be revealed by a positive Chvostek's sign—gentle tapping of the face with a tendon hammer just below the temporomandibular joint resulting in twitching of the corner of the mouth—but this may occur in a small proportion of normal subjects and is not a very reliable sign. Trousseau's sign is carpal spasm induced by occlusion of blood supply to the forearm using a sphygmomanometer cuff inflated above arterial pressure for up to 3 min. This can be a painful procedure and should not be pursued if unacceptable to the patient.

Prolonged mild hypocalcaemia leads predominantly to softening of bone due to osteomalacia. In children the condition is known as rickets and can result in stunting and bone deformity, particularly affecting the lower limbs causing either knock knees (genu valgum) or bowing of the legs (genu varum). In adults osteomalacia may present with pathological fractures, or pseudofractures evident on X-ray, loss of height due to vertebral compression and diffuse bone pain. Patients may have difficulty in walking or in rising from a chair unaided due to associated muscle weakness, especially a proximal myopathy.

Causes of Hypocalcaemia

The causes of hypocalcaemia are listed in Table 11.2. The commonest reason for a low serum calcium is probably due to a low serum albumin from whatever cause. The calcium in this situation is spuriously low due to the reduced calcium binding, and ionized calcium is normal. True hypocalcaemia is relatively uncommon compared with hypercalcaemia. In developed countries renal failure is probably now a more common cause of hypocalcaemia than dietary vitamin D deficiency, but the latter may still affect immigrant populations in northern latitudes and the elderly. Hypoparathyroidism as a complication of thyroid or other neck surgery is more common than other causes of hypoparathyroidism which are rare. These conditions will be considered in turn.

Renal failure

Hypocalcaemia may occur in acute renal failure and is usually found in chronic renal failure, as a result of an inability to produce 1,25-dihydroxy vitamin D in the kidney and is accompanied by phosphate retention. The typical biochemical picture is a low serum calcium, raised serum phosphate and raised alkaline

Table 11.2 Causes of hypocalcaemia

Spurious – Due to low serum albumin
Renal failure
Acute
Chronic
Vitamin D deficiency
Immigrants to northern latitudes
Elderly
Gastrointestinal disease
Liver disease
Pancreatitis
Anticonvulsant therapy
Vitamin D dependent rickets
Vitamin D resistant or hypophosphataemia rickets
Hypoparathyroidism
Post-surgery
Auto-immune
Pseudo hypoparathyroidism

phosphatase as well as raised serum creatinine. The hypocalcaemia and lack of 1,25-dihydroxy vitamin D induce secondary hyperparathyroidism and PTH levels, if measured, are raised and may lead to autonomous parathyroid function with tertiary hyperparathyroidism. The resultant bone disturbance is a combination of osteomalacia and changes due to secondary hyperparathyroidism known as renal osteodystrophy, whose radiological features include pseudofractures (Looser's zones), bone cysts and subperiosteal lesions. The vertebrae may show dense bands at the upper and lower margins with a more translucent middle zone which is described as a 'rugger jersey' spine (Fig. 11.4).

Treatment
Aluminium hydroxide is used to bind phosphate in the gut in order to prevent metastatic calcification, but absorption of aluminium can lead to aluminium toxicity which can itself cause osteomalacia. Calcium carbonate has been used as an alternative phosphate binder. 1,25-Dihydroxy vitamin D or 1-α-cholecalciferol may be given to try to correct the lack of 1,25-dihydroxy vitamin D production by the kidney, but they may not prevent the development of bone disease. When tertiary hyperparathyroidism develops parathyroidectomy is usually necessary.

Vitamin D deficiency

Vitamin D deficiency is no longer a major scourge in well-fed communities such as those of the UK, but it may still affect selected groups of the population, particularly the Asian community and the elderly. Deficiency of dietary intake of vitamin D is probably not the only contributory factor and lack of exposure to sunlight due to inability to get out of doors or customs and costumes which prevent skin exposure are also relevant. The condition is insidious in its development but should be suspected in patients in the at risk groups, who may complain of vague aches and pains and weakness. Bone pain is a relatively common feature in all age groups but deformities are usually only found in children or adults affected in childhood, or in the neglected elderly who may suffer pelvic and spinal deformities. Proximal muscle weakness may also contribute to difficulties in walking and cause the elderly to go 'off their legs'. Signs of tetany are uncommon.

Investigations
Vitamin D deficiency may be suspected, even in the absence of overt clinical features, from the biochemical picture of reduced serum calcium and phosphate concentrations and elevated alkaline phosphatase. The reduction in serum calcium is often only mild due to the compensatory effect of secondary hyperparathyroidism. The radiological findings depend on the severity of the

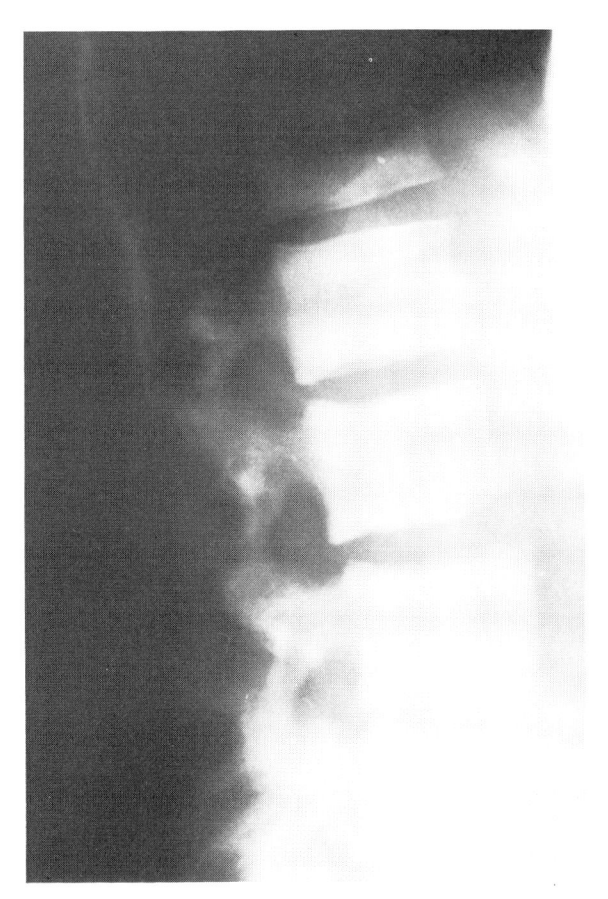

Fig. 11.4 The 'rugger jersey' spine of renal osteodystrophy.

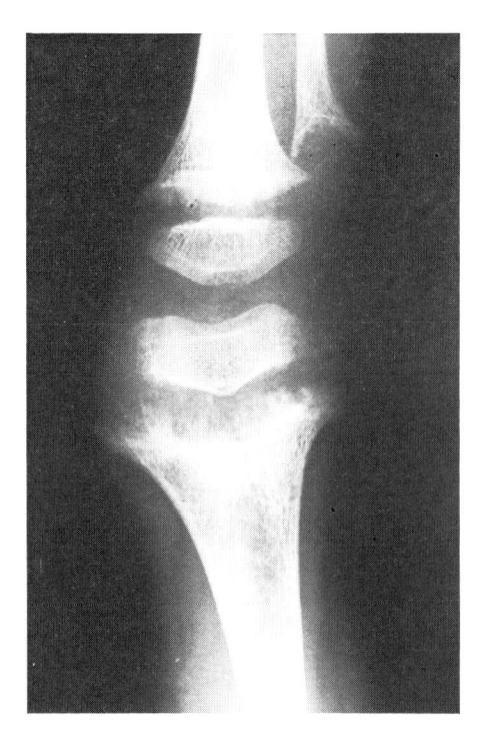

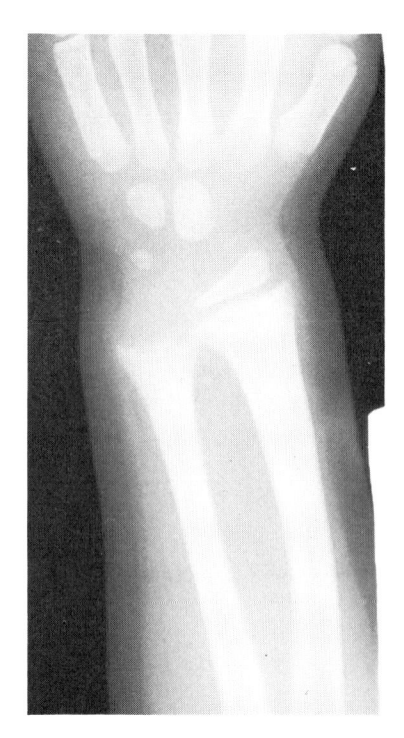

300 Calcium Metabolism, Parathyroid Hormone and Vitamin D

Fig. 11.5 (a, b) Metaphyseal changes in rickets.

condition, but when present they are characteristic. In children there is irregularity and widening of the metaphyses at the ends of the long bones (Fig. 11.5). In adults Looser's zones or pseudofractures are found typically in the pelvic rami, ribs and scapulae, and softening of the pelvic bones may result in severe deformity of the pelvis (Fig. 11.6).

Vitamin D deficiency may also result from malabsorption due to gastrointestinal disorders, pancreatic disease, liver disease or long-term anticonvulsant therapy. In malabsorption states there is decreased absorption of the fat-soluble vitamin D. Treatment is directed towards correcting the underlying cause but supplements of calcium and vitamin D in doses of up to 40 000 units daily may be needed to prevent osteomalacia.

Magnesium deficiency may also occur in severe gastrointestinal disease and induce secondary hypocalcaemia which is corrected with magnesium supplements.

In chronic liver disease, such as primary biliary cirrhosis, the mechanism of the osteodystrophy which can occur is less clearly understood.

The anticonvulsant drugs, particularly phenytoin and phenobarbitone, probably cause osteomalacia by induction of hepatic enzymes which result in conversion of vitamin D to its inactive metabolites rather than the active 1,25-dihydroxy vitamin D. The condition is nevertheless responsive to vitamin

D supplements. Where possible the patient's epilepsy should be controlled with other anticonvulsants that are less liable to induce osteomalacia.

Treatment of vitamin D deficiency
Prophylactic treatment with small supplements of vitamin D given daily to expectant immigrant mothers will protect both mother and child. No plain vitamin D tablet of this strength is available but tablets of calcium with vitamin D which contain 500 units of ergocalciferol (vitamin D_2) suffice. Established vitamin D deficiency sufficient to cause rickets or osteomalacia requires larger

Table 11.3 Vitamin D preparations

Calcium with vitamin D tablets	Calcium sodium lactate, 450 mg Calcium phosphate, 150 mg Ergocalciferol, 12.5 µg (500 units)
Ergocalciferol (calciferol, vitamin D_2)	Calciferol tablets, high strength, 250 µg = 10 000 units Calciferol solution, in oil, 75 µg = 3000 units/ml Calciferol injection, in oil, 7.5 mg = 300 000 units/ml

Alfacalcidol (1-α-hydroxycholecalciferol), 0.25 µg capsule or 1 µg capsule
Calcitriol (1,25-dihydroxycholecalciferol), 0.25 µg capsule or 0.5 µg capsule
Dihydrotachysterol, solution 250 µg/ml, tablet 200 µg

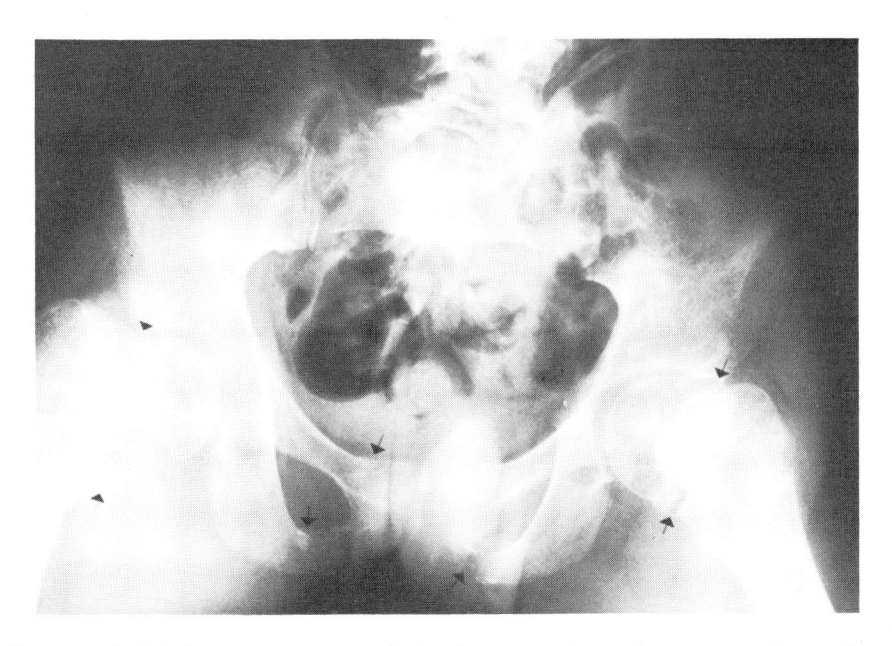

Fig. 11.6 Pelvis in severe osteomalacia. Arrows point to fractures and pseudofractures of femoral neck and pubic rami.

doses of vitamin D, up to 2000 units daily for several months. Vitamin D deficiency caused by intestinal malabsorption or liver disease usually requires pharmacological doses of up to 1 mg (40 000 units) daily. The hypocalcaemia of hypoparathyroidism may require doses of up to 5 mg (200 000 units) daily to achieve normocalcaemia and dihydrotachysterol may be used as an alternative.

1-α-Hydroxycholecalciferol or calcitriol should be used for patients with severe renal failure.

All patients receiving pharmacological doses of vitamin D should have serum calcium concentration checked at frequent intervals and whenever nausea or vomiting supervene (Table 11.3).

Vitamin D dependent rickets

This rare condition is inherited as an autosomal recessive and is due to deficiency of the 1-hydroxylase enzyme which converts 25-hydroxy vitamin D to 1,25-dihydroxy vitamin D. The clinical and biochemical picture is the same as for vitamin D deficient rickets but it fails to respond to the usual small doses of vitamin D. Large doses of 50 000 units per day result in healing, but the condition responds as to be expected to small doses, 1 µg daily, of 1,25-dihydroxy vitamin D.

Vitamin D resistant rickets or hypophosphataemic rickets

This rare condition is different from other forms of rickets in that it results from loss of phosphate rather than lack of vitamin D and may be due to a number of causes. It may be inherited as an X-linked or as a dominant disorder causing a defect in phosphate transport and increased renal phosphate excretion. It may also occur in defects of renal tubular function such as Fanconi's syndrome in which there is renal loss of phosphate, glucose and aminoacids. The serum calcium is normal but serum phosphate is low. Parathyroid hormone and 1,25-dihydroxy vitamin D levels are normal. Treatment is difficult and the condition does not respond well to large doses of vitamin D alone. A combination of 1-α-cholecalciferol and oral phosphate supplements is more effective.

Hypoparathyroidism

Surgical cause

The commonest cause of hypoparathyroidism is following thyroidectomy, and it may also occur after major resection for carcinoma of the larynx. It normally occurs a day or two after operation and may present with acute symptoms of hypocalcaemia, including paraesthesiae, tetany, positive Chvostek's and positive Trousseau's signs. It is important to monitor serum calcium daily post-operatively for the first few days. The hypocalcaemia may be mild, asymptomatic and transient, but if more severe or persistent it needs treatment with calciferol 100 000 units daily and calcium supplements. The therapy should be gradually reduced to the minimum needed to maintain normal serum calcium levels.

Other causes
Occasionally hypoparathyroidism is idiopathic. It may occur at any age and may be associated with auto-immune disorders such as primary hypothyroidism, premature ovarian failure and Addison's disease. Such patients are prone to severe chronic monilial infections. Other features include calcification of basal ganglia, extrapyramidal dyskinesis and papilloedema.

Pseudohypoparathyroidism

This condition has similar biochemical features to true hypoparathyroidism, with low calcium, raised phosphate and normal alkaline phosphatase, but the serum parathyroid hormone (PTH) level is raised. It is a rare inherited condition associated with resistance to PTH. Resistance can be demonstrated by the failure to increase cyclic AMP and phosphate excretion in the urine after injection of 200 units of bovine PTH. Clinically the patient may be mentally retarded, obese and have short stature with shortening of the 4th and 5th metacarpal bones exhibited by dimpling when a fist is made. Pseudo-pseudohypoparathyroidism is the term given to patients who present with the somatic features of pseudohypoparathyroidism but without the biochemical features. It may occur in families, others of whom exhibit the biochemical features of pseudohypoparathyroidism and patients may later develop hypocalcaemia and hyperphosphataemia suggesting that it may be a mild variant of pseudohypoparathyroidism.

Endocrine Aspects of Other Bone Disorders

Osteoporosis

Osteoporosis is the commonest disorder of bone and develops when bone resorption exceeds bone formation over a prolonged period of time causing thinning of bone trabeculae. This happens naturally with ageing after the fifth decade in both sexes but is more obvious in females after the menopause. It is likely to develop sooner in patients who suffer premature ovarian or testicular failure, whether primary or secondary to pituitary disease (Chapter 10), Cushing's disease or long-term steroid therapy for other conditions, and thyrotoxicosis. The morbidity of osteoporosis is considerable and includes vertebral collapse (Fig. 11.7) and a propensity for fractures following minor trauma, particularly to the wrist and hips.

If this is to be prevented then it is clearly appropriate to replace oestrogens or testosterone in patients with premature gonadal failure of whatever cause and

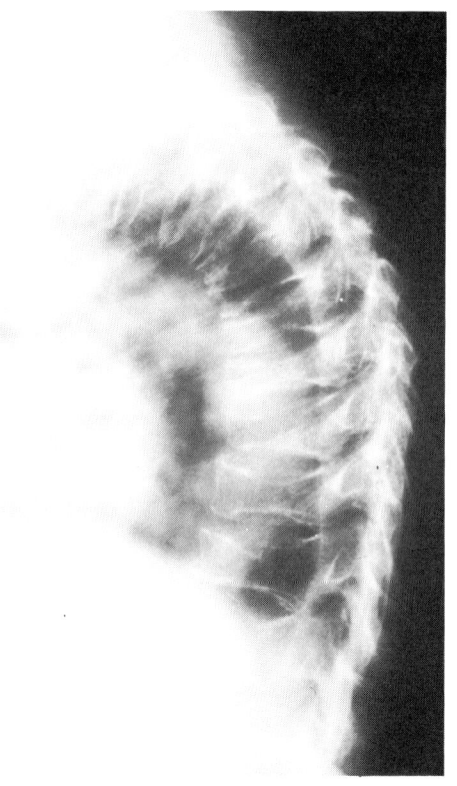

Fig. 11.7 Kyphotic spine in severe osteoporosis showing wedging and vertebral collapse.

this is common practice (Chapter 10). As oestrogen therapy delays or prevents osteoporosis following the menopause the question arises as to whether or not all women of menopausal age should be given hormone replacement therapy, and if so, for how long? The answers to these questions are still controversial. Long-term oestrogen therapy is not without risks although these may be reduced by the use of low-dose oestrogen/progesterone combinations and there may be contraindications such as hypertension and past history of venous thrombosis. The subject is discussed more fully under management of the menopause in Chapter 10. At present the authors feel that a woman of menopausal age should be given the option of hormone replacement therapy after an explanation of the advantages and disadvantages in her particular circumstances. If therapy is accepted then long-term follow up should be part of the agreement.

In patients presenting with established osteoporosis it is important to exclude the specific endocrine causes identified above. Osteomalacia may also co-exist with osteoporosis and will be evident from the serum biochemistry, whereas serum calcium, phosphate and alkaline phosphatase are all normal in osteoporosis *per se*. There is no clear evidence that vitamin D therapy has any benefit in osteoporosis in the absence of osteomalacia. Calcium supplements and cyclical oestrogens may be of therapeutic benefit or at least delay further progression of the osteoporotic process.

Paget's Disease

The aetiology of Paget's disease is not known. It is a common condition and is said to occur in about 5% of the population over the age of 50 years. It is often asymptomatic and may affect only one bone and be found incidentally on radiology of the spine, skull or pelvis. It may, however, be more extensive and cause bone pain and deformity. The commonly affected bones include the skull, clavicle, vertebrae, pelvis, femur and tibia. The patient may be noted to have an enlarged skull with frontal bossing and basilar invagination, and be wearing a deaf aid because of entrapment of the auditory nerve. An affected bone may be painful, tender and hot to touch compared with surrounding areas. This also raises the possibility of osteogenic sarcoma which is a recognized but rare complication of Paget's disease. Radiologically the features of Paget's disease are an abnormal trabecular pattern with a mixture of increased and decreased bone density, usually with expansion of the affected bone. The latter feature helps to distinguish it from metastatic malignancy which may cause sclerotic changes, such as carcinoma of the prostate, and can cause diagnostic difficulties particularly as both conditions can cause increased isotope uptake on isotopic bone scan.

Biochemically the serum calcium and phosphate are normal, while the serum alkaline phosphatase is not necessarily raised if the Paget's disease is confined to a small area of bone but is usually elevated in more extensive disease.

Treatment is indicated if the condition is painful. If simple analgesics do not suffice then endocrine therapy in the form of calcitonin or diphosphonate drugs should be considered. Salmon calcitonin in a dose of 100 units daily for several months has to be given by subcutaneous injection and may cause nausea and flushing. Sodium etidronate, a diphosphonate, is given orally in a daily dose of 5 mg/kg body weight for up to six months. Prolonged remission of bone pain can occur but the underlying condition persists and relapse is common (Fig. 11.8).

More recently bisphonates, which are synthetic analogues of pyrophosphate (a naturally occurring substance found in various body fluids which inhibits crystallization of calcium phosphate) have been developed. These agents inhibit osteoclast activity and reduce bone resorption. They are bound in the skeleton and taken up by osteoclasts during bone resorption and their action may persist for a long period after administration has ceased. Studies using 3-amino-δ-hydroxypropylidene-1, 1-bisphonate (APD) in 30 to 60 mg infusions repeated three times over two weeks have been shown to be effective in inducing remission of Paget's disease and the effect may last six months or more. Extensive Paget's disease may need larger doses repeated at six month

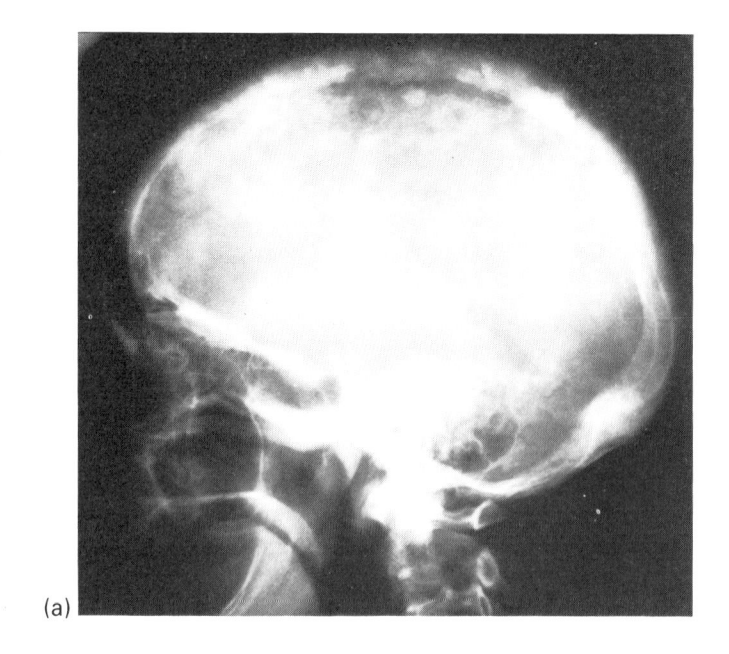

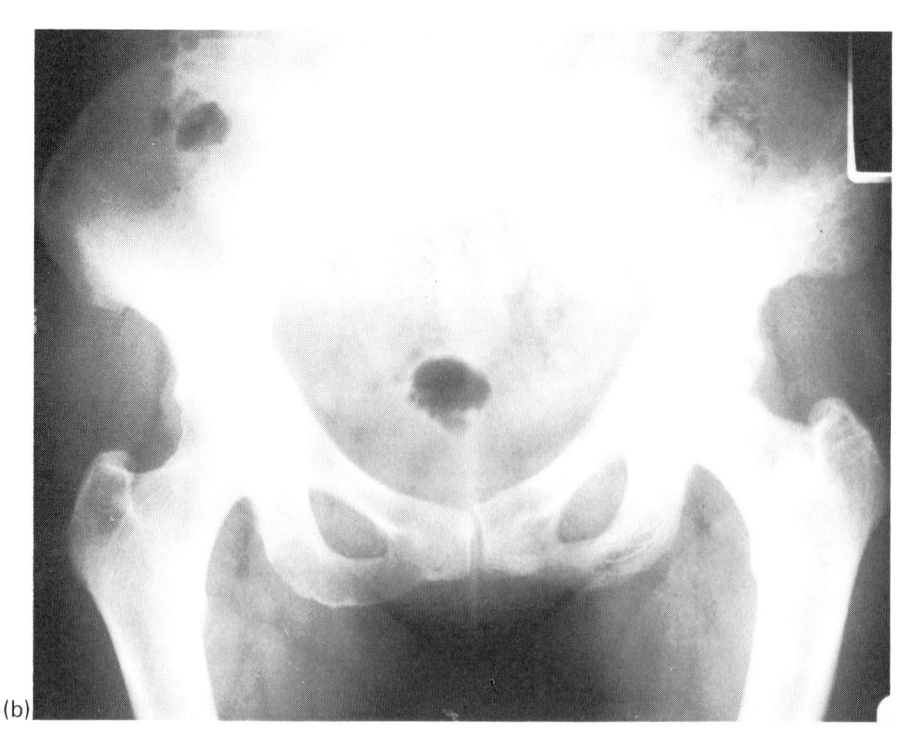

Fig. 11.8 Paget's disease of (a) the skull, (b) the pelvis.

intervals to induce remission. These agents offer real prospects for the prevention of progression to and effective treatment of advanced Paget's disease which can be a severely disabling and painful condition.

Further Reading

Francis, R.M. (ed) (1990). *Osteoporosis: Pathogenesis and Management.* Kluwer Academic Publishers, Dordrecht.

Heath, D.A. (1987). Treating Paget's disease. *British Medical Journal* **294**, 1048.

Martin, T.J. (ed.) (1988). Metabolic bone disease. *Ballière's Clinics in Endocrinology and Metabolism* **2**, No. 1. Ballière Tindall, London.

Mundy, G.R. (1989). Malignant hypercalcaemia. In: *Recent Advances in Endocrinology and Metabolism*, Volume 3. Edited by Edwards, C.R.W. and Lincoln, D.W. Churchill Livingstone, Edinburgh.

Nordin, B.E.C. (ed.) (1984). *Metabolic Bone and Stone Disease.* Churchill Livingstone, Edinburgh.

Smith, R. (1987). Osteoporosis: cause and management. *British Medical Journal* **294**, 329.

12
MULTIPLE CHOICE QUESTIONS

Indicate True (T) or False (F)

1. Knowledge of diabetes self-management:
   a) Needs regular review and reinforcement
   b) Is closely related to metabolic control
   c) Is easily gained during clinic/office consultations
   d) Is best obtained from specially prepared leaflets
   e) Has a major impact on motivation
2. Glycosylated haemoglobin:
   a) Is not found in normal people
   b) Is mostly formed by reaction with glucose during haemoglobin synthesis
   c) Will rise in percentage concentration with acute dehydration
   d) Is assayed on a plasma (heparin or EDTA) sample
   e) Is irreversible once formed until destruction of the erythrocyte
3. Serum cholesterol concentration in people with diabetes:
   a) Is often >6.5 mmol/l even if blood glucose control is good
   b) Should be monitored 5-yearly
   c) Should be controlled with bile acid sequestrants if high
   d) May be raised if hepatic VLDL synthesis is increased
   e) Is a useful measure of dietary compliance
4. The following are useful in the prevention of diabetes:
   a) Cyclosporin
   b) Control of free sugar intake
   c) Education of relatives of people with diabetes
   d) Education of relatives of people with ischaemic heart disease
   e) Public education about obesity
5. Audit of diabetes care:
   a) Should be performed 2-yearly by Health Authorities
   b) Requires the help of a qualified accountant
   c) Needs quantification of levels of retinopathy
   d) Requires sophisticated computer-based record systems
   e) Can help develop a case for further resources

6. Complications of diabetes:
   a) Are never seen before 16 years of age
   b) Are unrelated to blood glucose control
   c) Are the commonest cause of blindness in people under 65 years old
   d) May progress rapidly if diabetic control is tightened
   e) May regress rapidly if diabetic control is tightened
7. Diabetic maculopathy:
   a) Is the commonest cause of blindness in diabetes
   b) Does not respond to laser therapy
   c) Is easily detected if ophthalmoscopy is performed regularly
   d) Leads to traction retinal detachment if allowed to progress
   e) Is characterized by foveal retinal haemorrhage
8. Microalbuminuria:
   a) Responds to treatment with ACE inhibitors
   b) Progresses in 2–5 years to end-stage renal failure
   c) Is sometimes present at the time of diagnosis of diabetes
   d) May be caused by chronic pyelonephritis
   e) Is best detected after exercise
9. Diabetic foot problems:
   a) Lead to amputation in most patients
   b) Are reduced by effective diabetes education
   c) Are primarily due to occlusion of the skin microvasculature
   d) Are often secondary to Charcot-type joint degeneration
   e) Should be managed by early surgery
10. Myocardial infarction in people with diabetes:
    a) Is 10–15 times more common than in normal subjects
    b) Is usually preceded by worsening angina
    c) Is sometimes precipitated by hypoglycaemia
    d) Is caused by small vessel blockage and has a good outcome
    e) Is a common cause of death in Type 1 diabetes
11. Type 2 diabetes is characterized by:
    a) High plasma ketone body levels
    b) Absolute insulin deficiency
    c) Relative insulin deficiency
    d) Fasting hyperinsulinaemia
    e) Hypertriglyceridaemia
12. Diabetes can be diagnosed if:
    a) A single blood glucose concentration is 17.8 mmol/l in an asymptomatic patient
    b) Fasting blood glucose is 5.1 mmol/l and 2-hour (OGTT) is 11.5 mmol/l with symptoms
    c) In pregnancy, chance blood glucose concentration is 9.3 mmol/l
    d) Polyuria is reported, and chance plasma glucose is 7.3 mmol/l
    e) Polyuria is reported, and fasting blood glucose is 11.0 mmol/l

13. Recognized causes of islet B-cell damage include:
    a) Ionizing radiation
    b) Interleukin 1
    c) Islet cell complement-fixing circulating antibodies
    d) Viruses
    e) Therapeutic drugs
14. Diabetes commonly presents with:
    a) Weight gain
    b) Myocardial infarction
    c) Behavioural upset (in children)
    d) Necrobiosis lipoidica
    e) Oro-pharyngeal candidiasis
15. Pancreatic diabetes:
    a) May be associated with pancreatic calcification
    b) Is usually caused by a head of pancreas tumour
    c) May be exacerbated by insulin resistance due to cirrhosis of the liver
    d) May present before cardiopathy in haemochromatosis
    e) May be secondary to therapeutic drug-induced damage
16. Multiple endocrine neoplasia Type 1:
    a) Usually includes a phaeochromocytoma
    b) Is of recessive inheritance
    c) Generally presents in childhood
    d) Responds to treatment with streptozotocin
    e) May present with nephrocalcinosis and renal failure
17. Carcinoid tumours:
    a) May be managed surgically even with hepatic metastases
    b) Sometimes occur in the thyroid
    c) Are of neural crest origin embryologically
    d) Are usually highly malignant and metastasize to the lungs
    e) Are never large enough to cause mass effects
18. Hypoglycaemia
    a) May be fatal following high doses of sulphonylurea drugs
    b) May be reactive, causing coma 2–3 h after meals
    c) Can lead to a pleasant trance-like state if glucagon secretion is deficient
    d) Is often due to a missed insulin dose
    e) Is troublesome in patients with a somatostatinoma
19. Glucagonoma tumours
    a) Usually secrete pancreatic polypeptide
    b) Are sometimes found in the bronchial tree
    c) Are sometimes malignant
    d) Are associated with severely insulin-resistant diabetes
    e) May present with flushing and diarrhoea

20. Zollinger–Ellison (gastrinoma) syndrome:
    a) May present as pernicious anaemia
    b) Is usually associated with a pituitary adenoma
    c) Responds with reduced tumour mass to H_2 antagonists
    d) May be associated with a duodenal wall tumour
    e) Is commoner in smokers
21. In the management of ketoacidosis:
    a) Polymorphonuclear leucocytosis suggests a causative infection even without pyrexia
    b) 150 mmol of bicarbonate is beneficial if blood pH is less than 7.1
    c) Hyperosmolarity should be immediately corrected with hypotonic fluids
    d) Total body potassium deficiency may exceed 500 mmol
    e) Intragastric fluids may be given if a nasogastric tube is passed
22. In diabetic pregnancy:
    a) Early growth retardation may result in a small infant
    b) Most infants are macrosomic
    c) Islet cell antibodies commonly cross the placenta and damage the fetal pancreas
    d) Insulin dose requirements double in the first trimester
    e) Gestational diabetes may require sulphonylurea therapy
23. In Type 1 diabetes of childhood:
    a) The peak onset in winter is caused by viral islet damage
    b) Blood glucose monitoring is not preferred by children
    c) Family stress may lead to psychiatric problems in parents
    d) Microalbuminuria is rare
    e) Growth retardation suggests concurrent auto-immune anterior pituitary damage
24. Dyslipidaemia in diabetes:
    a) Is generally of the Fredrickson Type IV phenotype
    b) May be usefully treated with fish oil derivatives
    c) Is not found with good blood glucose control in the non-insulin-treated patient
    d) Is not found with tight blood glucose control in the insulin-dependent patient
    e) Is particularly common in patients with microalbuminuria
25. In the management of diabetes during surgery:
    a) Metformin should be stopped on the day of operation
    b) Glucose–insulin infusions should be stopped if blood glucose falls below 3.5 mmol/l
    c) Pressure mononeuropathies are more common
    d) Glucagon should be given if blood glucose falls below 1.5 mmol/l
    e) Reagent strip blood estimations may be affected by anaesthetic agents

26. In general blood glucose levels in insulin-treated patients:
    a) Are highest around breakfast
    b) Fall steadily overnight
    c) Have a consistent profile from day-to-day
    d) Rise during the day as non-esterified fatty acid levels increase
    e) Rise with mobilization of liver glycogen during exercise
27. Home blood glucose monitoring:
    a) Cannot be performed by the colour-blind
    b) Is not accurate unless a meter is used
    c) Occasionally causes finger pulp infections
    d) Is often recorded selectively by patients
    e) May be performed during the night after a change in evening insulin dose
28. Isophane (NPH) insulin:
    a) Was discovered by Collip shortly after Banting and Best's work
    b) Has a 24-hour duration of action
    c) Forms a loose complex when mixed with unmodified (soluble) insulin, delaying its absorption
    d) Is a complex of insulin with a foreign (animal) protein
    e) Is absorbed more rapidly than human lente insulin
29. Sulphonylureas:
    a) Are useful even after complete islet B-cell destruction
    b) May precipitate lactic acidosis
    c) Act directly on the post-receptor pathway of insulin action
    d) Were discovered accidentally in the search for anticancer agents
    e) Should be taken soon after meals
30. A modified fat diet:
    a) Must include very little cholesterol
    b) Should be low in monounsaturates
    c) Cannot be recommended for young children
    d) Increases the risk of colorectal malignancy in old age
    e) Should exclude some vegetable fats such as chocolate
31. In Cushing's syndrome:
    a) Approximately 10% of adrenal tumours are malignant
    b) A 9.00 a.m. plasma cortisol can be normal
    c) Plasma ACTH levels are usually normal in a patient with an adrenal tumour
    d) Peripheral neuropathy is a characteristic feature
    e) Bromocriptine effectively suppresses cortisol secretion
32. In acromegaly:
    a) A random plasma growth hormone estimation is a useful diagnostic test
    b) Growth hormone levels are suppressed to normal by bromocriptine
    c) The pituitary fossa is seldom enlarged
    d) 25% of patients have a normal glucose tolerance test
    e) Pituitary–gonadal function is usually intact

33. Serum total thyroxine levels are lowered:
    a) In pregnancy
    b) In the nephrotic syndrome
    c) By propranolol
    d) By phenytoin therapy
    e) In severe non-thyroid illness
34. Secondary amenorrhoea:
    a) Is a characteristic feature of Kallman's syndrome
    b) If associated with high FSH levels is due to primary gonadal failure
    c) Is responsive to clomiphene in untreated patients with anorexia nervosa
    d) Is due to a hypothalamic cause if there is no gonadotrophin response to clomiphene
    e) Has a recognized association with Addison's disease
35. Hypocalcaemia is a feature of:
    a) Chronic renal failure
    b) Pseudohypoparathyroidism
    c) Pseudo-pseudohypoparathyroidism
    d) Nephrotic syndrome
    e) Osteoporosis
36. Hyperprolactinaemia:
    a) Is invariably associated with amenorrhoea in young women
    b) May be due to stress
    c) Is decreased by dopamine antagonists
    d) May be due to chlorpromazine therapy
    e) May be due to cortisone therapy
37. Conn's syndrome is characterized by:
    a) Postural hypotension
    b) Increased pigmentation
    c) Hyperkalaemia
    d) High plasma renin levels
    e) Marked peripheral oedema
38. Recognized features of hyperthyroid Graves' disease include:
    a) Nodular goitre
    b) Proximal myopathy
    c) Limitation of upward gaze
    d) Menorrhagia
    e) Acropachy
39. Recognized features of untreated primary hypothyroidism include:
    a) Ataxia
    b) Ascites
    c) Normal tri-iodothyronine (T_3) levels
    d) An impaired TSH response to TRH
    e) Galactorrhoea

40. FSH levels are raised:
    a) In postmenopausal women
    b) In Klinefelter's syndrome
    c) In anorexia nervosa
    d) In Turner's syndrome
    e) In Kallman's syndrome
41. The syndrome of inappropriate ADH secretion is associated with:
    a) Squamous cell carcinoma of lung
    b) Peripheral oedema
    c) High urinary osmolarity
    d) Head injury
    e) Increased pigmentation
42. Presenting features of insulinoma include:
    a) Glycosuria
    b) Weight gain
    c) Abnormal behaviour
    d) Skin rash
    e) Peptic ulceration
43. Recognized features of osteomalacia include:
    a) Proximal myopathy
    b) Dermatitis
    c) Looser's zones on X-ray
    d) Elevated serum acid phosphatase activity
    e) Secondary hyperparathyroidism
44. Findings in Paget's disease of bone include:
    a) Normal serum alkaline phosphatase
    b) Paraplegia
    c) Lowered urinary hydroxyproline excretion
    d) Ewing's tumour
    e) Hypocalcaemia
45. Gynaecomastia is associated with:
    a) 5-α-reductase deficiency
    b) Klinefelter's syndrome
    c) Coeliac disease
    d) Spironolactone therapy
    e) Puberty in males
46. Recognized causes of hypoglycaemia include:
    a) Amanita phalloides (toadstool) poisoning
    b) Galactosaemia
    c) Addison's disease
    d) Leucine sensitivity
    e) Alcohol

47. Characteristic features of the ectopic ACTH syndrome include:
    a) Skin pigmentation
    b) Typical facial features of Cushing's syndrome
    c) Weight gain
    d) Peripheral oedema
    e) Suppression of plasma cortisol whilst on dexamethazone, 0.5 mg six-hourly

Multiple Choice Questions Answers

T = True   F = False

	(a)	(b)	(c)	(d)	(e)
1	T	F	F	F	F
2	F	F	F	F	T
3	T	F	F	T	F
4	F	T	T	T	T
5	F	F	F	F	T
6	F	F	T	T	F
7	T	F	F	F	F
8	F	F	T	F	F
9	F	T	F	F	F
10	F	F	T	F	T
11	F	F	T	T	T
12	F	T	F	F	T
13	F	T	T	T	T
14	F	T	F	F	F
15	T	F	T	T	T
16	F	F	F	F	T
17	T	F	F	F	F
18	T	F	F	F	F
19	T	F	T	F	F
20	F	F	F	T	F
21	F	F	F	T	F
22	T	F	F	F	F
23	F	T	T	T	F
24	F	F	F	F	T
25	F	F	T	F	F
26	T	F	F	F	F
27	F	F	F	T	T
28	F	F	F	T	F
29	F	F	F	F	F
30	F	F	F	F	T
31	T	T	F	F	F
32	F	F	F	F	F
33	F	T	F	T	T
34	F	T	F	F	T
35	T	T	F	T	F
36	F	T	F	T	F
37	F	F	F	F	F
38	F	T	T	F	T
39	T	T	T	F	T
40	T	T	F	T	F

	(a)	(b)	(c)	(d)	(e)
41	F	F	T	T	F
42	F	T	T	F	F
43	T	F	T	F	T
44	T	T	F	F	F
45	T	T	F	T	T
46	T	T	T	T	T
47	T	F	F	F	F

INDEX

Acromegaly 188–193
ACTH, *see* adrenocorticotrophic hormone
Addison's disease 248–252
Adrenal
  adenoma 258–259
  androgens 248
  antibodies 250
  carcinoma 258–259
  cortex 244–263
  failure 248–256
  gland 244–266
  hyperfunction 256–260
  medulla 263–266
  tumours 258–259
Adrenalectomy 260
Adrenaline 263–264
α-Adrenergic antagonists 102
Adrenocorticotrophic hormone 182–184, 198, 201, 246
Aldosterone 246–248
Alpha-adrenergic antagonists 102
Alpha-glucosidase inhibitors 110
5-Alpha-reductase deficiency 274
Amenorrhoea 194
Amiodarone 220
Androstenedione 248

Angiotensin 247
Antidiuretic hormone 205–207
Antithyroid drugs 228–230
APUD system 159–161
Autonomic neuropathy, *see* diabetic complications

Basement membrane thickening 34
Biguanide drugs 108–110
Bromocriptine 192–193, 195

Calcitonin 290, 305
Calcium metabolism 290–291
Carcinoid syndrome 172–174
Cardiopathy, *see* diabetic cardiopathy
Carnitine palmitoyl transferase inhibitors 102
Cheiroarthropathy 52
Childhood diabetes 139–143
Cholecalciferol 289
Chromosomal abnormalities 272–275
Chvostek's sign 297
Clotting abnormalities, *see* diabetic complications, clotting abnormalities

Congenital adrenal
    hyperplasia 252–256
Conn's syndrome 260–263
Continuous subcutaneous insulin
    infusion 130–132
Corticotrophin releasing
    hormone 181–184, 246
Craniopharyngioma 197
Cryptorchidism 275
Cushing's disease 256–257
Cushing's syndrome 256–260
Cyclosporin 63
C-peptide 12–13, 162, 164

De Quervain's thyroiditis 238
Dehydroepiandosterone 248
Dermopathy, see diabetic
    complications
Diabetes insipidus 205–207
Diabetes mellitus 1–158
    aetiology, see diabetes mellitus,
        Type 1, Type 2
    alcohol 101
    audit of care 85–87
    biochemistry 11–18
    blood glucose control 65–66,
        88–90
    carbohydrate intake 96–99
    care 61–91
    cataracts 41, 42
    childhood 139–143
    classification 2–5
    clinics 81–83
    complications, see diabetic
        complications
    contraception 136
    counter-regulatory hormones 14
    definition 19–20
    diagnosis 20, 22
    dietary fat 99
    dietary fibre 99
    dietary management 93–101
    dyslipidaemia 66
    education 67–77, 94–96
    elderly 143–146
    endocrine 10–11
    gestational 11, 139
    glucose tolerance test 19–20
    glycosylated haemoglobin 89

history 1–2
hypertension 53, 55–56
hyperglycaemic
    emergencies 146–151
hypoglycaemia 101, 104, 127–129,
    145
hypoglycaemic agents 101–110
infections 60, 157–158
insulin-dependent, see diabetes
    mellitus, Type 1
insulin, see insulin
ketoacidosis 21, 146–151
late tissue damage 24–61
malnutrition 4, 10, 11
metabolic control 65–66
monitoring 67–77
non-insulin-dependent, see
    diabetes mellitus, Type 2
pancreatic 4, 10, 11
pathogenesis 11–18
presentation 20–22
preventative medicine 61–64
prevention, see diabetes mellitus,
    Type 1, Type 2
pre-pregnancy counselling 136
pregnancy 134–139
    management 135–139
    problems 134–135
psychological aspects 142–143,
    70–72
screening 64
secondary 4, 10
self care 67
self monitoring 74–77
services 77–87
skin conditions 156–157
steroid therapy 11
surgery 151–154
syndromes 4
targets for control 64–67, 88–90
terminology 3–5
treatment 92–133
tropical 4, 10, 11
Type 1
    aetiology 5–7
    prevention 62–63
Type 2
    aetiology 5, 7–10
    prevention 63–64

Index 321

urinary tract infection 46
Diabetic complications 24–61
  autonomic neuropathy 47, 49–51
  cardiopathy 52
  chronic complications 24–61,
      66–67
    biochemistry 32–36
    capillary permeability 33–34
    classification 25–27
    clotting abnormalities 36, 54
    co-causation hypothesis 31–32
    genetics 27, 31
    glycosylation 35
    macrovascular 26
    metabolic hypothesis 28–31
    microvascular 26
    pathogenesis 27–36
    prevalence 24–25
    prevention 66–67
  dermopathy 52
  diarrhoea 50
  eye
    examination 39
    glaucoma 42
    retinopathy 36–42
  foot
    problems 56–61
    ulceration 58–60
  gastroparesis 51
  heart disease 52, 55
  macrovascular disease 53
    pathogenesis 53–54
    prevention 54–55
  maculopathy 36, 38, 41
  mononeuropathies 49
  nephropathy 43–47
    diagnosis 44
    management 44–46
    microalbuminuria 43–45
  neuropathy 47–52
    classification 47
    painful 48–49
  proximal motor neuropathy 48
  retinopathy 36–42
    management 40–41
    proliferative 36, 40–41
DIDMOAD syndrome 4
Dopamine 188
Dyslipidaemia 53–54, 154–156

Ectopic ACTH syndrome 259
Elderly with diabetes 143–146
Endocrine diabetes mellitus 10–11
Epinephrine 263–264

Follicle stimulating
    hormone 185–187, 202
  deficiency 199
Free thyroxine index 215
Fructosamine 89–90

Galactorrhoea 194
Gastrinoma 170–172
Gastrinomas, in multiple endocrine
    neoplasia 160
Genitalia, ambiguous 275
Gestational diabetes 11, 139
Gigantism 190
Glaucoma 42
Glucagon 167–169
Glucagonoma syndrome 167–169
Glucocorticoids 244–248
α-Glucosidase inhibitors 110
Glycosylated haemoglobin 89
Glycosylation 35
Goitre 239–243
Gonadal
  development 267–272
  dysgenesis 272–274
Gonadotrophin deficiency 199
Gonadotrophin releasing
    hormone 185–187
Gonads 267–287
Graves' disease 222–223
Graves' ophthalmopathy 224–225,
    231–232
Growth hormone 184–185,
    188–193, 199–201, 202
  releasing hormone 184–185
  release inhibiting
    hormone 184–185
Growth impairment 199–201
Gustatory sweating 51
Gut hormones 159–174

Hermaphroditism 274–275
Hirsutism 281
HLA immune response genes 5–6

322 Index

HMMA 263–266
Hormone replacement
    therapy 282–283
11-Hydroxycorticosteroids 248
17-Hydroxycorticosteroids 248
21-Hydroxylase defect 252–254
4-Hydroxy 3-methoxy mandelic
    acid 263–266
Hyperaldosteronism 260–263
Hypercalcaemia 291–296
  malignancy 295–296
Hyperglycaemic
    emergencies 146–151
Hyperinsulinaemia 54
Hyperosmolar state 146–151
Hyperparathyroidism 291–295
Hyperparathyroidism, in multiple
    endocrine neoplasia 160
Hyperprolactinaemia 193–196
Hypertension 53, 55–56
Hyperthyroidism 222–232
Hypocalcaemia 297–303
Hypoglycaemia
  alcohol 101
  causes 162–164
  elderly 145
  factitious 163
  insulin therapy 127–129
  presentation 161–162
  reactive 163–164
  sulphonylureas 104–105,
    145
Hypogonadism
  female 278–283
  male 283–287
Hypoparathyroidism 302–303
Hypophosphataemic rickets 302
Hypophysectomy 192, 260
Hypothalamic-pituitary-adrenal
    axis 181–184
Hypothalamic-pituitary-gonadal
    axis 185–187
Hypothalamic-pituitary-growth-
    hormone axis 184–185
Hypothalamic-pituitary-thyroid
    axis 180–181
Hypothalamus 175–209
Hypothyroidism 232–237
  congenital 236–237

Impotence 50, 194, 286
Inappropriate antidiuretic hormone
    secretion 207–209
Inhibin 186
Insulin 2, 12–18, 111–133
  absorption 119–122
  allergy 117
  deficiency 12–18
  dose adjustment 125–127
  hypersecretion 161–167
  infusion pumps 130–133
  injection site infections 118
  injection site lipodystrophy 117
  insensitivity 10, 16–17, 102
  oedema 118
  pharmacokinetics 119–122
  preparations 112–115
    extended acting 111, 113–115
    immunogenicity 113, 115–117
  receptor abnormalities 4
  receptor antibodies 4
  regimens 122–125
  resistance
    immunological 117
    see insulin insensitivity
  secretion 12
    abnormalities 17–18, 102
  synthesis 13
  therapy 111–133
    exercise 129
    illness 129–130
    intramuscular 132, 149
    other routes 132
    socio-psychological
      problems 118
    socio-legal consequences 130
Insulinoma 161–167
Iodine 214, 219–222
  deficiency 219, 222
  excess 219–220
Ischaemic heart disease 52, 55
Islet cell antibodies 7
Islet transplantation 133

Jodbasedow phenomenon 220

Ketoacidosis 21, 146–151
Ketone bodies 12, 15

Index 323

17-Ketosteroids 248
Klinefelter's syndrome 272–273

Lactic acidosis 108
Laron dwarfism 198
Lipid lowering agents 110, 156–157
Long-acting thyroid stimulator 223
Luteinizing hormone 185–187, 202
   deficiency 199

Maculopathy, see diabetic
      complications
Magnesium deficiency 300
Malnutrition diabetes 4, 10, 11
Medullary thyroid carcinoma 240, 243
Melanocyte stimulating
      hormone 182–183
MEN1 160–161, 292
MEN2 160–161, 292
Menopause 282–283
Menstrual cycle 270–271
Metyrapone 260
Microalbuminuria 43–45
Mineralocorticoids 246–248
Multiple endocrine
      neoplasia 159–161, 292
Myocardial infarction 52, 55
Myo-inositol depletion 35
Myxoedema 233
   coma 233, 236

Neonatal Graves' disease 225
Nephropathy, see diabetic
      complications
Nesidioblastosis 167
Neurohypophysis 205–209
Neuropathy, see diabetic
      complications
Non-esterified fatty acids 12, 15
Noradrenaline 263–264
Norepinephrine 263–264

Osteoporosis 303–305
Ovarian failure 279–280
Ovary 270
17-Oxysteroids 248

Paget's disease 305–307
Pancreas transplantation 132–133

Pancreatic diabetes 4, 10, 11
Parathyroid hormone 288–289
Peripheral vascular disease 56
Phaeochromocytoma 265–266
   multiple endocrine neoplasia 160
Photocoagulation 40
Pineal tumours 276
Pituitary gland 175–209
   anterior 188–205
   failure 197–205
   radiation 192, 196, 260
   radiology 176–179
   tumours 197, 259
   pressure effects 175–176
Polycystic ovaries 281
Polyol hypothesis 33, 34
Posterior pituitary 205–209
Precocious puberty 276
Pregnancy 134–139
Pretibial myxoedema 225
Proinsulin 12–13
Prolactin 188, 193–196, 199, 203
Proliferative retinopathy, see
      diabetic complications
Pseudohypoparathyroidism 303
Pseudoprecocious puberty 276
Puberty
   delayed 277–278
   female 272
   male 270

Radioiodine scans 220–221, 241
Radioiodine therapy 231
Reactive hypoglycaemia 163–164
Reaven's syndrome 53
5-α-Reductase deficiency 274
Reidel's thyroiditis 239
Renin 247
Retinopathy, see diabetic
      complications
Rickets 298–302
Rubeosis iridis 41

Sarcoidosis 292, 293, 296
Semen 269–270
Sheehan's syndrome 197
Somatostatin 169, 184–185
   analogues 193
   hypersecretion 169

Steroid therapy
  diabetes 11
  adrenal failure 250
Sulphonylurea drugs 103–108
Synacthen test 250

Testicular failure 284–285
Testicular feminization 274
Testis 186, 269–270, 284–285
Testosterone 186
Thyroglobulin 213
Thyroid
  acropachy 225
  autoimmunity 222–223
  crisis 226
  gland 210–243
    lingual 211, 221
    retrosternal 211, 221
  malignancy 242–243
  stimulating hormone 180–181, 199, 203, 216–217, 233–235
Thyroidectomy 230–231
Thyroiditis 237
Thyrotoxicosis 296
Thyrotrophin, *see* thyroid stimulating hormone

Thyrotrophin releasing
    hormone 180–181, 188
  test 227, 235
Thyroxine 213–216
  binding globulin 214–215
Toxic nodular goitre 221–222
TRH test, *see* thyrotrophin releasing hormone test
Triiodothyronine 213–216, 218
Tropical diabetes 4, 10, 11
TSH, *see* thyroid stimulating hormone
Turner's syndrome 272–273

Vasopressin 205–207
VIP 170
VIPoma syndrome 170
Virilization 280–281
Vitamin D 289–290
  deficiency 297, 298–302
  toxicity 291, 296
Vitrectomy 41
Vitreous haemorrhage 41

Wolff-Chaikoff effect 219

Zollinger-Ellison syndrome 170–172